Health and Health Care in Britain

HEALTH AND HEALTH CARE IN BRITAIN

Rob Baggott

MACMILLAN

First published 1994 by
MACMILLAN PRESS LTD
Houndmills, Basingstoke, Hampshire RG21 2XS
and London
Companies and representatives
throughout the world

ISBN 0–333–56295–X (hardcover)
ISBN 0–333–56296–8 (paperback)

A catalogue record for this book is available
from the British Library.

10   9   8   7   6   5   4
03   02   01   00   99   98   97   96

Printed in Great Britain by
Mackays of Chatham PLC
Chatham, Kent

To Mark, Danny and Melissa

Contents

List of Tables, Figures and Exhibits

■ *Tables*

■ *Figures*

▪ *Exhibits*

Preface

The term 'crisis' is so frequently used that as a description of a state of affairs it is often meaningless. Nowhere perhaps is this more true than in health care. The British health care system, and its central component, the National Health Service (NHS), is widely perceived as being perennially in crisis. Yet simply to accept, or deny, that this is the case does not take us very far. What is required is a better understanding of the complex combination of problems, circumstances and pressures that face the contemporary health care system.

Debates about health care are rarely conducted in an atmosphere of calm rationality. Take, for example, the 1992 General Election, where there was a lamentable lack of informed debate about the impact of more than a decade of reform in health care. Most attention centred upon a Labour Party broadcast which portrayed a 'two-tier' health service, highlighting the contrasting experiences of two girls needing the same ear operation. One was able to obtain private treatment, the other had to wait. The broadcast raised some important and relevant matters concerning access to health care, the role of private medicine, the determination of priorities, and the adequacy of health service funding. But these issues, and how they might best be resolved, were largely ignored in the political uproar which followed the broadcast. The public's attention was drawn instead towards the complex and contradictory details of the Jennifer Bennett case, upon which the film had been allegedly based, and focused upon those personalities involved in what was labelled by the media, 'the war of Jennifer's ear'.

Perhaps we should not be surprised that in matters concerning health and health care the heart tends to rule the head. After all, health issues are often highly emotive. Questions concerning the quality of life, and matters of life and death, should not be taken lightly. Health care debates can involve complex ethical issues, which prick the conscience and raise the temperature. Moreover, they increasingly involve controversial economic and resource issues. In view of this it is hardly surprising that health issues are politically sensitive. This is not necessarily a bad thing, providing that political debate is based on a clear understanding of the challenges and problems facing the health care system.

This book seeks to contribute to a better understanding of contemporary health care. The early chapters highlight the main issues facing the health care system. Chapter 1 explores health trends in Britain and seeks to locate them in an historical and global context. In this chapter the main health challenges which face many societies including our own are identified, such as the burden of the ageing population. In Chapter 2 the role of the medical profession is explored. Doctors have exerted a powerful influence over health and health care in modern societies, and in this chapter an attempt is made to explain why. This is followed in Chapter 3 by an analysis of the various critiques of the medically-dominated health care system, some of which have provided ideas for recent reforms.

Chapters 4 and 5 focus on health care in Britain. In Chapter 4 there is a discussion of the evolution of the British system of health care, which culminated in the creation of the NHS. This chapter also explores the problems faced by the NHS during its lifetime, along with some of the previous attempts to deal with these problems. This is followed in Chapter 5 by a more detailed description of the contemporary British health care system.

It is not sufficient merely to describe the features of the health care system and the challenges it faces. It is also important that recent reforms in this field are properly understood and their impact carefully analysed. With this in mind the latter half of the book concentrates on developments in health policy that have taken place since the Conservative government took office in 1979.

Chapter 6 examines the Conservatives' approach towards planning and management processes within the NHS. This chapter discusses the restructuring of the NHS in the early 1980s, the introduction of general management into the service, and the development of planning and review systems. Chapter 7 looks at health care resourcing and in particular at the impact of the growing private health care sector and government public expenditure policies upon the NHS. The introduction of internal markets and other related reforms are explored in Chapter 8. Chapters 9, 10 and 11 cover developments in three health policy areas which have been relatively neglected in the past. These are primary care, community care and public health. In recent years there have been a number of important initiatives in these areas of health policy. Each chapter analyses the background to these initiatives and their impact.

The book covers the broad canvas of contemporary health care, but it is something more than a descriptive account. Throughout the intention has been to provide an analysis of the contemporary health care scene, with an eye to possible future developments. The book will be of particular interest to those studying health and social policy, and to managers and professionals working within the field of health and social care.

I would like to thank my publisher, Steven Kennedy, for his help and encouragement while undertaking this project. I would also like to acknowledge the contribution of several anonymous individuals who have read complete drafts of the manuscript and whose comments have been extremely helpful. I am also grateful to a number of professionals working within the NHS, who should also remain anonymous, who have taken the time and trouble to comment on sections of the manuscript. I would also like to thank colleagues in the Department of Public Policy and Managerial Studies and the Department of Health and Community Studies at De Montfort University for their comments, advice and encouragement. Finally, I would like to thank my family for being very understanding and supportive throughout the course of this project.

ROB BAGGOTT

List of Abbreviations

AIDS	Acquired Immune Deficiency Syndrome
AHA	Area Health Authority
BMA	British Medical Association
BPA	Basic Practice Allowance
CHC	Community Health Care
CIP	Cost Improvement Programme
CMO	Chief Medical Officer
CNO	Chief Nursing Officer
DGH	District General Hospital
DGM	District General Manager
DoH	Department of Health
DHA	District Health Authority
DHSS	Department of Health and Social Security
DMT	District Management Team
DMU	Directly Managed Units
ECR	Extra Contractual Referral
EHS	Emergency Hospital Service
FHSA	Family Health Services Authority
FPC	Family Practitioner Committee
FPS	Family Practitioner Services
GHS	General Household Survey
GMC	General Medical Council
GP	General Practitioner
GPA	Good Practice Allowane
GPF	General Practitioner Fundholders
HAI	Hospital Acquired Infection
HCHS	Hospital and Community Health Services
HIV	Human Immunodeficiency Virus
HMC	Hospital Management Committee
HMO	Health Maintenance Organisation
HSSB	Health Services Supervisory Board
ME	Myalgic Encephalomyelitis
MHCO	Managed Health Care Organisations
MIT	Minimally Invasive Therapy
MOH	Medical Officer of Health
NAHA	National Association of Health Authorities
NAHAT	National Association of Health Authorities and Trusts

NAO	National Audit Office
NCT	National Childbirth Trust
NCEPOD	National Confidential Enquiry into Peri-operative Deaths
NCVO	National Council for Voluntary Organisations
NHI	National Health Insurance
NHS	National Health Service
NHSME	National Health Service Management Executive
NNS	Neighbourhood Nursing Service
OECD	Organisation for Economic Cooperation and Development
OPCS	Office for Population, Census and Surveys
PHCT	Primary Health Care Team
QALY	Quality Adjusted Life Year
RAWP	Resource Allocation Working Party
RCN	Royal College of Nursing
RCT	Randomised Controlled Trial
RGM	Regional General Manager
RHA	Regional Health Authority
RHB	Regional Hospital Board
RMI	Resource Management Initiative
SGT	Self-Governing Trust
SHA	Special Health Authority
SMR	Standardised Mortality Ratio
STD	Sexually Transmitted Diseases
STG	Special Transitional Grant
TQM	Total Quality Management
VFMU	Value for Money Unit
WHO	World Health Organisation
WRVS	Women's Royal Voluntary Service

■ *Chapter 1* ■
Health and Illness

Let us begin on a note of optimism. In terms of surviving to adulthood, life expectancy, and the chances of a living a life relatively free from the threat of fatal disease, the British people have perhaps never had it so good. Present standards of health are relatively high, not only in comparison with past generations, but also internationally. Britain in the 1990s is a comparatively healthy place in which to be born and to live.

However, this broad assessment is in many respects misleading. The focus upon overall standards of health can disguise important variations between different sections of the population, leading to complacency in the face of real health challenges that need to be confronted. Any judgement about health standards must be based on a more careful analysis of health and illness trends. This introductory chapter attempts to provide such an analysis, beginning with the concept of health. This is followed by a discussion of important variations in health and illness in Britain, within an historical and global context.

■ Defining health

There are two main ways of defining health; on the one hand the positive approach, where health is viewed as a capacity or an asset to be possessed, and on the other the negative approach, which emphasises the absence of specific illnesses, diseases or disorders (Aggleton, 1990, p. 5).

□ *Positive health*

The World Health Organisation (WHO) has defined health in a positive sense as 'a state of complete physical, mental and social well-being and not merely the absence of disease or infirmity' (World Health Organisation, 1946). As well as emphasising health in terms of positive attributes, this definition is also significant in placing stress on mental as well as physical aspects of health, and upon social as well as individual well-being.

This definition has been criticised for being utopian, though it is perhaps more appropriately viewed as being an ideal towards which health care

1

and other social actions may be orientated (Twaddle, 1974). Even so, there are also problems with the definition and measurement of well-being – a rather woolly notion – which raise further questions about the utility of the definition as a policy goal.

The WHO definition is an abstraction and fails to take into account that health is a relative concept. The health of individuals and groups in society has to be seen in relation to their environments, expectations, and capacities. A ninety-year-old would not expect, and would not be expected by others, to have the capacity to run a marathon. Yet he or she may well be healthy, relatively speaking, given society's expectations about nonagenarians. Seriously disabled people may live a full and fulfilling life, and therefore, in this sense, may be regarded as healthy.

Related to this is the idea that health is a type of strength or reserve. In a rather narrow sense, strength can be seen as being synonymous with physical fitness. Yet it has a wider meaning which goes beyond the simple ability to exert oneself physically. One can conceive of health as an inner strength which people may possess and develop in order to deal with the problems and stresses of life. Almost paradoxically, health may involve suffering as a creative way of dealing with destructive feelings (Wilson, 1975). Illich, in his critique of medicine (to be discussed further in Chapter 3), argues that health designates the intensity with which individuals cope with their internal states and environmental conditions. According to this view, a healthy environment is presumably one which encourages personal responsibility and the ability to cope with life's many problems.

To summarise, health in a positive sense can be seen as being a feeling of general well-being on an individual and social level. More specifically it can also be seen as a process of adaptation to the environment, a capacity to function, and a strength to cope both with specific illnesses and life in general.

☐ *The negative concept of health*

In terms of the negative concept of health, an individual is regarded as being healthy when not suffering from a particular illness or disease. The terms 'illness' and 'disease', although often used interchangeably, can be distinguished. Disease relates to a biological malfunctioning, diagnosed by doctors, while illness refers both to the personal experience of disease and its wider social implications (Kleinman, 1978). The concepts of disease and illness are explored in more detail during the next chapter.

The negative concept of health is closely associated with orthodox medicine, which is heavily focused on disease. It is often argued that doctors are not particularly interested in health in a positive sense and that the negative approach to health has tended to predominate (Gould, 1987).

☐ The measurement of health, disease and illness

The predominance of the negative approach, coupled with the difficulties of interpreting concepts such as 'social well-being', has implications for the measurement of health. Rather than indicating standards of health in a positive sense, official health statistics tend to measure how unhealthy we are. The emphasis is very much on mortality (death), morbidity (disease) and treatment or service statistics. Analysis of health trends is also usually confined to the changing prevalence of disease.

Yet it is possible to measure health in a positive sense. For example, life expectancy and infant mortality statistics (the latter is usually expressed as the number of deaths in children under one year of age per 1000 live births) are often used as indicators of the resistance of the population to disease.

Certain treatment statistics may also help us to build up a picture of the positive aspects of health. Immunisation rates, which indicate a community's potential resistance to certain diseases, can be viewed as an indicator of positive health. The growing use of mental health services and antidepressants, on the other hand, indicates the poor level of mental well-being in society, though it also reflects the greater willingness of sufferers to seek help and the wider availability of such therapies.

Finally, there are social surveys – such as the General Household Survey (GHS) – which ask individuals about their own attitudes to health, their lifestyles as well as their experiences of ill-health. These serve as indicators of positive health, making it possible to construct a less one-sided analysis of health trends.

■ Health trends and variations

The experience of health and illness can vary in several ways. There is often a variation over time, certain diseases being more prevalent in some historical periods than in others. Health and illness can also vary over one's lifetime, with individuals being more prone to particular illnesses at certain stages in their lives. There are also significant geographical variations in health and illness. Such variations can be found at the regional and local, as well as the international level. Finally, health and illness may vary according to the location of individuals in the social structure. There are differences in health between social classes, between the sexes, and between ethnic groups in the population.

☐ *Historical trends*

In 1901, average life expectancy in the United Kingdom (UK), at birth, was only 45.5 years for men and 49 years for women. In 1991 a newborn male could expect to live 73.2 years on average; a newborn female, 78.8 years. Over the same period, infant mortality has fallen from 142 to 7.9 per 1000 live births. These figures suggest a significant and remarkable improvement in the overall health of the population. But at the same time there has been an equally significant change in the burden of ill-health.

Perhaps the most marked trend this century has been the decline of the major infectious diseases which were widespread in the Victorian period: cholera, typhoid, measles, whooping cough and tuberculosis. Although medical interventions in the form of drug therapies and vaccination programmes were important in reducing morbidity and mortality related to these diseases, their decline was already underway due mainly to improved standards of living. However, medical intervention certainly played a much more significant role in the decline of many other infectious diseases, such as diphtheria and poliomyelitis. The contribution of medicine to the reduction of infectious disease is discussed further in Chapter 2.

The decline of the major infectious diseases has been offset to a considerable extent by a growth in the incidence of other, chronic, diseases. In the post-Second World War period for example, the number of measles cases in the UK declined from 632 200 (1951) to 15 600 (1990). Over the same period the number of deaths from lung cancer has increased from 13 800 to around 40 000. This illustrates the way in which lifestyle-related diseases have superseded the old infectious epidemics. Deaths caused by infectious diseases represent less than 1 per cent of the total number of deaths in England and Wales today, compared with 13 per cent only sixty years ago (Cm 1986, 1992). Currently, almost half of the mortality in England and Wales is due to circulatory diseases such as heart disease and stroke, with a further quarter of deaths attributed to cancers.

Much of the burden of morbidity and mortality today can be associated with modern lifestyles and environments. For example, a considerable proportion of circulatory diseases and cancers have been linked to lifestyle factors such as smoking, alcohol abuse, poor diet, stress and lack of exercise (Smith and Jacobson, 1988). It is now widely believed that action to promote healthy lifestyles and environments is needed to tackle the modern epidemics. These efforts are discussed in more detail in Chapter 11 in the context of the government's national health strategy.

A broader indication of the nation's health is given by large-scale surveys of health and fitness. In the findings of a survey of 9000 individuals reported by Blaxter (1990), 29 per cent of respondents claimed to have 'less than good health'. The General Household Survey (GHS) found that half the population do not indulge in active sports, games and physical activities (OPCS, 1992). It is therefore not surprising that as many as one-third of the population fail to reach basic fitness levels (Health Education Council, 1992), and that almost 90 per cent of adults have at least one risk factor for heart disease and stroke (DoH and OPCS, 1993a).

Surveys have also generated information on individual self-reported illness. One in three respondents reported long-term illness in the 1990 GHS survey (OPCS, 1992), and one in five claimed to have a long-standing illness which limited their activities; 14 per cent of the respondents claimed that illness had restricted their activities in the two weeks prior to the interview. The most common self-reported illnesses, revealed in an earlier GHS survey, are diseases and disorders of the musculoskeletal system, the heart and circulatory system, and the respiratory system (OPCS, 1990). It is clear from successive surveys that the proportion reporting a long-standing illness has increased significantly in all age and sex categories in recent years. In 1976, for example, only a quarter of respondents reported such illness, with 16 per cent reporting limiting long-term conditions and less than one in ten claiming to have restricted activity. It has been estimated that there are over six million adults in Great Britain having at least one form of disability (OPCS, 1988). This represents approximately 15 per cent of the adult population.

The burden of chronic illness and disability should not produce complacency about the relatively low levels of infectious disease. Older infectious diseases such as tuberculosis and hepatitis have recently made an alarming comeback. Food poisoning notifications almost quadrupled during the 1980s, while other infectious diseases, including Legionnaires' disease and meningitis, have represented a growing threat to health in recent years.

Reported cases of sexually transmitted diseases (STD) have risen dramatically during the post-Second World War period. In 1951, 73 000 cases of STD were reported. By 1990 this figure had risen to well over half a million (DoH, 1992a). Forecasts of a world AIDS (Acquired Immune Deficiency Syndrome) epidemic have done much to stimulate concern about STD. There have been over 7000 cases of AIDS in the UK, of which over half have died. Yet over twice this number are known to be HIV positive (human immunodeficiency virus) and may develop AIDS. The actual number of HIV positives is thought to be significantly higher than the number of reported cases.

The extent of mental illness is also a cause for concern. Trends are very difficult to establish, however, as the interpretation of mental illness has varied considerably between different historical periods (Scull, 1979). In recent years the growing use of mental health services and antidepressant drugs are believed to indicate deteriorating levels of mental health. But, as mentioned earlier, such statistics reflect the availability of such therapies as well as changing perceptions of need.

Certainly, the level of mental illness represents an enormous social problem today: 15 per cent of general practitioner (GP) consultations concern mental health problems. Around 70 per cent of women and 50 per cent of men will at some time during their lives consult their GP regarding their mental health, while at least 3 per cent of the adult population suffer from a depressive disorder and over 2 per cent suffer from anxiety states (Cm 1986, 1992, p. 81).

It should be pointed out that mental and physical illness are often related, though often in ways which are poorly understood. Serious physical illnesses, such as cancer, can have wide-ranging psychological implications, not only for the sufferer but also for his or her closest relatives. Mental illness can lead to physical illness, injury and even death. Skin diseases, such as psoriasis, which affects about 2 per cent of the population, are thought to be related in some cases to mental health. Addiction problems, such as smoking, alcohol and drug abuse, are linked to physical diseases. Suicides (of which there are around 5000 every year in England) and injuries due to unsuccessful suicide attempts, are also often related to underlying mental illness.

☐ Life cycles and demographic change

Not only does health (and ill-health) vary over time, it also varies over an individual's lifetime. There is a kind of life-cycle in operation, with people being prone to certain illnesses at particular times in their lives. Figure 1.1 illustrates the main causes of death in different age groups for men, showing that the main causes of mortality in younger men are quite different from the diseases which kill middle-aged and elderly males. Violent death, accidents and injury (both external and self-inflicted) are major causes of death in younger people. Around 15 000 people a year die from accidents or violent incidents every year in Britain. A third of these deaths are road-traffic-related, 40 per cent of these involving the under-25s. Circulatory diseases, cancers and respiratory diseases are the most common causes of death in the older age groups.

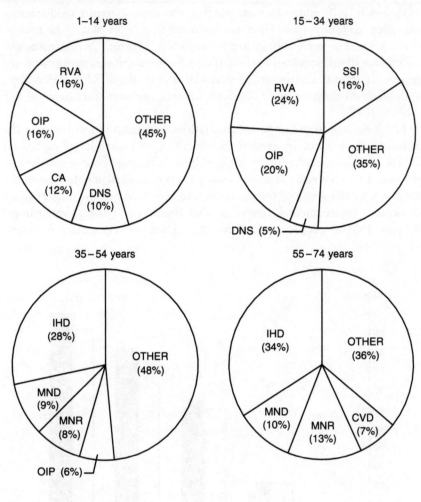

Key

CA	Congenital anomalies
CVD	Cerebro-vascular disease (stroke)
DNS	Diseases of the nervous system and sensory organs
IHD	Ischaemic heart disease
MND	Malignant neoplasm (cancer) of digestive system
MNR	Malignant neoplasm (cancer) of respiratory and intra-thoracic organs
OIP	Other causes of injury and poisoning
RVA	Road vehicle accidents
SSI	Suicide and self-injury

Note: Percentages indicate the proportion in each age category dying of the disease.

Source: DoH, Chief Medical Officer, *On the State of the Public Health 1991*, London, HMSO 1992.

Figure 1.1 *The main causes of death in selected age groups, males, 1991 (England)*

Studies of self-reported illness confirm the chronic nature of disease in the older age groups. The GHS survey found that in the oldest age groups, those reporting such illness are a majority. Figure 1.2 illustrates the differences in self-reported chronic illness between the various age and sex groups. It should also be noted that almost two-thirds of disabled men, and nearly three-quarters of disabled women, are over sixty years of age (OPCS, 1988).

There are also some important variations in mental illness between the different age groups. In general the elderly have higher levels of mental illness. Depression is common in the elderly, affecting about one in five of the over-65s. Dementia is also a major form of mental illness among the elderly. One in twenty of the over-65s, and one in five of the over-80s, has dementia. Severe mental illness is also found in younger age groups. Around 150 000 people in the UK suffer from schizophrenia, an illness

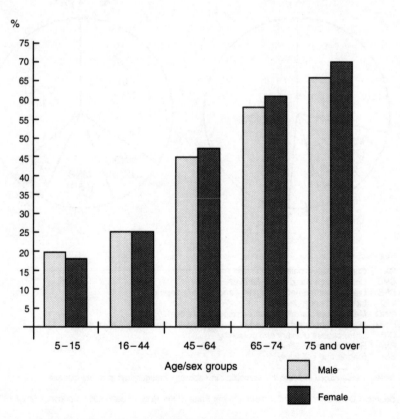

Source: OPCS, General Housing Survey 1990 (HMSO, 1992).

Figure 1.2   *Respondents reporting long-standing illness, 1990, (Great Britain)*

which tends to develop in young adults. Suicide, which as noted earlier is often the result of underlying mental illness, is a major cause of death among the both the old and the young. Although suicide rates are highest among the elderly, particularly elderly men, there has been in recent years a sharp increase in suicide rates among younger males.

The discovery that older people are more likely to die from chronic disease and to have long-standing conditions and disabilities should come as no surprise. Yet it does raise questions about the implications of an increasing elderly population – a trend which is being faced by most developed countries today. The projected growth of the elderly population in the UK is shown in Figures 1.3 and 1.4. Figure 1.3 shows that, following a sharp rise in the elderly population in the 1960s and 1970s, something of a plateau has now been reached. This situation is expected to persist until the early years of the twenty-first century, when there will be a further significant rise in the proportion of elderly people in the UK, reaching almost a fifth of the total population by the year 2030. Figure 1.4 also illustrates the growth in the very elderly population over the same period. By 2030 one in twenty of the population will be over aged eighty.

The growth of the elderly population is more spectacular in some countries. It is estimated that by the year 2030 Switzerland will have the highest proportion of over-65s – 29 per cent of its population. In the same

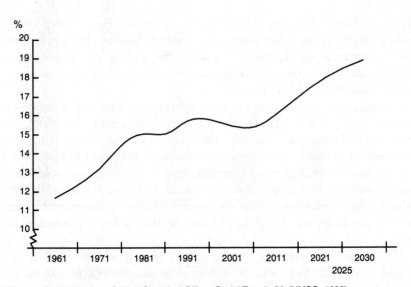

Source: Calculated from Central Statistical Office, *Social Trends 22*, (HMSO, 1992).

Figure 1.3 *The increase in the elderly population (UK), percentage of total population over 65 years old*

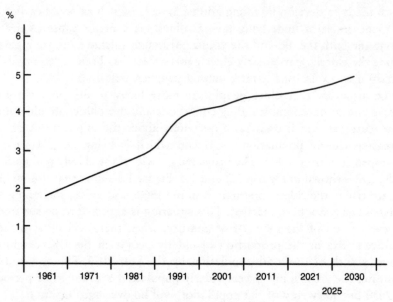

%

Source: Calculated from Central Statistical Office, *Social Trends 22*, (HMSO, 1992).

Figure 1.4   *The increase in the elderly population (UK), percentage of total population over 80 years old*

year it is likely that the elderly will account for over a fifth of the populations of Sweden, Germany, Italy, Austria, Norway, France, Finland, The Netherlands and Canada. The increasing elderly population, while affecting all the main industrialised countries, is therefore likely to have a greater impact on some than on others.

The growing proportion of elderly people in our society is not a problem in itself. Rather, it is the likely consequences of this growth for health care provision and other social services which causes concern. Relative to other age groups, the elderly, and particularly those over the age of 75, are heavy users of health care. Figure 1.5 illustrates the relatively high levels of health care expenditure accounted for by the elderly, and in particular by the very elderly. The implication is that the growth of the elderly population, all other things being equal, will produce an escalation in the costs of health care.

The rising cost of caring for the elderly is only a problem if society cannot afford it. Yet there is a fear that the growth in the elderly population will not only add to the cost of care but that it will also prevent society from generating the necessary resources (Johnson, Conrad and Thomson, 1989). Indeed, it does seem that the growth of the elderly population will place a greater onus upon the rest of society. In 1961 there

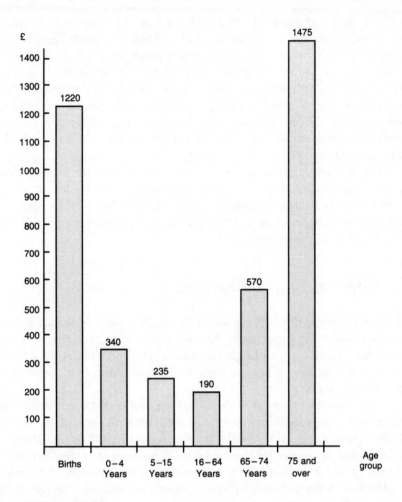

Source: HM Treasury (1988).

Figure 1.5   *Health and social care costs by age group (England), current costs per head in £s*

were almost six people of working age for every person aged over 65. By the year 2011 this ratio will be less than four to one. This implies that the working population will face an increasingly heavy burden of providing the resources necessary for the care of the elderly.

This gloomy scenario has been challenged. Some have pointed out that dependency ratio (the ratio between those of working age and the rest of the population) is remarkably stable over time (Thane, 1987). This argument is based on a prediction that the growth in the elderly population will be offset to some extent by changes at the other end of the age structure. A decline in the numbers of children and young people in the future through falling birth-rates could result in savings on spending programmes such as education, for example. These resources could be reallocated towards the provision of social care for the increased elderly population. It has also been suggested that people are more resistant to illness than in the past and may not need such varied and prolonged care in the future, thus reducing to some extent the burden on those of working age (Bosanquet, 1975).

Despite these arguments, concern about the growth of the elderly population remains. Even if people live healthier lives for longer periods, they will at some stage require care and support. Health care systems face an enormous challenge in accommodating the new and varied needs which this trend will undoubtedly produce.

☐ *International variations*

Countries such as Britain have had considerable success in reducing disease and increasing life expectancy. But some countries, particularly those in the Third World, are still fighting battles which in the developed world were won long ago. When studying health and illness one cannot ignore the global context.

It is a tragic fact that out of the 50 million deaths that occur in the world each year, almost a third are of children below the age of five (WHO, 1990). Most of these child deaths are due to infectious diseases. Diarrhoea-related diseases alone are associated with between four and five million deaths of children under the age of five every year. Another four million children die from respiratory diseases, mostly pneumonia. Diseases such as poliomyelitis, tetanus, measles, diphtheria, whooping cough and tuberculosis kill a further three million children.

Infant mortality is high in the developing world. But poor standards of health are found among adults as well as children. The climate of many developing countries also produces an environment which can be damaging to health. Over two-fifths of the world's population live in areas threatened by malaria and around 100 million actually suffer from the disease. Other tropical diseases, such as schistosomiasis (a water-borne parasitic disease), affect twice this number.

High levels of infectious disease in Third-World countries are not simply due to the environment. Poverty and deprivation, which some attribute to the world economic system, undermine the health of many people in these countries (George, 1976). In some cases the situation is made worse by unstable political and economic conditions, leading to civil war and famine. Such a combination of circumstances can lead to massive public health disasters, as the recent cases of Ethopia and Somalia have graphically shown.

Nevertheless, there have been significant improvements in health in many Third-World countries during the post-Second World War period. Death rates in virtually all of these countries have fallen significantly (Phillips, 1990). This has been due in part to better medical facilities and public health programmes in these countries. But general improvements in living standards have also played a major (and some would say the main) role.

Economic development, however, often brings new problems. There is increasing evidence that Third-World countries are now having to bear a much heavier burden of chronic and degenerative diseases than before. This is partly due to the adoption of lifestyles found in the developed world. Take tobacco smoking, for example, which is associated with a range of cancers and circulatory diseases. Rates of smoking are growing 7 per cent faster than the population in Asia and Latin America, and 18 per cent faster than the population in Africa. Developing countries are now responsible for 52 per cent of tobacco consumption, and the proportion is increasing (Jacobson, 1983). Some countries – notably China and India – have experienced a considerable rise in tobacco-related diseases in recent years. It is not surprising, therefore, that tobacco is now being regarded as one of the most serious threats to the health of the Third World (Nath, 1986).

Diseases of poverty and affluence tend to coexist in Third-World countries, along with diseases of climate and those which are 'man-made'. Furthermore, as if this is not enough, AIDS has disproportionately affected many of these countries, particularly in Africa. By the end of 1990, out of the estimated 995 000 cases of AIDS world-wide, two-thirds are in Africa (Blaxter, 1991). It is expected that in the future Asia will take over from Africa as the centre of the AIDS epidemic (Mann, 1993).

Although the picture looks bleak for many of the developing countries, one must be careful to avoid over-simple generalisations. The Third World is not as uniform in terms of health and health care as is often assumed. Indeed there are many different 'worlds', consisting of groups of countries in particular regions (Latin America, Africa and so on), or at similar levels of economic development. Notably, the least developed countries (as designated by the United Nations General Assembly) have a much higher average infant mortality rate (125 per 1000) than those which have become more economically developed (70 per 1000). In the poorest countries 22 per cent of infants can be expected to die before they reach five years of age. This is roughly twice the mortality rate of the 'better off' category of developing countries (WHO, 1990).

☐ *The industrialised countries*

In comparison with the Third World, the developed countries suffer relatively less from infectious diseases and more from chronic and degenerative diseases. Over half the deaths in the developed world each year can be attributed to heart disease, strokes and cancer (WHO, 1990). Moreover, the trend towards chronic disease in these countries is continuing (OECD, 1987).

These broad trends mask a considerable variation in health and illness within industrialised countries. Infant mortality rates vary considerably, even within European countries, from just over 6 per 1000 in Finland to just over 17 per 1000 in Hungary. Life expectancy at birth also varies significantly, from 66 years in Hungary to 74 in Greece and Switzerland. Mortality rates from various categories of disease also vary substantially within Europe. Mortality from infectious disease in Italy, Czechoslovakia and Austria is less than half the rate found in France, Switzerland and Poland. Death rates from cancer are roughly 50 per cent higher in Hungary, Czechoslovakia and Denmark than in Romania, Bulgaria, Greece and Portugal. Mortality rates from circulatory disease are considerably lower in France, Switzerland and The Netherlands than in Finland, Ireland and most of the former 'Eastern bloc' countries.

Compared with other European countries the UK has a comparatively low mortality rate from infectious diseases. However, it does have a higher than average mortality rate from cancer and in the case of circulatory disease UK mortality is about average. One should bear in mind, however, that the overall statistics for the UK (and for that matter, other countries as well) tend to obscure the fact that some parts of the country and some sections of the population have higher rates of death and illness than others. These important variations will be explored later.

Variations in general and specific mortality rates and in rates of illness between industrialised countries may be interesting to observe, but are they significant? Some of the variations between countries undoubtedly reflect specific local conditions such as differences in climate, demography, physical geography, and social and economic conditions. They may also relate to differences in the diagnosis of disease by the medical profession in each country, as we shall see in the next chapter. To some extent variations are due to differences in the accuracy of information systems which record illness and death. Variations in health and illness between countries may also reflect other factors, such as the method of organising health services, the funding of the health care system, and wider health and social policies. Used with caution, such variations can provide a basis for judging both the comparative effectiveness of health care systems and national health strategies. This in turn raises the possibility of countries learning from those which have achieved success in improving the health of their populations.

□ *Regional and local variations*

As suggested earlier, there are important variations in health and illness within industrialised nations. Scotland, Wales and Northern Ireland have higher infant mortality rates than England as a whole. Scotland has a much higher death rate from cancers and strokes than other parts of the UK. Scotland and Northern Ireland have higher rates of heart and circulatory disease compared with England and Wales. In 1985 coronary heart disease rates in Scotland and Northern Ireland were 25 per cent higher than in England and Wales.

Within England many areas also have relatively poor levels of health, with the northern regions being as bad in many respects as Scotland and Northern Ireland. A general North–South gradient has been identified with the northern regions having a higher death rate for men and married women (adjusted for the age of the population) than the southern regions (Townsend, Davidson and Whitehead, 1988). The general health of the population is also worse in the North and Midlands than in the South.

However, the immediate local environment is regarded as a more important determinant of health than the region in which one resides. In the North one can find areas where the population's health is good, while some localities in the South have very poor levels of health. Much of the North-South 'divide' results from the greater concentration of poor environments in the North. (Blaxter, 1990, p. 87).

Finally, it should be pointed out that regional, local and indeed other forms of inequality are not confined to the UK (Fox, 1989). In the United States, for example, the infant mortality rate for non-whites in Washington DC is more than double the national average. Many other developed countries, such as Italy for example, have considerable regional inequalities in health. In the Third World the problem of geographical inequalities is even more striking, with wide differences in health between rural and urban environments (Phillips, 1990).

■ Social structure and health

□ *Social class, deprivation and health*

Interest in the relationship between social class and health was stimulated by the Black report which found considerable inequalities in health status between different socioeconomic groups (DHSS, 1980; Townsend, Davidson, Whitehead, 1988). Although an official report, this document was disowned by the government of the day, for reasons which will be discussed in later chapters. Further studies of health inequalities have confirmed many of the findings identified in the Black report and have provided additional evidence of widening health inequalities since its publication (Whitehead, 1987; Smith, Bartley and Blane, 1990).

There are considerable differences in mortality between the social classes (Delamothe 1991). This is illustrated by the fact that 62 of the 66 major causes of death in men are more common in social classes IV and V (unskilled and semi-skilled manual workers) than in other social classes. Also, of the 70 major causes of female deaths, 64 were more common in women married to men in social classes IV and V than in the other social classes. Stillbirths, infant mortality and deaths of children are all more likely in these social classes. A child born into a family where the father is an unskilled worker has twice the risk of being stillborn or of dying in infancy compared with one born into a professional family.

Class differences can be expressed in the form of Standardised Mortality Ratios (SMRs). SMRs are a technique which can be used to compare the health of populations having a different age and sex structure (see Exhibit 1.1).

SMRs are expressed as index numbers. If a population subgroup has an SMR over 100 this means that it has a higher than average mortality, even after taking into account age and sex differences. An SMR of under 100 reflects a lower than average level of mortality. Figure 1.6 illustrates that in the case of both men and women, the 'non-manual' social classes have a lower than average SMR, and the 'manual' social classes have higher SMRs. Indeed, the SMR for unskilled men (social class V) is two and a half times that of professional men (social class I).

Social class differences for males are considerably wider when mortality is expressed in terms of number of years of potential life lost due to premature death (Blane, Smith and Bartley, 1990). In 1981 mortality among males in the 20–64 age group led to the loss of 114 years of potential life per 1000 population in social class V. This is almost three times the number of years lost by the population in social class I (39 years per 1000).

There is also a significant variation in morbidity between the classes, based on self-reported illness statistics (OPCS, 1992). Rates of self-reported long-standing illness in men and women vary considerably with social class. This is most evident in middle-aged people. For example, 40 per cent of middle-aged men in non-manual occupations (social classes I, II and IIIN) reported long-standing illness in 1990 compared with 50 per cent of manual workers(social classes IIIM, IV and V).

Exhibit 1.1   Standardised mortality ratios

The Standardised Mortality Ratio (SMR) is a useful technique for comparing the health of different sections of the population. The SMR adjusts for differences in the composition of a section of the population and the population as a whole.

The SMR expresses the actual number of deaths in a section of the population (e.g. professional men) over a given period as a proportion of the number of expected deaths. This is then expressed as an index number by multiplying by 100.

$$\text{SMR} = \frac{\text{Actual Deaths}}{\text{Expected deaths}} \times 100$$

The number of expected deaths is calculated as follows. The number of people in each particular age group is multiplied by the overall death rate for that age group. The expected number of deaths for each age group are then added together to produce the total number of expected deaths.

A simplified worked example is show below:

Age	(a) Social Class I Number of Males (1000s)	(b) Male death rate per 1000 (general population)	Expected Deaths (a × b)
Under 1	3	20.0	60
1–14	30	0.5	15
15–44	60	1.0	60
45–64	80	14.0	1120
65 and over	60	80.0	4800

Total expected deaths	6055
Actual deaths among males in social class I	5075

$$\text{SMR} = \frac{5075}{6055} \times 100 = 83.8$$

If the SMR is less than 100 (as above) then this section of the population has a low death rate and is regarded as being relatively healthy. An SMR greater than 100 indicates that it is less healthy than the general population.

SMRs can be used to compare the relative mortality of social classes (as in the worked example). They can also be used to compare other population subgroups, such as those living in different localities and ethnic groups.

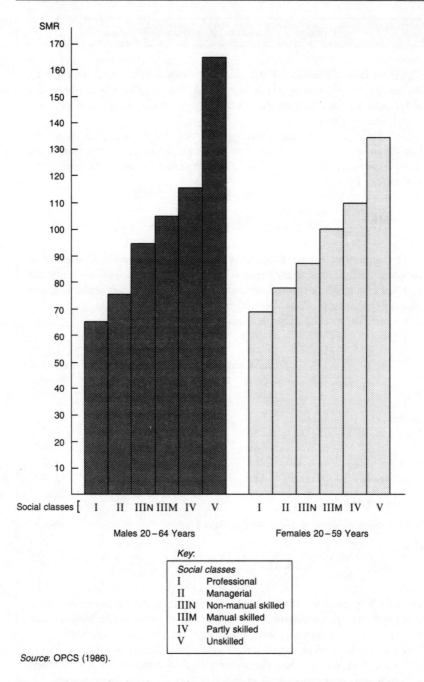

Figure 1.6   *Standardised mortality ratios (SMRs) (Great Britain), 1981*

Further evidence of social class differences has been found in occupational studies such as that undertaken by Balarajan (1989) into the mortality rates of male NHS workers. This study found mortality rates significantly higher among the lower paid 'manual' occupations (porters, ambulancemen, for example). Significantly lower mortality rates were found among the professions which enjoy higher pay and status – for example, doctors, dentists and opticians. Research into the health of civil servants at different grades has also revealed that employment grade and salary is strongly related to both objectively measured and self-reported health status (Marmot *et al.*, 1991).

These variations in morbidity agree with data produced by health and lifestyle surveys, where the focus is on health as well as illness. The survey reported by Blaxter (1990) for example, found that at all ages and in each aspect of health measured, health experience was poorer as social class declined. The survey found that differences between social classes did exist at the start of adult life but that they were small and not always quite regular. However, the effect of social circumstances was more noticeable as people grew older. By middle age, class differences in health had become wider, particularly among men. Among people aged over 60 (and especially among those over 70) it was found that the social class differences became even greater in terms of the individual's subjective assessment of their own health. Yet, paradoxically, in terms of actual disease the health of classes appeared to converge in old age. This was presumably due in part at least to the 'healthy survivor' effect. The least fit and healthy among the manual classes had, in fact, died before reaching old age, leaving only the more resilient who were by the very fact of their survival more healthy.

A brief review of the evidence on health inequalities indicates a clear class gradient, particularly in middle age. Yet the underlying causes of these variations in health, morbidity and mortality have been the subject of much controversy. The precise nature of these arguments will be explored in Chapter 11, alongside the strategies which have been suggested as a means of tackling health inequalities. For the time being it is sufficient to make the point that health inequality on the scale shown here presents a considerable challenge to the health care system and to health policy-makers. Unless and until these inequalities are reduced, it will be difficult if not impossible to achieve improvements in the overall standards of health of the population as a whole. This is because the health status of those social groups which suffer disproportionately from ill-health in effect prevents the average rates of illness from falling further.

□ *Other social inequalities*

Ethnicity

Most ill-health suffered by ethnic groups in Britain is common to the rest of the population. However, there is evidence to suggest that certain diseases occur more frequently among ethnic groups than in the general population (DoH, 1992a; Marmot *et al.*, 1984; Rathwell and Phillips, 1986). For example, the Asian community is more likely to suffer from coronary heart disease. The coronary heart disease mortality rate for those originating from the Indian subcontinent is 36 per cent higher for men and 46 per cent higher for women when compared with the national average (Balarajan, 1991). Asians are also more at risk from other circulatory diseases such as strokes, as indeed are those born in the Caribbean and in Africa.

Those originating from the Indian subcontinent have an above-average rate of infection from tuberculosis and certain cancers (such as liver cancer) although it should be noted that cancer mortality overall is lower among all the immigrant groups compared with the general population. There is a disproportionately high incidence of diabetes in West Indian and Asian communities (Nikolaides *et al.*, 1981). There are higher reported rates of mental illness in the Caribbean community, the incidence of schizophrenia, for example, being higher than among the general population. In addition, there are a number of diseases which are rarely found in Britain outside certain ethnic groups, such as rickets (in Asians) and sickle cell disease (in Afro-Caribbean people). Finally, perinatal and infant mortality is significantly higher among the Asian, African and West Indian communities (Bhat *et al.*, 1988).

So there is evidence that illness among ethnic minority groups differs significantly from the general population. Yet systematic and detailed evidence on the health needs of these groups does not exist. Little is known about why these health differences persist and how they could best be tackled. There have been some recent attempts to formulate health strategies for the ethnic minorities at a local level, but these efforts have so far been piecemeal and tentative.

Gender

The gender gap in health is neatly summarised by Agnes Miles (1991): 'Women live longer but suffer from more health problems in their lifetime and many of these problems are specific to the female gender.' In 1991 the life expectancy of a woman at birth was 78.8 years (over 5 years longer than for a man). The death rates for women are lower than for men in every age group, and for most disease categories. Yet the rates of self-reported long-standing illness for women – 35 per cent in the 1990 General Household Survey (OPCS, 1992) are slightly higher overall than for men (33 per cent). However, this gap is due to differences between the male and female rates in the older age groups (see Figure 1.2). Indeed, among children the rate of self-reported long-standing illness is higher among males. The finding that older women are more likely than older men to report such illness could reflect the fact that more women than men survive to reach the ages where greater levels of long-standing illness are experienced.

The health and lifestyle survey reported by Blaxter (1990) also found that women were more likely both to report illness and to experience lower levels of what could be termed 'well-being'. This was partly attributed to the greater willingness of women to admit to illness. But it was also believed that physiological differences – pregnancy, menopause and menstruation – meant that on average women were likely to suffer more often from pain and dysfunction than men.

Breast cancer and cancers of the genito-urinary system are major causes of death in women. Every year, around 15 000 women in Britain die from breast cancer. It is the biggest cause of death from cancer among women. A further 2000 women a year die from cervical cancer. Other diseases are found more commonly in the female population, such as osteoporosis and cystitis. Women also appear to suffer disproportionately from mental illness. There is a significant variation among women in this respect which should be noted. Married women and women living in urban areas seem to suffer above-average levels of anxiety and depression. Also working-class women are far more likely to suffer from depression than are middle-class women (Brown and Harris, 1982).

During the twentieth century the role of women has undergone a dramatic change, particularly in relation to the world of work. Over the past few decades the pace of change has, if anything, increased. Two-thirds of married women now have jobs outside the home. Given that surveys have consistently found housewives to have more health problems than women in paid employment, one would expect this trend to have a beneficial impact upon women's health (Warr and Parry, 1982). In reality it has had a differential impact depending on other social circumstances. Paid employment is generally associated with more illness for working-class women with children but less for middle-class women having the same family responsibilities (Blaxter, 1990, p. 101). Much of the impact on women's health seems to depend on the extent to which women have to combine the responsibilities of work and home (Shimmin *et al.*, 1981).

It is also apparent that social changes are leading many women to adopt traditionally male lifestyles and habits. Around a third of women under the age of 50 smoke, the same proportion as men in this age group. The increase in smoking among women has been associated with the recent growth in female lung cancer rates (Jacobson, 1981). Lung cancer is now the second largest cancer killer of women (it remains the largest cause of death by cancer in men). Alcohol consumption among young women is also increasing and this has been paralleled by an increase in drink-related problems.

■ Conclusion

Inequalities of health in terms of gender, ethnicity, class and region are important. Further improvements in general levels of health can only be achieved by improving the health of sections of the population that are currently below average. There is a need to understand these inequalities and minimise them wherever possible. In addition, health services should be geared to the different needs of the various sections of the population. This is particularly important in the case of women and ethnic minorities, who have specific health needs different in many ways from those of the general population.

Yet health inequalities represent only one category within a range of challenges facing contemporary health care. As we have seen, the increasing elderly population is likely to have considerable implications for the health care system. This development will probably require some increased expenditure on health and welfare services. At the very least a redirection of health care will be required to meet the needs produced by this demographic change.

This survey of health trends has pinpointed the growing burden of chronic and degenerative disease in our society. It has also revealed the extent of premature death, accidents and violent death – a waste of life on an alarming scale. All these trends require an appropriate response from health policy-makers and service providers. However, the emphasis on chronic disease should not produce complacency about the threat of infectious disease, even in the UK, which has a comparatively good record in this area. Nor should one concentrate exclusively on physical illness. Mental illness exists on a large scale, and requires an appropriate response.

There are a number of economic and political questions raised by this survey of health trends. For example, how can the health care system respond to changing needs? What are the financial implications of this? How can we tackle the broader social, environmental and lifestyle factors which lie behind many contemporary health problems? Later chapters explore the extent to which the British health care system has responded to important questions such as these. But first we must examine the crucial role of the medical profession in relation to health and health care, the subject of the next chapter.

■ *Chapter 2* ■

Medicine and the Medical Profession

Medicine, as a profession and as a body of scientific knowledge, exerts so much influence over health care that observers often speak of medical hegemony – a domination of health care by medical ideas, concepts and practices. This chapter investigates medical hegemony, beginning with a discussion of the nature of orthodox medicine. This is followed by an examination of alternative medical approaches and perspectives. The status of the medical profession and the roots of its power are then explored, both in relation to health care and with regard to the wider social context. Finally, the challenges to medical hegemony and the prospects of its future survival are discussed.

■ Medicine

Modern medicine is a subtle combination of art and science. Medicine is an art in the sense that its practice involves a wide range of mental and physical skills. These run from the dexterity of the surgeon to the ability to communicate with patients in a sensitive way. Medicine is also regarded as an art because it requires personal capacities for judgement and understanding. When doctors actually diagnose and treat patients such capacities are at least as important as scientific knowledge.

Modern medicine is strongly underpinned by scientific methods, principles and disciplines. It is heavily based on what has become known as the biomedical model or biomedicine (Engel, 1977). The main features of this model and its development are discussed below.

☐ *Medicine as a science: the development of biomedicine*

Biomedicine is based on a belief that the only satisfactory basis for medical practice is scientific experimentation, observation and discovery. From this

24

perspective, medicine is the accumulation of a body of scientific knowledge and its subsequent application to the diagnosis and treatment of disease.

Important discoveries in anatomy and human physiology during the seventeenth and eighteenth centuries laid the foundation for the development of biomedicine. These discoveries included the circulation of the blood, the functions of organs, and the impact of disease and external agents upon these organs. Scientific experimentation gradually became accepted during the nineteenth century as the legitimate source of medical knowledge. Experiments became more sophisticated and important discoveries were made about disease processes. In particular, there were great advances in the understanding of the bacterial causes of disease. Experiments by scientists, such as Louis Pasteur and Robert Koch, led to the identification of the infectious agents which caused major diseases such as cholera and tuberculosis. The focus of medicine therefore increasingly emphasised germ theory – that diseases were largely caused by specific infectious agents in the environment.

Medical knowledge of the body's structure and composition also improved a great deal during the nineteenth century. Advances in microscope technology enabled the study of cell biology. This in turn led to the work of Rudolf Virchow on cellular pathology, the study of the actual cell changes which result from disease.

A further area of medical advance came from a better understanding of body chemistry. It was discovered that chemical processes were responsible for regulating a wide range of the body's activities, and that diseases could be attributed to deficiencies in these processes. This was to lead to the discovery of hormones, such as insulin, and vitamins, which have a crucial role in the maintenance of health.

Advances in medical knowledge led ultimately to the development of new techniques and interventions. Diagnosis benefited from the development of instruments to measure blood pressure, blood flow and heartbeat. Surgery improved with the advent of antiseptics, pioneered by Joseph Lister. The emergence of effective anaesthetics not only made surgery more bearable for patients, it also gave surgeons extra time to perform operations, thereby facilitating the development of more complex surgical techniques. Furthermore, the increasing institutionalisation of health care in hospitals provided doctors with better conditions, both for observing disease processes and for applying new medical technologies.

Meanwhile, the growing knowledge of bacterial causes of disease led to the development of vaccines to prevent these diseases, and so-called 'magic bullets' to cure them. An example of the latter was the discovery by Paul Ehrlich in 1910 of Salvarsan as a treatment for syphilis. This was followed by the development of antibiotics, beginning with the discovery of penicillin by Alexander Fleming in 1928. The early part of the century also saw attempts to treat diseases caused by hormone deficiencies, such as diabetes (see Exhibit 2.1), and those caused by vitamin deficiencies, such as rickets.

These medical interventions were based on scientific knowledge and methods. In exploring the disease process, medicine increasingly focused upon specific aetiology. Put simply, this means that diseases can be attributed to specific biological causes and processes. The aim was, first of all, to reveal through scientific means the nature of the disease process, then, on the basis of this understanding, to discover how this process could be reversed or limited.

Yet it should be pointed out that intervention has not always taken place on the basis of a firm understanding of the relationship between cause and effect. Action has often followed as a result of experiments, which, although scientific, only demonstrate an association between two events.

Exhibit 2.1   Diabetes mellitus

Aetiology

This disease occurs as a result of a deficiency in the production of insulin, a hormone secreted in the pancreas, which regulates sugar levels in the body. The deficiency leads to an accumulation of sugar in the blood, which in turn produces a range of symptoms (see below). The relationship between these symptoms and insulin deficiency was discovered by empirical observation and scientific experimentation. Particularly important were experiments conducted by Frederick Banting and Charles Best in the 1920s. The pancreatic ducts of dogs were blocked in order to reproduce the symptoms of diabetes. When the accumulated pancreatic secretions were subsequently injected back into the animals (and later into humans), the symptoms were alleviated.

Diagnosis

The common presenting symptoms of diabetes mellitus are increased thirst, a frequent urge to pass urine, weight loss and a propensity to infections. The longer-term complications include nerve damage, producing a loss of sensation in the limbs, and damage to other organs including the kidneys and the eyes. Tests for sugar in the blood and urine will confirm the diagnosis.

Treatment

The patient may be given insulin to counteract the deficiency. He or she may have to observe certain dietary restrictions.

The classic example is Edward Jenner's experiment with inoculation in the eighteenth century. Jenner was able to prevent smallpox by inoculating people with material taken from cowpox sufferers. Yet the disease process which led to this outcome was not fully understood until the following century. Similarly, John Snow's identification in 1854 of contaminated water supplies as being the factor responsible for outbreaks of cholera preceded the identification of the cholera organism by almost thirty years. Yet by the time Koch had made this discovery, efforts to improve water supplies and sanitation were well under way. Intervention on the basis of partial evidence of disease processes is a particular feature of the public health model of medicine discussed later.

☐ *The features of biomedicine*

The development of medicine as a scientific exercise means that the focus is now upon the disease process itself, rather than on the sufferer. Biomedicine concentrates mainly on biological changes which can be defined, measured and isolated. It is directed towards the dysfunction of the various organs and tissues of the body rather than the condition of the patient as a whole. Indeed, biomedicine is identified as a negative perspective on health because it views health more in terms of the absence of disease than the possession of healthy attributes.

Biomedicine has resulted in improved knowledge and understanding about disease. In many cases it has produced practical improvements in the treatment of patients, so improving the length and quality of life. Yet in spite of its achievements, biomedicine has been subjected to considerable criticism in recent years. Some feel that its domination of modern medicine is in many respects inappropriate to the health problems of today (Inglis, 1981), while others cast doubt on the extent to which the rational scientific principles are actually employed in medical practice today.

☐ *Is modern medicine scientific?*

The idea that doctors operate within the narrow confines of the biomedical model has been rejected by some supporters of modern medicine, as well as its critics. A number of doctors have rejected the strict application of the biomedical model, claiming it to be an abstraction which has limited application in practice (Black, 1984). They argue that modern medicine is not wholly focused on disease but is eclectic, taking into account wider influences on health such as lifestyle and emotional factors (Brewin, 1985). Some see medical practice as being less dominated by the biomedical model than in the past. According to Tudor-Hart (1981), doctors are increasingly concerned about health promotion, the environment and public health, and as a result are more likely to intervene at a social and political level in order to promote health in a broader and more positive sense.

Certainly, the biomedical model does not describe the approach of every medical practitioner in every single situation. It perhaps applies less to general practitioners and community-based doctors than to their hospital colleagues. The model is also probably more applicable to the older rather than to the younger generation of doctors.

It is also the case that the biomedical model cannot be entirely insulated from the culture in which it is being applied. Doctors are influenced by non-medical models of health. Both medical and lay models are shaped to some extent by the culture in which they operate (Helman, 1990; Herzlich and Pierret, 1985). Doctors may also retain lay assumptions about illness that remain with them after clinical training. These assumptions can supplement the orthodox approach in practice (Gaines, 1979).

The extent to which the process of identifying disease is influenced by culture is explored in a comparative study of medicine and health in West Germany, France, Germany and the USA by Lynn Payer (1989). She claims that the choice of diagnoses and treatments is not a scientific process, for two main reasons. First, most consultations are about health problems – such as, fatigue or anxiety, for example – for which there are no scientific solutions. Second, cultural factors, which vary from nation to nation, have a great impact on the treatment of disease, and upon the diagnosis of illness. Payer gives a number of examples to back up her case. She notes, for example, that blood pressure considered high in the USA might be considered normal in the UK. While low blood pressure, considered to be a problem by German doctors, is not regarded as such by their British and American counterparts.

☐ *Subjectivity*

Modern medicine may not be as scientific as many doctors claim. It has been pointed out that doctors cannot even agree on the meaning of a fundamental term such as 'disease' (Campbell *et al.*, 1979). Confusion within the medical profession surrounding the concept of disease, and a variation in the way in which disease concepts are applied, means that medicine is far more subjective than has been commonly supposed. Doctors operate within a framework of medical knowledge which focuses upon specific diseases. They may be tempted to pigeonhole patients' illnesses into convenient categories in order to make the situation more manageable. Indeed, according to Payer (1989) some doctors use so-called 'wastebasket diagnoses'. These diagnoses are used when patients are presenting ambiguous symptoms and the doctor is unable to give a clear diagnosis. For example, a patient complaining of fatigue actually may be suffering from one of a number of possible illnesses. Yet it may be convenient for the doctor simply to tell the patient that he or she has a 'virus', 'anaemia' or even 'depression' without further elaboration.

Diseases are deviations from normality. Yet, with the exception of extreme cases, deviations from normality are inherently ambiguous (Twaddle, 1974). Health status changes do not therefore follow automatically from biological changes. Instead, the latter are events requiring interpretation, which depend on medical judgement, which is in turn influenced by a variety of cultural and social factors.

Kennedy (1981) claims that doctors make two sets of judgements when diagnosing patients. First, they must assess whether the patient's problem or condition represents a deviation from what would be considered normal. Second, they have to make a judgement about the deviation itself, and whether this constitutes an illness. According to Kennedy such judgements are not objective but subjective. Doctors are not insulated from social and cultural values and expectations. Kennedy gives as an example the American Psychiatric Association's debate over the definition of homosexuality as an illness. From this point of view, medical practice is a political enterprise with medical judgements reflecting doctors' beliefs about social order.

The case of obesity further illustrates the subjectivity of medicine. Obesity is seen by many doctors as a major public health problem (Garrow, 1991; Royal College of Physicians, 1983a). It is defined objectively – in terms of a Body Mass Index (calculated from an individual's weight and height ratio). Yet the extent to which an individual's body weight is judged to deviate excessively from the norm is in turn related to cultural values and expectations. Dutch doctors, for example, are far more likely to diagnose obesity than are British doctors (Payer, 1989).

Doctors are not insulated from these social and cultural influences. Therefore medical concern with obesity may be a reflection of Western society's current obsession with slimming, rather than being wholly based on the health implications of being overweight. This argument is supported by evidence that moderate obesity does not necessarily cause ill-health (Mann, 1974; Noppa *et al.*, 1980). Moreover, an individual's bodyweight may have less to do with eating habits and more to do with metabolism (Hirsch and Leibel, 1988), suggesting that dieting and slimming is inappropriate for some. Indeed, it has been suggested that serious psychological disorders related to dieting, such as anorexia nervosa and bulimia nervosa, are in part the product of social pressures, particularly on young women, to be slim (Cataldo, 1985). Doctors, in recognising obesity as a disease, may be legitimising these social pressures, rather than helping to alleviate them.

This is not to deny that extreme obesity is linked with chronic illness. Individuals should pursue a recommended balanced diet, provided there is a sound empirical foundation for these recommendations. The point being made here is that the identification of obesity as a medical condition may be as much the result of social and cultural values as objective, scientific fact and that the same reasoning may apply to other conditions which have a clear social dimension.

□ *Difficulties of diagnosis*

The scientific basis of medicine may be undermined by the fact that some diseases are difficult and in some cases impossible to diagnose. Signs and symptoms may be highly ambiguous. A patient complaining of a persistent headache could be suffering from one of a number of possible conditions from a migraine to a brain tumour. Furthermore, many diseases do not have objective conditions or signs. This often leads to disputes about whether, in fact, the disease exists at all.

Such controversy has surrounded myalgic encephalomyelitis (ME), an illness with influenza-like symptoms followed by chronic physical and mental fatigue. ME sufferers are in no doubt that they are ill, but doctors have been reluctant to accept their condition as a genuine illness, largely because there is no objective way of testing for the disease (see Exhibit 2.2).

An additional problem for the biomedical model is that a disease may have multiple causes. Alzheimer's disease, for example, is now thought to be caused by environmental as well as genetic factors. Many cancers result from a complex interaction of factors. Doctors accept that the causes of illness are increasingly complex. However, the acceptance of a number of possible causes for a particular illness does leave much more scope for doubt and ambiguity, and thereby subjectivity also.

Critics argue that the kinds of factors discussed above render the biomedical approach inappropriate in the present context (Kennedy, 1981; Inglis, 1981). They claim that the biomedical emphasis of modern medicine is misdirected, and that doctors are hiding their subjective judgements behind a smokescreen of pseudo-science. Some doctors react defensively by upholding the sanctity of the biomedical model. Others, as we have seen, argue that although modern medicine remains scientifically based, medical practice is far more eclectic and is able to incorporate new theories and concepts which improve our understanding of the causes of illness.

Exhibit 2.2   Myalgic encephalomyelitis

ME initially gives rise to influenza-like symptoms, followed by chronic physical and mental fatigue. Other symptoms include vertigo, ringing in the ears, blurred vision, muscle spasms, memory impairment, excessive sweating and an inability to concentrate. The illness can be long-term, lasting over ten years in a quarter of sufferers.

Yet the medical profession has been reluctant to acknowledge ME as a genuine illness. In 1955 an outbreak of ME at the Royal Free Hospital was later identified by doctors as a form of mass hysteria. The majority of doctors do not recognise the illness, preferring to believe that sufferers are neurotic or malingering.

Those suffering from ME feel stigmatised. They have difficulty in obtaining the social support and understanding which the sick normally expect. Moreover, they find that doctors cannot offer much help in the way of advice, care or treatment. A number of doctors, some of whom have suffered from ME, have tried to promote awareness and understanding of the illness, both within the profession and in the wider community.

One of the main difficulties in obtaining recognition for ME is that there is no clear test to confirm diagnosis, as in diabetes mellitus for example. Although new research has identified the presence of a virus in a number of sufferers, an objective test for ME does not exist at present.

Modern medicine, however, remains strongly wedded to the guiding principles of the biomedical model. This is reflected by the failure of alternative models to displace this orthodoxy.

☐ *Other medical models: public health medicine*

Public health has recently been defined as 'the science and art of preventing disease, prolonging life, and promoting health through the organised efforts of society' (Cm 289, 1988). McKeown's work (1979), the definitive statement of the modern public health perspective, argues that modern medicine focuses primarily upon the disease process within the individual and ignores the wider social, economic and environmental factors relevant to health.

Much of McKeown's argument is based on historical evidence which challenges the conventional view of the contribution of modern medicine. Diseases such as measles, whooping cough and tuberculosis were in decline well before the introduction of immunisation and effective medical treatment. McKeown identifies better nutrition and rising standards of living as the key factors in the reduction of morbidity and mortality since the late nineteenth century. Improvements in health are also partly attributed to better hygiene during the Victorian era (Wohl, 1984).

McKeown also points out that the major causes of ill-health and death today – cancer, heart disease and circulatory disease – are largely the result of individual behaviour and the environment. Orthodox medicine is viewed as providing an inappropriate response to these problems. It is reactive, waiting for illness to happen. It also requires conclusive evidence of a specific disease process. Modern health problems frequently involve a complex combination of factors and 'action is often needed to protect and promote health in circumstances where the evidence is less than complete' (McKeown, 1979).

While many of McKeown's conclusions are supported by others (Dubos, 1959; Fuchs, 1974; McKinlay, 1979; Powles, 1973), some have challenged aspects of his thesis. Szreter (1988) accepts that modern medicine cannot be credited with the decline in mortality over the past century, but disputes that rising nutritional and living standards were the main reasons for falling mortality rates. He argues that the medical profession played a key role in improvement of health through their involvement in the Victorian public health movement. They were also active in promoting local preventive measures, including the establishment of community health services.

Sagan (1987), while sharing McKeown's cynicism about the impact of medical care, rejects the argument that public health measures or nutrition were responsible for declining mortality. Sagan identifies the reduction in family size and modern parenting behaviour as the main reasons for the improvements in health. He identifies the social support function of the family unit as being particularly significant in the maintenance of mental and physical health.

Finally, McKeown's thesis has been attacked for not appreciating the full contribution of modern medicine. For example, it has been pointed out that improvements in the quality of life do not always show up in mortality and morbidity indicators. Hip replacements are a commonly cited example (Morris, 1980).

In the nineteenth century the public health model was highly regarded and provided much of the rationale for such interventions as sanitary improvements, housing reforms and vaccination. For most of the twentieth century it has been very much the junior partner to the biomedical model. There are, however, signs that this may be changing. As noted earlier, some doctors are paying more attention to the wider causes of ill-health. Furthermore, during the late 1980s the Chief Medical Officer in the Department of Health signalled his concern by undertaking the first review of public health in England for over a hundred years (Cm 289, 1988). More recently, the government has outlined a national health strategy aimed at tackling some of the main causes of illness and death. This is discussed in Chapter 11.

☐ *Alternative medicine*

In addition to the public health model there are alternative medical approaches based on different theories of health and illness (Sharma, 1992; Saks, 1992). The main forms of alternative medicine are shown in Exhibit 2.3.

The distinguishing feature of alternative therapies is their marginal standing in relation to the medical establishment and the health care system rather than any common content. Alternative medicine covers an enormous range of therapies based on a variety of theories and methods. Moreover, some alternative therapies have features which are not radically different from some aspects of the biomedical approach. Osteopathy and chiropractic, for example, are aimed at correcting the body's mechanical functions just as (by different methods and using different theories) the biomedical approach has tended to emphasise physical dysfunction. Homeopathy uses drugs aimed at clearing up specific disorders, though it takes a different view of the causal processes at work. Also, many of the plants used in herbalism have been exploited by orthodox medicine as remedies for specific diseases.

In addition to these similarities and overlaps there are a number of more general points to make about the relationship between alternative and orthodox medicine. First, most of the alternative therapies are, in fact, interventionist – they involve some form of treatment for specific disorders. Second, they are often focused on the individual, though some take into account relevant background factors in a more systematic and comprehensive manner.

A further point is that alternative therapies are not necessarily in competition with conventional medicine. A survey of patients using alternative therapy revealed that many patients had not lost total confidence in orthodox medicine (Moore *et al.*, 1985). Furthermore, many qualified doctors are now taking a greater interest in alternative therapies. According to Stanway (1986) 300 fully qualified British doctors practice homoeopathy. Osteopathy is also practised by a small but growing number of doctors in this country. Around fifty British medical practitioners are also qualified osteopaths and 700 doctors are members of the British Medical Acupuncture Society (Saks, 1992). One in twelve of all general practitioners (GPs) in the UK are members of complementary medical bodies (Fulder, 1992, p. 169).

Exhibit 2.3　*Alternative medicine*

Acupuncture

This practice, developed in ancient China, is based on the theory that there is a connection between body organs and body surface. Acupuncture involves using needles to stimulate acupuncture points under the skin in an attempt to influence the related organs. It is also claimed that acupuncture has a more general effect in promoting relaxation and relieving pain.

Homoeopathy

A system of medicine based on the principle that agents which produce certain signs and symptoms in healthy people cure the same signs and symptoms of disease. The more a particular drug is diluted, the more potent it will be as a cure. Furthermore, the treatment given will be tailored to the individual, rather than to the characteristics of the disease as is generally the case in mainstream biomedicine.

Chiropractic

This is a manipulative therapy designed to maintain the spinal column in a good state of health, without the use of drugs. The therapy is aimed at dealing with specific disorders such as back and neck pain, and headaches.

Osteopathy

This is similar to chiropractic in that it involves the manipulation of the spine in order to remedy disease. However, osteopaths' manipulative techniques are based on different theories of the causes of illness from those adopted by chiropractors.

Herbal medicine

The use of plants and herbs to deal with specific illnesses and to maintain health. A related therapy – aromatherapy – involves body massage using oils extracted from plants.

Hypnotherapy

The inducement of trance has been used to combat a variety of psychological disorders such as anxiety, phobias and insomnia. Hypnotherapy is sometimes used by individuals who are trying to change unhealthy lifestyles such as smoking. Hypnotherapy has also been used in the treatment of conditions with physical symptoms where there may be an underlying psychological cause.

Given this level of participation, some doctors now believe alternative medicine is a misleading term, preferring instead 'complementary medicine'. If more orthodox doctors adopt these therapies in future, one may see greater incorporation of alternative techniques into mainstream medicine. However, there has been some resistance from the medical establishment. In the early 1980s the British Medical Association (BMA) established a working party to look into the question of alternative medicine. The report of this working party adopted a negative tone. It criticised the lack of a rational scientific base for many of the alternative therapies and rejected the theories which underpinned them (BMA, 1986b).

The BMA working party argued that unconventional techniques could be incorporated within mainstream medicine if they were properly subjected to evaluation. It also maintained that where alternative therapies were of value, they should only be undertaken by suitably qualified persons operating within an approved system of qualification and registration and under the direction of the medical profession. More recently the BMA position on alternative medicine has become less hardline. In 1993 it produced a further report which was far more positive about the role of alternative medicine, but which still stressed the importance of evaluation and qualification.

The alternative therapies continue to flourish. The latest estimate is that there are over 10 000 alternative therapists in the UK (Fulder, 1992, p. 168). This figure excludes faith healers, of which there are a further 20 000. The number of therapists has increased rapidly in recent years, as more people have turned to alternative medicine, with the biggest growth being in acupuncture and homoeopathy.

A survey undertaken by MORI (*The Times*, 13 November 1989, p. 15) revealed a high level of public interest in alternative therapies. A minority – less than a quarter of those asked – said they would not consider using any of these therapies. There was also evidence of considerable satisfaction among those who had tried alternative therapies. For example, in the case of homoeopathy, where 11 per cent of those questioned had undergone a course of treatment, four-fifths expressed satisfaction.

It is believed by some that alternative medicine may benefit from the recent funding changes in the NHS (see Saks, 1990). Under this new system many GPs now have their own budgets and may have greater incentive to refer patients to alternative therapists because of their relatively low cost and increasing popularity. But there are also factors which are likely to constrain the growth of this sector of care, not least the continued opposition of the orthodox medical establishment. A particularly serious threat is posed by moves towards further European integration. This has created pressures for uniformity in the standards of health care qualifications. As a consequence, the rights of alternative therapists to practise may be reduced or removed.

☐ *Lay models of health and illness*

There is a rich and growing literature exploring the different ways in which ordinary people view health and illness. Orthodox medicine does seem to exert a considerable influence upon lay views (Calnan, 1987). However, the latter are notoriously complex and have a certain independence (Fitzpatrick, 1984, p. 11). Moreover, while orthodox medicine is supreme in terms of its formal domination of health care, lay health beliefs, knowledge and behaviour regarding illness can have an impact on health care in practice. This can occur in a number of ways.

First, the individual's health beliefs may influence the decision to seek treatment. If individuals do not perceive themselves to be ill, their symptoms are unlikely to be presented to doctors. As a result, their illness will probably remain hidden and the condition will not come to the attention of the doctor (Mechanic, 1961; Robinson, 1971).

Second, even if the individual sees a doctor and is diagnosed as having a particular disease, this does not guarantee that the patient will agree with the diagnosis. Neither does it ensure that he or she will comply with the prescribed course of treatment (Ley, 1982; Thompson, 1984).

There are ways in which the medical profession can circumvent such attitudes and behaviour. Screening programmes can be used to detect illness. Compulsory treatment has been used in the past, particularly in the areas of mental illness and immunisation. But at the end of the day, lay perspectives still retain a character of their own, influenced in part by the medical profession itself but also by the deeper cultural and ideological influences within society.

■ The medical profession

☐ *Medicine as a profession*

There is much disagreement between sociologists over the precise meaning of the term 'profession' (see Johnson, 1972; Wilding 1982). However, most would agree that medicine has most of the features commonly associated with a profession, involving the application of a body of expertise, knowledge and skills. It operates within a framework of licensing, where only those sufficiently qualified can practise legitimately, following a considerable period of approved education and training. There is a system of self-regulation and a well-developed sense of service standards. Furthermore, as with other professions, those who practise medicine tend to be drawn from middle-class or upper-middle-class backgrounds. Finally, medicine is well organised by a range of bodies which take responsibility for education, licensing, the maintenance of standards and the representation of interests.

According to Freidson (1988, p. xv) 'it is useful to think of a profession as an occupation which has assumed a dominant position in a division of labour so that it gains control over the determination of the substance of its own work'. Medicine, as will become clear later in this chapter, has successfully monopolised important areas of work and insulated itself to a large degree from outside interference.

Within health care, medicine enjoys a superior status. The way in which alternative therapists have been successfully marginalised by the orthodox medical profession has already been noted. Other health care professions act for the most part under medical direction and instruction. They have less autonomy than medicine and are weaker in terms of their political organisation and leverage.

Nurses, for example, despite their popularity with the general public, have much less control over health care than do doctors (Salvage, 1985). Much of their workload is routine and, according to many nurses, their contribution to the care of patients is not maximised. Politically, nurses are less well organised than the medical profession (Hayward and Fee, 1992). They also tend to be drawn from less exclusive social class backgrounds – the working class and lower middle class.

Tension between nurses and doctors, though common, has tended to be implicit rather than overt. Even when there has been open conflict between the paramedical professions and the medical profession, the latter has invariably won. An often cited example is the struggle between doctors and midwives over childbirth and maternity care, a conflict which continues today (Donnison, 1988).

According to Armstrong (1990) the status of paramedical professions has improved during the twentieth century, through registration, education, self-discipline and licensing. While paramedical skills have achieved professional recognition, however, the core of medical dominance has not been eroded (Larkin, 1983). Medicine continues to determine the overall division of labour in health care, and doctors remain the dominant profession in this sector.

□ *Doctors, patients and the public*

Doctors are also in a dominant position with respect to the patient. Most studies of the doctor–patient relationship emphasise the power of the former and the weakness of the latter (see, for example, Byrne and Long, 1976; Tuckett *et al.*, 1985). Consultations for most episodes of illness tend to follow the guidance–co-operation model (Szasz and Hollender, 1956), where the doctor is in a superior position to the patient and where the participation of the latter is low.

There are a number of reasons why this is the case. It has often been argued that patients are somewhat afraid of doctors. In a survey of patients in the mid-1970s, over a quarter of the respondents said they often or always felt nervous about seeing their doctor (DHSS, Fitton, and Acheson 1979). Reasons for this included the patients' own temperaments, the doctors' manner, and awe of doctors in general.

Patients are traditionally passive, and particularly so in the UK. This may be due, perhaps, to the long history of charitable health care in this country, which placed most patients in a highly dependent position. An alternative explanation is that the absence of a health care market in the UK in the post-Second World War period has undermined the development of the kind of health care consumerism one finds in the United States. Yet even in the USA a minority of patients are believed to indulge in consumerist behaviour (Hibbard and Weekes, 1987). Moreover, the consumer model is not necessarily the best way of enhancing patient participation, as we shall see in later chapters. The passivity of patients in the UK could also be related to our deferential culture. It is conventional wisdom that the British have a traditional respect for authority, and that it is alien to the British culture to complain. But even those patients wishing to complain about the standards of service have faced difficulties. Complaints procedures are complicated and intimidating. Compensation and redress are difficult to obtain. Furthermore, patients have a general disadvantage in terms of knowledge and information (Association of Community Health Councils, 1992).

There are signs that the traditional passivity of patients may be changing. There has been a greater focus on the importance of the patients' views, particularly in general practice. Some doctors have attempted to alter the style of consultation in order to improve communication with their patients (Savage and Armstrong, 1990). In addition, the past decade has seen a number of health care reforms such as internal markets, the patient's charter and greater access to medical records, which have attempted to instil a consumerist philosophy into British health care. The impact of these reforms is examined in later chapters.

The medical profession enjoys considerable social status beyond its dominant position in relation to patients and other health professions. The evidence of public opinion surveys points to a high degree of satisfaction with the work of doctors. In the British Social Attitudes Survey of 1988/9, for example, which was undertaken at a time when the state of the NHS was the subject of public concern, just under 80 per cent expressed satisfaction with local doctors and GPs (Jowell *et al.*, 1989). There is also evidence of a high level of respect for doctors, compared with those in other occupations and professions (Harrison, 1988a, p. 89). This seems to be universal and is not confined to the UK. Even in the United States, where one might expect the high financial rewards of doctors to create an atmosphere of envy and hostility towards the profession, doctors are nevertheless held in fairly high esteem by the public (Ginzberg, 1990).

□ *Internal hierarchies and specialisation*

Medicine itself is an arena for professional conflict and battles over status. Indeed, the status of doctors varies considerably. Compare, for example, the prestige enjoyed by the consultant with the humble position of the junior doctor. Traditionally, hospital doctors have enjoyed higher status than those working in the community and in general practice (Honigsbaum, 1979). Even within hospital medicine, certain specialities are regarded as being more prestigious than others. Surgeons, particularly those who specialise in the vital organs (brain, heart and so on) appear to have the highest status, while those specialising in the care of low-status social groups, such as the psychiatrists who treat the mentally ill, and geriatricians who treat the elderly, tend to have correspondingly lower status themselves.

Stars can rise and fall. Surgery, for example, has greatly improved in status during this century, due partly to the development of new surgical technology. In previous centuries the physicians were the most prestigious wing of the profession (Parry and Parry, 1976). General practice, which at the turn of the century was regarded with great inferiority, has gradually lost most of its humble image. Its status is likely to continue to rise in view of the greater emphasis on primary care today and with the emergence of GP fundholding, both of which have given important new responsibilities and roles to general practitioners.

□ *Explaining medical hegemony*

Four factors appear to be associated with the status of medicine, both in relation to health care and in society at large. These are: the social composition of the medical profession; its role in legitimising health and illness; the autonomy doctors have in relation to their work; and the political organisation of the profession.

☐ Social composition

The social status of the medical profession as whole can be attributed in part to the exclusive social background of its individual members. There are three common beliefs about the composition of the medical profession. First, that it is male-dominated. Second, that doctors tend to come from 'medical families', where at least one parent has a medical background. Third, that it is largely restricted to those from upper-middle class backgrounds. These features will now be examined in turn.

It is true that women are in a minority in the medical profession. Just over a fifth of doctors in the UK are female, compared with 10 per cent in the USA (but 70 per cent in Russia). Women are in an even smaller minority in the higher clinical grades – only 15 per cent of UK consultants are female.

Women are also under-represented in the more prestigious specialities. They are, however, more strongly represented in those branches of the profession which are increasing in importance, such as general practice. Women have also made greater inroads into hospital medicine, with the proportion of female hospital doctors doubling over the past twenty years. Furthermore, the proportion of women studying medicine has also doubled over the same period. Half of all medical students are now female.

Turning to the second popular belief, it is not true to say that most doctors come from 'medical families', though a proportion do. A study of a sample of doctors by Allen (1988) discovered that 17 per cent had followed either one or both parents into the profession.

The same study confirmed that doctors are drawn from the upper middle classes. Three-quarters were from families in social class I (professional) and social class II (managerial). This proportion has not varied significantly over time or between the sexes. The evidence appears to support the view that medicine is to a large extent a socially exclusive profession. However, it is not impossible for those with working-class backgrounds to break into the profession. Allen's analysis showed that the proportion of newly-qualified doctors from manual family backgrounds had increased in recent years.

☐ Legitimation of health and illness

Medical knowledge is regarded as an important source of power in itself (Foucault, 1973; Turner, 1987). This power is not only political (in terms of enabling doctors to dominate patients and other professionals) but is also social in the sense that it carries within it the power to define and redefine the social meaning of various conditions and states. Medicine has the authority to label people's conditions as illnesses and can therefore create illness as a legitimate social status.

According to Parsons (1951), the function of medicine in legitimising illness is particularly important. Parsons regarded illness as a form of social deviance that had the potential to undermine the social system. Such deviance had to be controlled, with the instrument of control being the medical profession: doctors certify who is genuinely ill and who is not. The genuinely sick (as certified by the medical profession) are absolved of responsibility to fulfil social obligations, while those whose sickness is not legitimised are labelled as malingerers and are subjected to social disapproval and sanction. In this way the extent of deviance is controlled through the 'sick role', and the social order is preserved.

Parsons' analysis is, superficially at least, attractive. The power of the medical profession over the definition of illness apparently springs from its gatekeeper role. The sick role also further explains the dependence of the patient upon the doctor.

Yet the simplicity of this explanation has been challenged on a number of grounds (see, for example Turner, 1987). It has been argued that exemption from social obligations can vary according to particular types of illness and according to the social position of those suffering from illnesses. Even when an illness is recognised by the medical profession as being genuine, sufferers may be stigmatised if their condition is seen as a continuing threat to the social order (Goffman, 1968). The consequences of such social disapproval are not confined to malingerers. Indeed, individuals suffering from genuine illnesses may be deprived of privileges and rights. The mentally ill, for example, may be deprived of their liberty. Individuals who have been identified as being HIV positive may be discriminated against in the markets for jobs and housing.

Moreover, in some cases, society may believe that the individual has brought the problem on himself in some way. Hence the assumption that the sick role removes responsibility from the individual may in some circumstances be incorrect. For example, drug addicts and alcoholics are often blamed for their particular illnesses.

In spite of all these flaws, Parsons' analysis has proved useful. The focus upon the function of medicine in legitimising illness provided at least a partial explanation of the role of the medical profession in modern societies and also stimulated others to further explore and clarify this important role.

☐ *Autonomy and self-regulation*

The privileges of self-regulation and clinical autonomy are important symbols of medical power and status. Yet they are more than just symbolic. They give doctors an advantage over both patients and other health professionals in the clinical setting.

The autonomy of the medical profession takes two main forms: clinical autonomy and self-discipline. Doctors are resistant to direction in clinical matters. As professionals they believe they should be allowed to use their own judgement to guide diagnosis and treatment. Yet there is often disagreement on what constitutes a clinical decision. Williams (1988) has noted the difficulties in distinguishing between strictly clinical factors and other extraneous yet important factors such as the availability and use of resources. Doctors themselves agree that clinical decisions cannot be taken in a vacuum, detached from personal, moral, ethical, legal and economic constraints (Hoffenberg, 1987).

Nevertheless, doctors resent interference in matters concerning the admission and treatment of patients. Even peer review (the monitoring of medical work by doctors themselves in an attempt to maintain and promote good practice) is still viewed with suspicion by many within the profession, while the thought of supervision and direction being undertaken by people with a non-medical background, is anathema to them.

Doctors in the UK have enjoyed a high level of clinical autonomy compared with their counterparts in the USA, for example (Harrison and Schulz, 1989). In recent years, as we shall see in later chapters, there has been pressure for greater accountability.

In addition to clinical autonomy the medical profession also treasures the power of self-discipline. In the UK the body responsible for regulating the profession is the General Medical Council (GMC). The GMC maintains a register of doctors and regulates the fitness of doctors to practise. It investigates complaints about doctors from the public, the police, the NHS and from other doctors. Ultimately, doctors found guilty of serious professional misconduct can be suspended or removed from the register, but only about two dozen doctors a year are actually subjected to such a fate out of a thousand complaints on average every year.

The GMC is dominated by doctors. Only a small minority (just over 13 per cent) of its members are lay people. Most of the pressures for reforming the GMC have come from within the profession itself (Stacey, 1989). In the 1970s such pressures led to an inquiry into the regulation of the medical profession (Cmnd 6018, 1975) and subsequently a number of new measures were introduced. These included a new procedure to deal with doctors whose performance was impaired by illness. Changes were also made to the composition of the GMC. The proportion of the GMC elected by the medical profession (as opposed to those appointed by the medical establishment) became a majority of the total for the first time.

Nevertheless, the GMC has resisted radical change. Richard Crossman, a former Labour health minister, complained in his diaries of his inability to influence the regulation of doctors (Crossman, 1977). More recently, Parliament has attempted to put pressure on the GMC to investigate cases of medical incompetence and unacceptable behaviour by doctors. The GMC has responded by proposing changes in its procedures to deal more effectively with poor performance. Radical change is unlikely, but cannot be ruled out in the future. Indeed, the Labour Party is committed to the abolition of the GMC, while the Department of Health is exploring the possibility of new procedures to monitor the professional competence of doctors working in the NHS.

☐ Political power, politics and the state

The medical profession has established its pre-eminence with the help of the state (Freidson, 1988; Larkin, 1983). The superior position of medicine within health care has been granted by the state largely as a result of the effective political organisation of the profession. The major landmark was the Medical Act of 1858, which established the GMC and established a register of qualified medical practitioners. Since then the profession has been able to maintain its position through effective political organisation.

The GMC, as we have seen, is dominated by the medical profession. The other principal medical organisations are the British Medical Association (BMA) and the Royal Colleges of Medicine (see Watkins, 1987). These are briefly discussed below.

☐ The British Medical Association (BMA)

The BMA is the main representative organisation for British doctors. It has a long-established reputation as an effective pressure group (Eckstein, 1960; Grey-Turner and Sutherland, 1982). Around three-quarters of practising doctors are members of the BMA and it has few rivals. However, during the 1970s a number of splinter groups representing consultants, junior doctors and others with special interests did attract some support, and some of these (such as the Hospital Consultants and Specialists Association) continue to exist today.

The BMA lobbies on public health issues such as smoking and road safety, and has even campaigned in recent years against boxing, on health grounds. But most of its activity is concerned with sectional issues such as doctors' pay and conditions of work. The craft committees, which operate under the auspices of the BMA, are recognised bodies which negotiate with the Department of Health on behalf of each branch of the profession: hospital consultants, junior doctors, doctors specialising in public health; and general practitioners.

During the post-war period, the BMA has been regarded as a powerful group, accepted by the government and possessing extensive and close political contacts. Over the years it has enjoyed the privilege of being consulted by government on a wide range of health policy matters. More recently, the BMA's relationship with the government has been less harmonious for reasons which will become clear in later chapters.

☐ *The Royal Colleges of Medicine*

The Royal Colleges (such as the Royal College of Physicians, the Royal College of Surgeons and so on) proclaim themselves to be non-political. Their main responsibility lies in the accreditation and training of specialists. They are, however, consulted by the government on a wide range of health issues.

The Royal Colleges usually operate with a much lower public profile than does the BMA. Yet they are in regular contact with the Department of Health, putting forward their views on a range of issues. The Royal Colleges have representation alongside the BMA on the Joint Consultants' Committee, which since its creation in 1949 has met regularly with officials at the Department of Health. The Royal Colleges are also represented on the Standing Medical Advisory Committee, an official body which advises the Department of Health on a wide range of medical matters.

Over the past few decades, the Royal Colleges have begun to raise their public profile to some extent. In the 1960s, for example, the Royal College of Physicians began to publicise the health dangers of tobacco and called for action to reduce smoking. Along with the Royal Colleges of Psychiatrists and General Practitioners, it has called for action on alcohol abuse. The Royal Colleges of medicine have been involved in the creation of anti-alcohol and anti-tobacco pressure groups in recent years, while in 1987, three Royal College presidents became further involved in public controversy, this time over the funding of the NHS.

☐ *Medical power in decline?*

The medical profession is certainly well organised. Although there are a number of groups representing the profession, they tend to complement rather than conflict with each other, and present a relatively united front. This has not always been the case, as the divisions between the Royal Colleges and the BMA at the time of the creation of the NHS illustrate. But generally there appears to have been less overt conflict and rivalry between the main medical organisations than between, say, the nursing unions, which are very fragmented. The overall solidarity of the medical organisations has been a considerable source of strength.

The past decade has been a challenging one for the medical profession. As suggested earlier, its relationship with the government seems to have deteriorated considerably. Public exchanges between ministers and representatives of the profession have been vitriolic on occasion. The privileges of medical advice and consultation, while not totally withdrawn, have been more limited in recent years. For example, the BMA and the Royal Colleges were not consulted on major issues such as the NHS White Paper of 1989 (Klein and Day, 1992).

These developments must be seen in perspective. Hostility between the government and the doctors has broken out on a number of occasions in the post-war period. During a contractual dispute in 1965 general practitioners threatened mass resignation from the NHS. In the 1970s there was an enormous dispute between the government and the medical profession over the phasing out of pay beds in the NHS.

Klein and Day (1992) argue that the disputes of the 1980s have been of a different order from those of the 1960s and 1970s. Yet they also point out that they are not new. Similar structural upheavals in health care took place in 1911 (the introduction of national health insurance) and again in 1945 (the creation of the NHS). In both cases, the government of the day confronted the profession and introduced structural change in spite of opposition. Klein and Day also note that that the period following such reforms has tended to be more constructive, with the government working once again with the profession in an atmosphere of co-operation.

The re-establishment of what Klein (1990a) has elsewhere called 'the politics of the double bed' looks increasingly likely. Since the departure of Prime Minister Margaret Thatcher, the protagonist of the latest round of health service reforms, the medical organisations have reported an improvement in their relations with the government.

Alternatively, the latest dispute over the NHS reforms can be seen as a stage in the long-term decline of medical power (Armstrong, 1990). It has been argued that doctors have suffered greater blows to their autonomy in recent years compared to other professions such the legal profession (Brazier *et al.*, 1993). Certainly, the fortunes of the medical profession compare adversely with the predominantly private sector professions in an era when the public sector has been under attack (Perkin, 1989), though doctors have perhaps suffered less than many other public sector professions in this period (Deakin, 1991).

Doctors in the UK now face greater restrictions on their freedom, particularly when speaking to the media about the condition of the NHS. The emergence of self-governing trusts (SGTs) is likely to encourage such restrictions on grounds of commercial secrecy. There also appears to be an increasing use of NHS disciplinary procedures to remove and suspend doctors from their posts, which undermines to some extent the tradition of self-regulation.

Furthermore, doctors in the UK have since the early 1980s been subjected to a barrage of reforms designed to make them more accountable. These reforms include the introduction of general management, which has led to the creation of a professional management hierarchy (Loveridge and Starkey, 1992) to counterbalance the power of the medical profession. Other specific reforms have included measures to monitor and evaluate clinical activity and resource-use, such as medical audit and resource management. Finally, the creation of an internal market in health care represents a further discipline to which doctors are being compelled to respond (Flynn, 1992). The introduction of market forces into health care also threatens to undermine the solidarity of the medical profession by setting hospital against hospital and doctor against doctor.

The challenge to the medical profession is not confined to the UK, however: it appears to be fairly universal (Moran and Wood, 1992; Godt, 1987; Freddi and Bjorkman, 1989; Wilsford, 1991). Indeed, in some countries, notably the USA, the challenge has perhaps been even greater, with some claiming that medical autonomy has been seriously eroded (Armstrong, 1990; Ginzberg, 1990).

Alford (1975), in attempting to make sense of power relations in the US health care system, has devised a model of structural interests which has wider significance in the debate about medical power. According to Alford, the health care system comprises three structural interests. The dominant interest is the *professional monopoly* of the medical profession. The subsidiary interest is that of the *corporate rationalisers*. These are the politicians and managers of health care (and in, the American context, the private funders of health care). These interests seek to challenge the professional monopoly by introducing planning and forms of cost control, with the aim of limiting medical autonomy. As spending on health increases, these challenging interests become more influential. Finally, there is the *community interest*. This is the repressed interest, which lacks coherence and a power base, and which as a result exerts little influence over health care.

Health care systems, including that in the UK, are currently in a state of flux. It is difficult to see what exactly the position of the medical profession will be when the dust has settled. The profession has accumulated considerable status and power over the years and its representative bodies are powerful defenders of their self-interest. It has been argued that medicine can still draw on many sources of power to prevent or divert pressures for change (Coburn, 1992). Indeed, observers of the US health care scene indicate that the medical profession can, when under pressure, retain sufficient professional power to enable it to dominate, if not control, the health sector (Bjorkman, 1989 p. 72). Medicine may have lost some of its clout in recent years. It may have more to lose in the future. But for the moment it remains a formidable profession at home and abroad.

■ Conclusion

The medical profession has built up a dominant position within the health care system. During the twentieth century it has consolidated this position, enjoying a great deal of control over the provision of health care. Yet, as we have seen, this medical hegemony has been under pressure on several fronts.

The domination of health care by orthodox medicine has been increasingly criticised. Criticism has been levelled at the biomedical model. Paramedical professions have seen an improvement in their status, and alternative medicine has grown in popularity. Orthodox medicine's 'poor relation', the public health approach, has been revived. There has also been a greater interest in lay perspectives of health and illness.

During the 1980s medical organisations lost influence over important policy developments. Their relationship with the government became less stable and more acrimonious. Doctors also voiced fears that their independence and autonomy were under attack because of government reforms. Later chapters, in which the impact of these reforms is explored, assess the consequences for the medical profession in greater detail.

Yet these developments, and the challenges they pose for the profession, have to be seen in the context of the pre-existing medical hegemony. They have not as yet seriously undermined those factors which underpin the power of orthodox medicine, which remains the dominant form of health care knowledge today. For this reason the medical profession, for the time being at least, continues to exert a powerful influence within the health care system.

■ *Chapter 3* ■

Critical Perspectives on Health Care

Contemporary health care has been criticised from a variety of perspectives. As shown in the previous chapter, there has been criticism of orthodox medicine from alternative practitioners, other health care professions and even from within the medical profession itself. To these one may add a number of broader critical perspectives. These include the economic critique, the views of the technological pessimists, the Marxist perspective, the feminist critique, and, finally, the medicalisation thesis. This chapter explores these perspectives on health care, the problems they identify, and their proposals for change.

■ The economic critique

The rising costs of health care have prompted a growing interest in the use of resources. Economists and other business-related professions, such as accountants and management consultants, have played a major role in promoting a greater emphasis on efficiency within the NHS. This economic approach has attracted wider support: from among the new breed of NHS managers, from some doctors, and from politicians, particularly those on the right of the political spectrum.

□ *Efficiency and effectiveness*

In health care, an effective procedure is one which produces a desirable health outcome, for example, patients who recover from an operation. In practice, however, the judgement of effectiveness is not as simple and is often disputed. According to some, the medical profession tends to judge the effectiveness of a treatment mainly on the basis of its success in saving lives (Kennedy, 1981; Illich, 1975). They argue that the effectiveness of treatment which saves lives but which severely reduces the quality of life is highly questionable. For them, the quality of life should be regarded as an equally important standard of effectiveness when judging the value of health care.

Efficiency can be distinguished from effectiveness. In simple terms, efficiency is achieved where output is maximised from a given input of resources. In reality, the concept is far more complex (Culyer, 1991). There are at least four types of efficiency in relation to health care. These are shown in Exhibit 3.1.

Exhibit 3.1 Types of efficiency

1. Providing only services that are effective (i.e. where there is clear evidence that patients enjoy better health as a result of care).
2. Providing effective services at minimum cost.
3. Concentrating resources on effective services, provided at minimum cost, that offer the most benefits in terms of health.
4. Providing a mix of effective services at minimum cost and on such a scale that the benefits to society of providing more services are outweighed by the additional costs.

Source: Culyer (1991).

It is possible for a medical procedure to be effective but not efficient. This could happen for a number of reasons. Patients may be cured following medical intervention, but at an unjustifiably high cost relative to the benefits of the treatment. Or there may have been an alternative treatment available which could have cured at least the same number of patients at a lower cost. From an economic point of view it is not sufficient that health care is effective: it must also be efficient.

☐ *Inefficiency in health care*

Cochrane (1971), a strong advocate of evaluation within medicine, has identified four main aspects of inefficiency in health care: the use of ineffective therapies; the inappropriate use of effective therapies; the inappropriate use of health care settings; and incorrect lengths of stay in treatment facilities.

Later in this chapter, discussion of Illich's (1975) concept of clinical iatrogenesis reveals evidence of the use of dangerous therapies. Other therapies, while not positively harmful to patients, may simply be ineffective and therefore a waste of resources. To remedy this, Cochrane urged the use of the Randomised Controlled Trial (RCT). The RCT randomly allocates patients to one of two groups. The first receives the treatment which is under evaluation. The second (the control group) is given a placebo (that is, a pill with no active ingredients); or left untreated; or in some cases given an alternative treatment. The outcomes for the two groups are then compared.

RCTs can be useful in evaluating the effectiveness of a new technique or drug. They have also been used to evaluate different forms of prevention and aftercare. When RCTs were applied to the care of patients who had suffered a heart attack, no significant difference was found in the mortality rates of those admitted to hospital and those who were allowed to recover at home (Hill *et al.*, 1978).

Greater use of RCTs may well improve both efficiency and effectiveness. However, there are problems associated with their use, the most important of which are ethical. For example, it is often difficult to justify entering patients in a trial, thereby refusing them treatment which could improve their health or save their lives. Indeed, doctors are reluctant to evaluate by RCT when there is a strong likelihood that the treatment will be effective, when there is no alternative treatment available, and where the known side-effects of treatment are minimal.

☐ *Inappropriate use of effective therapies*

What about the inefficiency associated with the inappropriate use of effective therapies? There is much evidence that medical services are over-produced and over-supplied. Diagnostic tests are a common target for criticism. It has been found that one-third of a sample of patients with trauma to the skull were unnecessarily subjected to an X-ray examination (Bell and Loop, 1971). Routine tests may also involve considerable waste. One study found that routine tests on blood and urine contributed to only 1 per cent of diagnoses, though they did reveal significant undiagnosed coexisting diseases in around 10 per cent of cases (Sandler, 1979). Another found that routine microbiological tests were largely unnecessary and that in 60 per cent of the cases studied patients were discharged before the results of the tests were available (Hashemi and Merlin, 1987).

There is also a tendency to over-diagnose illness. This tendency is not new, as a study in the USA during the 1930s demonstrates. In a sample of eleven-year-olds, 61 per cent had already had their tonsils removed. The remainder were examined by a group of doctors, who recommended that 45 per cent of these children required tonsillectomy. A different set of doctors then examined the remaining children who had not so far been recommended for treatment. Again, just under half were diagnosed as being in need of the operation. A third round of examinations produced a similar result (Bakwin, 1945).

There is a considerable variation in diagnosis and treatment between countries. Overall, surgical rates in the USA are twice those of the UK (Vayda *et al.*, 1982). Rates in Canada are 1.8 times higher for men and 1.6 times higher for women when compared with England and Wales (Vayda, 1973). Differences in surgical rates are even higher for some operations. For example, three times as many hysterectomies are performed on average in the USA compared with England and Wales (McPherson *et al.*, 1981).

The accuracy of such studies can be challenged on methodological grounds. It is particularly difficult to establish beyond doubt that variations in surgical rates are unrelated to the prevalence and severity of illness in the general population. The pitfalls of international comparisons should always be remembered when interpreting such data. One should also take note of variation in surgical rates within countries as well as between them.

There are several possible explanations of why doctors might over-provide medical services, and why this may vary between countries. Some believe that doctors simply prefer intervention to inaction (Illich, 1975; Kennedy, 1981). According to Payer (1989) this dominant interventionist philosophy is more deeply ingrained in the profession in some countries (such as the USA) than in others (for example, the UK).

Doctors may over-provide services if they fear the consequences of litigation. Failure to intervene may be construed as negligence. It is easier to prove medical negligence than incompetence or malpractice. Legal factors may partly explain the variation between countries. Litigation by patients is more common and generally more successful in the USA than in the UK.

The system of remunerating doctors may also encourage over-supply. In the USA, many doctors receive a fee based on the actual work done. In an attempt to restrain health care spending, the Americans have introduced tighter regulation of fees and new forms of health care provision. In the UK, doctors' incomes have not until recently been tied to the performance of specific tasks.

☐ *Other aspects of inefficiency*

It will be remembered that Cochrane (1971) noted that medical treatment was often given in inappropriate settings and that this could be unnecessarily expensive. He believed that certain conditions could be treated more efficiently outside hospital, perhaps in the GP's surgery, or at home. Cochrane also pointed out that patients were often kept in hospital for much longer periods than necessary, again adding to costs.

Costs can be reduced by reorganising health care so that patients spend less time in hospital and more time in the community (Audit Commission, 1990, 1992b). The expansion of day surgery, made possible by new surgical techniques, discussed later in this chapter, is an important development in this respect. One should not forget, however, that other significant costs may be incurred in caring for patients outside hospital. The burden of care may fall more heavily upon the family or on social services. These factors should always be taken into account when calculating the balance of costs and benefits of transferring care from hospital into the community.

☐ *Priorities and rationing*

The gap between health needs and the provision of services may be partly satisfied by securing greater efficiency in the provision of services. Other possible ways forward are to prioritise health care or ration it more effectively (see Weale, 1988; Cochrane *et al.*, 1992). Prioritization and rationing are not new concepts in health care. After all, waiting lists, a constant feature of the NHS, are a form of rationing. Furthermore, since the late 1970s priorities have been set for the NHS. What is new is making the criteria for priority-setting and rationing explicit.

In an attempt to establish such criteria, economists have devised techniques to help evaluate the costs and benefits of health care. One technique in particular, the Quality Adjusted Life Year (QALY), has attracted considerable attention (Williams, 1985; Carr-Hill, 1991). The benefits of health care, measured in QALYs, are calculated from estimates of the length and quality of a patient's life following treatment. The costs of treatment are then expressed in terms of a cost per QALY (see Exhibit 3.2). The QALY can be used to compare the relative cost-effectiveness of different treatments for the same illness. More controversially, the technique has potential as a rationing tool, facilitating the expansion of treatment of certain illnesses (those that achieve QALYs at a lower cost) at the expense of others (those that achieve QALYs at high cost).

There is strong opposition from health care professions to the use of cost–benefit criteria in this way. Doctors claim that QALYs undermine their clinical judgement (Smith, A., 1987). Williams (1988), a pioneer of the QALY in the UK, denies this, arguing that the technique will only lead to more accountability for the use of resources. Loewy (1980) has criticised

Exhibit 3.2   QALYs (Quality Adjusted Life Years)

QALYs can be used to compare the relative benefits of different forms of care and treatment. Each year which the patient is expected to survive following a course of treatment is weighted by a factor reflecting the patient's quality of life. The quality of life weighting is in turn calculated from a table representing different levels of disability and distress (such as Rosser's Index). Once the number of QALYs generated by each treatment is calculated, it is then possible to compare the relative costs in order to find out which treatment has the lowest cost per QALY. A simple worked example is shown below:

Treatment A

Cost = £10 000 per patient
Life expectancy after treatment = 10 years
Quality of life   (No Distress;
(Rosser's Index)   Slight Social Disability) = 0.990

Treatment B

Cost = £5000 per patient
Life expectancy = 20 years
Quality of life   (Mild Distress;
(Rosser's Index)   Slight Social Disability) = 0.986

Treatment A

$$QALY = \text{Life expectancy} \times \text{Quality of life}$$
$$= 10 \times 0.990$$
$$= 9.9$$

$$\text{Cost per QALY} = \frac{10\,000}{9.9} = £1010.10 \text{ per QALY}$$

Treatment B

$$QALY = \text{Life expectancy} \times \text{Quality of life}$$
$$= 20 \times 0.986$$
$$= 19.72$$

$$\text{Cost per QALY} = \frac{5\,000}{19.72} = £253.55 \text{ per QALY}$$

In the light of this simple calculation, treatment B appears to be more cost-effective than treatment A.

the ethics of QALYs, commenting that optimisation of survival and not optimisation of cost-effectiveness is the only ethical rule to follow. Others have attacked QALYs for their discriminatory impact on vulnerable groups such as the disabled and the elderly (Jones and Higgs, 1990; Crisp, 1989). The benefits of treatment (in terms of survival and externally-assessed quality of life) for these groups are likely to be estimated as being below average. As a result, they may be denied treatment on the basis of an economic calculation.

The calculations themselves are rather crude. It is difficult to reduce the quality of life to a single index as individuals differ widely in their judgements about this. Furthermore, it is difficult to calculate the long-term costs of health care, particularly those that fall on families, other social services and the wider community.

The application of QALYs to health care decision-making is at an early stage in the UK, but interest in their use has been stimulated by the introduction of the NHS internal market. A number of health authorities in the UK have considered withdrawing funding from so-called 'low priority' treatments such as fertility services, the removal of wisdom teeth, treatment of varicose veins, and the removal of tattoos and benign cysts partly on cost-benefit grounds, as we shall see in later chapters.

In some other countries, notably the USA, explicit rationing has gone a stage further. A number of states have expressed concern about large numbers of people who are not covered either by state or private health insurance schemes and who have difficulty in obtaining access to care. One state, Oregon, responded by formulating a plan to ration public expenditure on health care. The idea was to expand access to state-funded health care to include the uninsured, while restricting the range of treatments paid for by the state (see Exhibit 3.3). The plan has been agreed to for a five year trial.

☐ *Accountability*

Calls for a more explicit approach to rationing have been accompanied by a plea for more accountability in health care (see Weale, 1988). Accountability has a variety of meanings (Day and Klein, 1987). In a narrow sense, better accountability means improved financial management. Those who deliver health care – professionals and institutions – being held to account for the financial aspects of their activities. Accountability can also be interpreted more broadly, as a responsibility upon health care providers to answer for the decisions they make. This type of accountability can also occur on an individual and an

Exhibit 3.3 The Oregon experiment

In the late 1980s Oregon, like many other states in the USA, faced two main health care problems: rising health care costs, and large numbers of uninsured people. The state government therefore decided to try a different approach towards the allocation of health care resources. Plans were set out to alter the coverage of Medicaid, the state-run system for funding the care of poor people (and also the blind, the disabled, and children in foster care). The main idea behind the plan was to extend Medicaid to a larger proportion of those on low incomes without private health insurance, while at the same time restricting the range of treatments funded by the programme.

With this in mind the state began collecting cost–benefit data with respect to the various treatments available. An initial ranking of treatments was produced but it was subsequently withdrawn after criticisms of the data collection process.

A second list was then produced and at this stage the public were consulted on their views of the benefits of treatment. The top five conditions listed were:

- Pneumonia;
- Tuberculosis;
- Peritonitis;
- Foreign body in throat; and
- Appendicitis.

Also appearing in the top half of the rankings were treatment for cancer of the uterus, heart bypass operations and treatment for the early stages of HIV-related disease.

In the light of this revised ranking, the Oregon legislature approved the funding for the first 587 treatments listed (out of a total of 709). Had the plan gone ahead at this stage, the Medicaid system would have been extended to an additional 120 000 individuals currently excluded from the programme. At the same time, public funding for the treatment of many 'low-priority conditions', including those listed below, would have ended.

- Varicose veins;
- Bronchitis;
- Cancers where treatment will not result in 10 per cent of patients surviving for 10 years;
- Uncomplicated haemorrhoids;
- AIDS (Terminal Stage HIV); and
- Extremely low birthweight babies.

In order to proceed, the Oregon government required approval from the Federal Government in Washington. This approval was initially withheld following pressure from organisations representing the disabled. Further negotiations between state and federal officials produced a number of concessions (including an agreement that treatment for AIDS patients would not be withdrawn). Subsequently, permission was granted which enabled Oregon to introduce its plan for a five-year trial period.

Source: Honigsbaum, 1992.

organisational level. On an individual level, it would be facilitated by a greater openness in the making of clinical judgements. This could be brought about by making explicit the criteria used by health care professions when making decisions about treatment. On an organisational level, accountability would be enhanced by clarifying the responsibilities of institutions within the health care system – hospitals, health authorities and government agencies. Better accountability would also result from greater openness at the organisational level, with decisions being subjected to wide public scrutiny.

It is often claimed that the providers of health care, particularly in the UK, are not accountable to the user – the patient (Green *et al.*, 1990). Patients tend to be passive, have little information, and have few rights of redress. In recent years there has been an emphasis on the patient as a consumer of health services. There has been considerable attention given to the the so-called 'supermarket model', which focuses mainly on customer relations, performance targets and better information for patients. But a number of other models have been identified as having greater potential to increase patient power and professional accountability in health care (Winkler, 1987). Some of these are shown in Exhibit 3.4 below.

Exhibit 3.4   Models of consumer power

1. *The Community Health Councils model.*

   Consumers are represented by an organisation which monitors local services on their behalf and which may take up individual cases.

2. *The Democratic Accountability model.*

   Consumers elect representatives on to the bodies which manage local services.

3. *User Power model.*

   The consumers decide for themselves the care they require. Health professionals then supply the necessary pattern of care.

4. *Partnership.*

   Health professionals and consumers of health come together to decide what action is best. This can operate at an individual level (doctor and patient) or at an institutional level (between health agencies and patient representatives).

□ *Markets*

Some believe that efficiency, more effective rationing and prioritisation, and better accountability will result from a greater use of market forces in the provision of health care. Economic theory predicts that greater competition between suppliers will in the longer term drive down prices and improve efficiency.

Yet even among the ranks of economists, few favour unrestrained markets in health care. Health care is not a public good in the economists' strict sense of the term: where one person's consumption of a good does not exclude others from consuming the same good (Alchian and Allen, 1974). Yet it does have certain special characteristics which lead some to believe that it would be inefficiently provided or under-provided if left entirely to the private market (Normand, 1991).

There has been greater support in recent years for combining the state's role in health care with market forces in the form of an internal or managed market. Some economists argue that effective competition between providers can take place within a publicly-funded health care system. This, it is argued, will generate considerable benefits in the form of a downward pressure on costs, and greater efficiency (Enthoven, 1985). The enclosure of market forces within a clear framework of regulation is designed to rule out any sharp practices and to ensure that the system is in harmony with publicly-stated policy objectives, such as fair access to services.

Markets are seen by many economists and by right-wing politicians as an antidote, not only to what they regard as inefficient state health care bureaucracies, but also to the power of the health care professions (Gladstone, 1992). Professional bodies are seen as being monopolistic producers, controlling the supply of labour and thereby keeping wages (and costs) high. Markets in health care undermine this monopoly by forcing professionals to compete against each other. At the same time, measures can be taken to reduce the control of professional bodies over the supply of labour – by introducing competition from overseas or from less skilled or less well-qualified practitioners.

Despite the theories of the economists, the consequences of markets in health care are not always as predicted. This will become clear in later chapters, in the context of privatisation and internal markets in the NHS.

□ *Criticism*

Most broadly support the movement towards greater efficiency in health care, better evaluation of the effectiveness of treatment, prioritisation on the basis of need, and a greater emphasis upon financial, professional and political accountability. Yet there is a great deal of suspicion about the means which have been suggested to achieve these laudable aims, not least from within the health care professions.

There are two main worries. As we have already seen, there is doubt about some of the techniques suggested to improve efficiency. There is also concern that the emphasis on efficiency is part of a hidden agenda, in two senses. First, it is seen as a means by which the political right-wing are seeking to undermine the welfare state. Second, while economists may have a useful supplementary role in the allocation of health care resources, there are worries that they seek to occupy a more strategic role (Klein 1989a). The 'efficiency agenda' could represent a strategy for professional advancement by economists, and other business and management-related occupations. Indeed, health economists have been characterised as being imperialists seeking to colonise the minds of health care practitioners (Ashmore *et al.*, 1989). Along with other professional groups, such as accountants, management consultants and NHS managers, they may be seeking to subvert the existing medically-dominated structure of professional power, replacing it with a system commanded by their own expertise.

■ Technological pessimists

A second critical perspective focuses on the dependence of modern health care on high technology. It is difficult to define high technology in a simple way, and its meaning is often taken for granted (Richman, 1987). In the context of health care, high technology essentially means the use of complex machinery and advanced techniques in the diagnosis and treatment of patients. Examples would include magnetic resonance imaging (MRI), which can produce detailed cross-sectional images of the body, and the new minimally invasive therapies (see p. 59 below). Pharmaceutical products manufactured and developed on the basis of advanced research may also be regarded as high technology.

A number of reasons have been advanced to explain why health care has become more dependent on high technology (Reiser, 1978). First, high technology has been supported by the medical profession, largely because doctors believe it introduces a scientific precision into clinical practice. Second, medical education, training and research have all emphasised technological medicine. Third, particularly in the USA, doctors have often felt compelled to use high technology as a defensive mechanism against claims of negligence. Fourth, the public is fascinated by medical technology, and generally supports its use. A fifth reason may be added to this list. According to Jennett (1986) doctors increasingly see the development of high technologies as a symbol of their own success.

Despite the general support of the public and the medical profession, high technology has been criticised on a number of specific grounds: that it is inefficient and ineffective; that it subjugates and depersonalises the patient; and that it creates ever more complicated ethical problems.

☐ *Efficiency and effectiveness*

Critics of high technology often point out the scale of both capital and running costs (Council for Science and Society, 1982). A heart transplant costs about £26 000. The expense of new technology may be justified if the benefits to patients are considerable. But the problem in the past has been that many new technologies have not been evaluated, either in terms of their efficiency or their effectiveness (Stocking and Morrison, 1978; Jennett, 1986; Stocking, 1988).

New technology can, however, be both efficient and effective. Some technologies are relatively cheap and yet effective. Take, for example, hip replacements, which are of enormous benefit in improving the quality of life and which cost around £4000 each. Some technologies raise the possibility of reducing costs as well as improving the quality of care for patients. Minimally invasive therapies (MITs) have been heralded as a great leap forward in both respects. Take, for example lithotripsy – the crushing of stones such as those found in the kidney or gall bladder, by using ultrasound waves. This is a relatively quick treatment which reduces hospital stays for the patient by around a third compared with conventional surgery. There is also less chance of infection following the operation. The lower costs of recovery and convalescence have clear resource implications (Audit Commission, 1990, 1992b).

Other techniques are also believed to cause less injury to the body than conventional techniques and therefore imply shorter hospital stays, a shorter period of convalescence and a better chance of a complete recovery for the patient. Doctors are increasingly adopting endoscopic surgery – where instruments are passed into the body through the mouth, other natural orifices, or through small incisions ('keyholes') in the skin.

Laser surgery is a further technique which has attracted attention in recent years: using electromagnetic radiation, doctors can tackle a range of problems from the treatment of cancer to delicate eye surgery.

Despite the potential benefits of MITs and other new techniques, it is important that their use is carefully monitored. Indeed, there have been worries in recent years about the side-effects of 'keyhole' surgery, lithotripsy and laser therapy, and around 10 per cent of hip replacements have to be repeated. But doctors are often reluctant to countenance evaluation of techniques which they feel are unambiguously beneficial.

☐ *Doctor–patient relationship*

Some have identified a technological imperative in medicine, whereby technical skill and progress is seen as being more important than interpersonal skills and the patient's interests (Kennedy, 1981). It is often claimed that although the use of high technology often has public support, it alters the doctor–patient relationship in an adverse way. Reiser (1978) has commented that machines direct the attention of both doctor and patient to the measurable aspects of illness and away from personal and social factors relevant to health. Technology can reinforce the disease orientation of biomedicine, discussed in the previous chapter, and may further weaken the position of the patient.

A further problem is that the use of technology may absolve doctors from blame. Illich (1975), among others, has claimed that the depersonalisation of diagnosis and therapy has transformed malpractice from an ethical into a technical problem. The machine also becomes the carrier of bad news and can take the blame when things go wrong.

High technology can also be regarded as inhumane. It will be many years before we can evaluate the contribution of those pioneers of heroic medicine, particularly in the area of transplants. As Gould (1987) has observed, the quality of life for many of these patients has been very poor. As for the terminally ill, high-technology treatment may perhaps be less humane than the 'low tech' care provided by the hospice movement.

Medical technology has also been blamed for increasing the power of the doctor over the patient. The use of technology, it is often argued, confirms the role of the doctor as expert. 'The more decisions are made by experts, the less they can be made by laymen' (Freidson, 1988, p. 336). As knowledge becomes more technical, doctors and other experts can dominate ever more spheres of activity. For example, the medical domination of childbirth has been assisted by the emergence of birth technologies introduced by doctors (Oakley, 1980, 1984).

However, it is also possible that the reliance on technology might actually work in the opposite direction, effectively de-skilling the medical profession. As the interpersonal and diagnostic skills of doctors are replaced at least in part by new technologies, it is possible that they could become merely intermediaries between the patient and other technical experts (Reiser, 1978).

☐ *Ethical problems*

The final area of concern about high technology in health care relates to ethical dilemmas raised by many new technologies. Medical interventions such as organ transplants, genetic engineering, screening and testing for disease raise a variety of ethical issues. For example, under what circumstances should organ donation be permitted? To what extent should genetic manipulation be allowed to alter the characteristics of unborn children? Should patients be screened for diseases which may lead to them being discriminated against by employers, insurance companies and so on? A further set of ethical questions is raised by the availability of life-saving care and treatment, where previously patients would be allowed to die. How should these scarce and expensive services be allocated? Should treatment be withdrawn from those who are unlikely to regain consciousness?

Such ethical questions are not easily resolved. They often produce a controversial debate, frequently polarised on the basis of firmly-held moral and religious convictions. These issues also increasingly raise complex questions of law, bringing health care more closely into the realm of legal decision-making.

☐ *Dealing with new technology*

Those who are pessimistic about health care technologies are themselves often attacked for wanting to stop progress. Yet even critics of high technology accept that 'it can confer substantial benefits when appropriately employed' (Jennett, 1986, p. 141). Few would wish to prevent the emergence of potentially effective treatments.

Nevertheless there is unease about the rapid progress of high technology. Clearly, new technologies must be carefully evaluated, and not merely on narrow economic cost–benefit grounds. Evaluation should take into account other important criteria, such as the impact on professional competence and the doctor–patient relationship. It should also take into account the moral and ethical issues raised by the use of new technology.

■ The Marxist perspective

Marxists analyse contemporary health care in terms of the class structure of capitalist societies, the search for profits, and the role of the state in ensuring both capitalist domination and capital accumulation (see Navarro, 1978; Doyal, 1979; Waitzkin, 1983).

To fully understand the Marxist perspective let us begin with the original views of Marx, writing in the nineteenth century. For Marx, capitalist societies consisted of two main classes: the capitalists – who own the means of production (factories, machines and so on), and who seek to make profits; and the workers, who sell their labour for wages. He argued that there was a powerful tendency for the capitalists to exploit the workers in an attempt to increase profits and accumulate more capital. He identified three main consequences of this process: inequality, as the material conditions of the workers decline relative to the capitalists'; crisis, as the capitalist system finds it more difficult to continue exploiting labour in the long term; and conflict between the classes, leading ultimately to socialised control of the means of production.

The implications for health from the unbridled capitalist system were evident during the nineteenth century. Poverty and material deprivation were widespread, and the conditions endured by the working classes were a breeding ground for disease. Although the wealthy were not immune from the infections created by these social and economic conditions, the poor suffered disproportionately (Smith, 1979). There were also wide inequalities in the standards of health care received by the different social classes (Abel-Smith, 1964).

Since the time that Marx was writing, capitalist societies have become more complex. The clear division of interest between employers and workers has been blurred by the emergence of new occupational groups such as public-sector workers, the new professions, and the managerial classes.

Capitalist states have also responded to the social problems and economic tensions of capitalism in ways unforeseen by Marx. They have intervened in the economy to moderate economic crises: replaced capitalist production with public ownership in many areas; and created welfare states to cushion the impact of capitalism. Yet Marxists have refused to accept that the beast is dead. They argue that the state has merely protected capitalism from extinction by expedient short-term intervention. The state, in their view, is a defender of capitalism, not a guardian of social welfare. It is this general principle which guides their analysis of health care in capitalist states.

☐ *Inequalities, class and capitalism*

In Chapter 1 a number of significant inequalities in health and illness were identified. Marxists attribute the persistence of such inequalities to the material inequalities generated by capitalism. Certainly, specific social conditions allied to deprivation are associated with ill-health, such as bad housing and unemployment. Though there are a number of possible explanations for the class gradient, it is undoubtedly true that material conditions are important factors in health. Yet it is not clear to what extent health inequalities are directly, exclusively or wholly a product of capitalism. Indeed, health inequalities vary considerably between capitalist countries (Fox, 1989). Moreover, it is now known that social inequalities persisted under Communism in the post-war period.

Marxists identify inequalities in the provision of health care as a feature of capitalism. They point out that such inequalities are greater in health care systems where private enterprise has a larger role, such as in the USA and that health care inequalities will also be a feature of state health systems in capitalist societies.

There is some support for this. The inverse care law states that areas where health needs are greatest – generally the poorest areas – will be the least likely to receive high-quality care (Tudor-Hart, 1971). This is not just a feature of market-led health systems, though the law is more accentuated in such systems. A number of studies of the NHS have found that areas where the poorer classes are concentrated tend to have poorer health services and that the higher social classes get more health care resources relative to their level of need (West and Lowe, 1976; Noyce, Snaith and Trickey, 1974; Le Grand, 1978). These findings are not universally accepted, however. The validity of the inverse care law has been challenged (Powell, 1990). In addition, a number of recent studies have not found evidence of significant inequalities in the use of the NHS between the various social classes and income groups (Collins and Klein, 1988; O'Donnell *et al.*, 1991).

Marxists believe that the health care system is a microcosm of the capitalist society in which it operates. They see a clear class bias in the production of health care. For them, the upper classes and upper-middle classes are in a position to decide on key questions of resource allocation and the organisation of care. State health care systems operating within capitalist societies are not regarded as special cases. Marxists identify a class bias in the NHS, with upper and middle classes (and increasingly, businessmen) dominating health authorities. They also believe that the medical profession, as the most socially exclusive in health care, is part of the general conspiracy.

As we shall see in Chapter 6, it is true that health authority membership is not representative of society. But to equate socioeconomic class with support for capitalism is rather crude. Many health authority members have themselves opposed the moves to commercialise the NHS. Similarly, the fact that doctors are drawn from higher social classes does not necessarily make them allies of capitalism. British doctors have been broadly supportive of the NHS, though they have been opposed to certain models of state ownership. Moreover, one should note that the government's internal market – the most explicit attempt yet to introduce capitalist values into socialised medicine – has been strongly resisted by most doctors and other health professionals.

☐ *Profits and capital accumulation*

From a Marxist perspective, state health care may have moderated to some extent the health problems caused by the capitalist system, but it has been unable to counteract them. Marxists point out that state health services still allow some scope for private enterprise, and the profit motive has never been totally eradicated, even in nationalised health care systems such as the NHS. When the NHS was created consultants retained the right to treat private patients. General Practitioners also secured their status as independent contractors, though they had little scope for private practice. The profit motive has survived in many areas vital to health care such as the supply of medical equipment, in pharmaceuticals, and in hospital building and construction: the so-called medical–industrial complex (McKinlay, 1979).

In recent years private sector involvement in UK health care has increased substantially, with the privatisation of ancillary services and the growth of private health care. Moreover, the introduction of business-style management processes and market mechanisms into the NHS has placed new emphasis upon commercial motives and judgements.

Marxists also argue that state health services assist capital accumulation in other ways. They make more palatable the problems which arise from capitalist production. Industrial pollution, accidents and injuries, and stress-related illness are seen by Marxists as side-effects of the quest for profits. Health problems associated with consumption of commercially-produced goods such as alcohol, tobacco and junk food can be viewed in a similar way. Arguably, it would be better if these problems were tackled at source. Marxists believe that the people are fooled into thinking that 'what is politically and collectively caused can be individually and therapeutically cured' (Navarro, 1978). Individuals who suffer ill-health can obtain treatment from state-financed health services in a such a way that public awareness of the root causes of illness is prevented. Protest is thereby neutralised, allowing capitalists to continue making their profits at the expense of public health.

Yet the existence of health services has not neutered public protest nor prevented support for public health campaigns. Governments in capitalist states have been persuaded to take action against pollution, accidents at work, alcohol and tobacco and so on, even where this has offended vested interests. Commercial organisations have formidable lobbying powers, but they are not invulnerable.

There are a number of other ways in which health services may assist profit-making and capital accumulation. Modern capitalism needs high-quality labour in order to thrive. Marxists argue that the productivity of labour can be maintained by protecting the health of key workers (that is, of skilled and technical workers) Moreover, the quantity of labour available to capitalists can be increased by providing social support systems. When workers are needed they can be relieved of at least some of their caring duties. At the same time, health services become the dumping ground for the 'economically unproductive' (the mentally and physically ill; the elderly) who cannot be used by the capitalist production process.

This process appears now to be operating in reverse. A major strand of policy in recent years has been to reduce state responsibilities for health and health care. Informal carers increasingly shoulder the burden of looking after the sick and elderly. The government has also encouraged self-care and private health care expenditure.

Marxists explain these new trends by arguing that we have entered a new phase of capitalism (O'Connor, 1973; Offe, 1984). This takes the form of a crisis, the main features of which are rising tax burdens, high inflation, trade union militancy, and a stifling of capitalist activity. In response, the state adopts policies to curb welfare expenditure and to encourage private enterprise. This leads to a reinvigoration of capitalism, but also produces greater social conflict and inequality.

☐ *The contribution of the Marxist approach*

The value of the Marxist perspective, rather like the public health approach discussed in Chapter 2, lies in its focus upon the social and economic roots of ill-health. The Marxist emphasis on inequalities in health care also reminds us that we should never assume that access to health care will always be equitable, even in state systems. Marxists help to explain the motives of private health care providers. Indeed, the expansion of private care and the application to the NHS of management practices similar to those used in business enhances the relevance of the Marxist approach today. Finally, Marxism also sheds light on why commercial activities harmful to health may be tolerated to some extent by governments.

There are, however, a number of general criticisms of the Marxist approach (see, for example, Hart's (1982) review of Doyal, 1979). The Marxist critique of the NHS is perhaps less than fair. The NHS has done much to improve health care in the UK, and is widely judged as being an improvement on the system of health care which existed previously. Furthermore, as we have seen, the Marxist approach to class relations in the NHS is flawed and the evidence of class inequalities in health care is ambiguous.

Another general criticism is that Marxists are long on analysis but short on specific recommendations for improving health care. Hard-line Marxists are not satisfied with a state-owned health service. They point out that health and health care will only improve significantly when the general social and economic organisation of society is changed; that is, when the capitalism itself is superseded. However, evidence suggests that health services in communist systems are in many respects worse than those in capitalist countries (*Economist*, 1990). Furthermore, as already noted, health and health care inequalities persisted under Communism. Communist countries also appear to have a worse record on industrial pollution, alcohol and tobacco-related problems, and other public health problems linked with industry and industrialisation.

■ The feminist critique

Contemporary health care can also be viewed from a feminist perspective (see Miles, 1991; Graham, 1984). There are two main strands to this critique. First, it is often claimed that the delivery of health services is dominated by men. Second, and arising out of this, there is criticism of the way in which the health care system, and in particular the medical profession, view female patients and their health problems.

In traditional societies women were invariably cast in the role of healer. As societies developed, healing became professionalised and male-dominated (Leeson and Gray, 1978). Where women were still allowed to undertake health care roles, they were subservient to the male medical profession. This domination continued even where female health care roles became professionalised, as illustrated, for example, by the emergence of the 1902 Midwives Act (Donnison, 1988). This Act established state regulation of the midwifery profession and was the product of a protracted battle between doctors and midwives over who should control childbirth.

The (male) doctors won the day, the Act introducing a number of safeguards to protect the doctors' role and limit midwives. During the latter part of the nineteenth century, nurses also successfully pressed for professional recognition, but again on terms acceptable to the doctors (Abel-Smith, 1960).

The professionalisation of nursing and midwifery enhanced the social status of these occupations but did not challenge the power of the medical profession, which in turn strongly resisted the entry of women. Even today women are still under-represented in the ranks of doctors and find it difficult to penetrate the higher echelons of medicine, as discussed in Chapter 2. Women have made considerable progress in the professions allied to medicine: physiotherapy, occupational therapy, radiography, dietetics, speech therapy, and so on. But these occupations, like nursing and midwifery are subservient to medicine.

Women therefore tend to perform health care roles which place them in a subservient position relative to men. Medicine is male-dominated: nursing (which is 90 per cent female) and other non-medical health professions are predominantly female. Moreover, non-professional health occupations are also mainly female. Seventy per cent of ancillary workers in the NHS are women. In addition, almost two-thirds of those who provide informal care for relatives at home are women (Green, H., 1988).

It is argued that the male domination of medicine and health care leads to a failure to understand women's health care needs. This is often seen as a historical, and in particular a Victorian, legacy. During the Victorian period the health of women, particularly those in the upper and middle classes who had access to health care, was defined by male doctors very much in terms of reproduction. Many social and psychological problems experienced by women were attributed to disorders of the sexual organs. Some women were treated for these conditions by surgical 'cures' such as the removal of the sexual and reproductive organs (Dally, 1991).

Doyal (1979) argues that doctors still take a particular view of female health problems. This view is shaped by the belief that men are normal and women abnormal in respect of intellect, emotion and physical functioning. Abnormalities in women are still associated with their reproductive role. Doctors assume that motherhood and the maternal instinct is the main driving force in women's lives, and that a denial of this instinct causes depression and so on. Doctors are also more likely to see women as being neurotic and emotionally unbalanced (Miles, 1988).

Some complain that the medical profession has failed to take into account in the organisation and delivery of services, the particular needs of women (Jenkins, 1985; Roberts, 1992). A commonly cited example is childbirth, where it is claimed that the medical domination of procedures has led to the subjugation of women (Oakley, 1980; 1984). Women feel they have lost control of the birth process, which is treated as if it were an illness. This process, as noted earlier, has been assisted by the use of technology. By the mid-1970s induction of births rose to over 40 per cent of the total. Most births now take place in controlled conditions in hospital, the seat of medical power and technology. Women have questioned the effectiveness and efficiency of this technology, suspecting its main function to be one of control.

The treatment of breast cancer is another issue where women have felt that their views were not being heeded by doctors. Radical mastectomy (the removal of the breast) can have a damaging psychological impact on patients. There have been criticisms, not only of the practice of removing the breast – which in some cases may be necessary to preserve the life of the patient – but also of the absence of counselling facilities and the failure to explain beforehand the nature of the operation.

☐ *Feminist solutions*

Feminists blame the failure of the health care system on the wider social processes of male domination. The overall solution proposed is to change society by strengthening the position of women.

Within health care, the position of women could be improved through greater participation in medicine and medical decision-making. There has been in recent years a considerable increase in the proportion of women training as doctors. However, this alone will not guarantee that women will stay in medicine, or that they will rise to the highest echelons (Allen, 1988).

The situation for women could also be improved by shifting the balance of power in health care away from doctors and towards those professions where women predominate. This could be secured through greater professional autonomy for midwives, nurses, and professions allied to medicine. Women are also likely to benefit from moves which give them, as patients, more choice in health care. The 'consumer' movement in childbirth is one example. Self-help approaches enable women to retain control over their own bodies (Phillips and Rakusen, 1989).

Although attempts to improve the role and status of women in health care are to be applauded, it is important to realise that some changes may not provide clear benefits for all women. It is possible that the type of limited self-help and consumerism has only introduced benefits for middle-class women, who are more articulate, more vociferous and more highly motivated to do something about the problems they face. This raises the possibility of the emergence of a two-tier system of care, to the disadvantage, perhaps, of working-class women.

It is also ironic, as we noted in Chapter 1, that many of the illnesses from which women now suffer increasingly have arisen from the adoption of male lifestyles. Many women are also nowadays expected to combine the traditional role as mother/housekeeper with that of worker, which for some is stressful and possibly harmful to their overall health. So while there is no logic in the male domination of society, it must be said that the health consequences of a changing role for women are far from straightforward.

■ Iatrogenesis: Illich's thesis

It is one thing to argue that contemporary health care is inefficient, inconsiderate or misdirected; to argue that the medical establishment is a direct threat to health is far more radical. Yet this is precisely the argument advanced by Illich (1975) in his examination of the nature and extent of iatrogenesis – illness caused by medicine. Illich identifies three dimensions of iatrogenesis: clinical, social and cultural, and each will now be examined in turn.

□ *Clinical iatrogenesis*

Clinical iatrogenesis occurs when illness is caused by diagnosis or treatment undertaken by medical practitioners. Illich begins by claiming that the successes of modern medicine are overrated. In accordance with those who support the public health approach, he observes that better housing, better nutrition and an improved environment were more effective in reducing mortality and morbidity. He then goes on to argue that a number of aspects of medical treatment are actually useless and ineffective, while others are positively dangerous. He identifies several types of clinical iatrogenesis: diagnostic errors, accidents during the course of treatment, and the side-effects of treatment.

There is growing evidence of clinical iatrogenesis. Anecdotal evidence – fairly commonplace – about professional incompetence and negligence is not really satisfactory. But there is a growing body of more systematic evidence which provides considerable support for Illich's argument. Misdiagnosis appears to be a serious problem. In one study, autopsies confirmed clinical diagnoses in only 61 per cent of the cases (Cameron and McGoogan, 1981). Another study found an even higher rate of error, clinical diagnoses being confirmed in less than half the cases considered (Mercer and Talbot, 1985). This study also found that in 13 per cent of the cases doctors had not diagnosed treatable diseases.

Evidence concerning illness directly caused by medical diagnosis and treatment is more difficult to obtain, though there are plenty of case studies of adverse effects in drug therapies – such as with Opren and Thalidomide (Collier, 1989). In recent years, however, attempts have been made to measure clinical iatrogenesis more systematically. The Harvard Medical Practice Study (1990), for example, found that 4 per cent of admissions to hospital in New York experienced adverse events. In a quarter of these cases doctors had actually been negligent. An earlier study, however, suggests that the extent of clinical iatrogenic illness may be greater than most would believe. A study of a general medical service in an American University hospital found that 36 per cent of the patients studied had an iatrogenic illness. In 9 per cent of admissions, the incident was life-threatening or produced a serious disability, and in 2 per cent of all cases, the incident was believed to have contributed to the death of the patient (Steel *et al.*, 1981). Furthermore a Canadian study has found serious deficiencies in the work of between 8 and 15 per cent of family doctors and 2 per cent of specialists (McAuley and Henderson, 1984).

Recent studies of hospital acquired infections (HAI) in the UK have been estimated at worryingly high levels. According to one report, over 10 per cent of surgical patients were affected by HAI (*Independent*, 4 September 1990, p. 5). Emergency readmissions to hospital, which some regard as crude indicator of clinical iatrogenesis, are also increasing (Henderson *et al.*, 1989).

Alarming new evidence concerning the extent of clinical iatrogenesis in the UK was further revealed by the report of a National Confidential Enquiry into Perioperative Deaths, NCEPOD, (Buck *et al.*, 1987). The overall death rate from surgery was low, at 0.7 per cent and most of these deaths were due to the fact that the patients in question were elderly or suffered from other medical conditions. Nevertheless, the inquiry found that death was avoidable in 22 per cent of the cases. The surgical intervention itself was an associated factor in 30 per cent of the deaths, and was wholly responsible for 7 per cent of the deaths. The inquiry found evidence of inappropriate operations, poor pre-operative management, a failure to apply knowledge, and in some cases operations being undertaken by inexperienced and under-qualified doctors. In addition, 2 per cent of deaths were associated with anaesthesia.

☐ Social and cultural iatrogenesis

Turning from clinical to social iatrogenesis, Illich argues that health is undermined by the impact of medical organisation on social life. Illness is created as more and more social and individual problems are labelled as medical problems (see also Zola, 1975).

Illich argues that this process of medicalisation is harmful because it gives the medical profession enormous power to judge others. As individual conditions and experiences are defined as illnesses, they fall within the judgement and control of the medical profession. Social iatrogenesis is therefore a kind of medical imperialism, with doctors identifying illness in ever more aspects of an individual's life.

A further reason why Illich believes medicalisation to be harmful is that it moves the focus away from activities which deal more effectively with the problems faced by society and the individual. It also stifles lay initiatives which otherwise might arise to tackle these problems.

The third type of iatrogenesis identified by Illich is cultural. Medicine seeks to alleviate pain. Most people would agree that this is a noble aim. However, Illich argues that pain is an important part of human experience. To overcome suffering, to cope with pain, to face and accept death, are not necessarily negative experiences. By denying these experiences and turning them into technical matters, medicine therefore undermines the individual's spirit and personal capacities. Moreover, because most pain and suffering in industrial society is man-made, there are wider implications. Illich argues that the alleviation of pain and suffering leads to the neutralisation of political forces which might otherwise arise to prevent the underlying causes of illness.

☐ *Illich's solutions*

Attempts to assert political control over medicine and therefore redirect health care are doomed to failure, according to Illich. Moves to increase consumer control of health care and to impose a more rational organisation of health care will, in his view, also be ineffective in reducing medical power and may indeed worsen the situation. He also argues against a public health approach, because individuals are presumed ill until proved otherwise, and because medical influence will spread to other areas of social and economic life, thus causing more social iatrogenesis.

Illich does accept that health and health care may be improved by focusing on equity, which in turn raises questions about the social and economic causes of illness. But he goes on to argue that iatrogenesis will not be checked if the concern with equity is confined to matters of health service provision. The only real solution is therefore to limit the scope of professional monopolies and to extend personal responsibility for health. In his own words 'that society which can reduce professional intervention to the minimum will provide the best conditions for health' (Illich, 1975, p. 274).

□ *Challenges to Illich*

Illich's thesis arises out of a more general critique of industrialisation, institutionalisation and professional power in modern societies, but his arguments have not gone unchallenged. Doctors argue that much clinical iatrogenesis is an inevitable consequence of the advancement of medical science. According to this view, the frontiers of knowledge can only be moved forward by attempting new treatments, some of which may prove initially to be harmful to the patient. This is the price to be paid for long-term success. The failure to try new therapies, doctors argue, would have kept medicine in the Dark Ages.

A further counter-argument is that much clinical iatrogenesis is due to patient ignorance. For example, the failure to follow medical advice properly, particularly in the taking of drugs, is a well-known source of adverse reactions. From this viewpoint, clinical iatrogenesis may be reduced through doctors educating patients and communicating with them more effectively, increasing rather than reducing the scope of professional responsibility.

A further point is that Illich ignores the positive aspects of medicine. Though iatrogenesis has to be recognised and reduced, modern medicine has contributed to the improvements in health, particularly by improving the quality of life for many sufferers. Illich's thesis can therefore be criticised as being polemical and unbalanced in that he does not appear to accept that modern medicine has any redeeming features.

Illich is also criticised for being utopian. The processes of industrialisation, institutionalisation and professionalisation, which are the main causes of the problems he identifies, cannot simply be rolled back. It could be argued that professionalism combined with self-regulation and peer review are the most effective safeguards against malpractice in an industrialised society, given the complex division of labour and the diversity of knowledge and expertise. It may be better to reform health care rather than dispense with it altogether. The introduction of systems of quality control and medical audit, discussed in later chapters, may be less radical but yet provide a more practical way of reducing clinical iatrogenesis.

■ Conclusion

The various perspectives explored in this chapter, along with the critiques of orthodox medicine discussed previously, highlight a range of problems and issues facing modern health care systems. These include: the lack of accountability in health care; the dominant role of orthodox medicine and the medical profession; the lack of responsiveness to consumer wants and patient needs; the thorny questions of priorities and rationing; the need to evaluate the quality and cost-effectiveness of health care in general, and the contribution of new technologies in particular; the problems of health and health care inequalities; and the need to tackle the wider social, economic and environmental causes of ill-health. All health care systems in the developed world are confronting these issues and defining their own particular response to them.

Critical perspectives on health care have also provided a wealth of ideas for would-be reformers of the health care system. Some of the ideas and arguments may be regarded as extreme – certainly to the defenders of the status quo. Some are flawed and have attracted criticism. But this has not stopped them from infiltrating debates about the future of health care, nor has it prevented policy-makers from drawing on these ideas when reforming health care policies and programmes, as we shall see in subsequent chapters.

■ *Chapter 4* ■

The Evolution of the British Health Care System

An understanding of how the British health care system evolved is necessary in order to place contemporary developments in context. We begin by looking at the system of health care which existed before the emergence of the NHS. This is followed by an examination of how and why the NHS was created. The experience of the NHS in the post-Second World War period up to the Royal Commission's inquiry in the late 1970s is then considered. Finally, there is an analysis of the distinctive approach of Margaret Thatcher's Conservative government, which inherited the problems identified by the Royal Commission, and which in many respects posed a challenge to the ideas which underpinned the post-war health care system.

■ The health care system before the NHS

Before the creation of the NHS, Britain's health care system was a rather disorganised and complex mixture of private and public services (Webster, 1988; Abel-Smith, 1964). The private sector consisted of voluntary hospitals, private practitioners, and other voluntary and commercial organisations. The public sector comprised municipal hospitals and community health services run by local government. In addition local government was responsible for sanitary and environmental health services and health-related services such as housing. Let us now look in more detail at these sectors and how they evolved.

□ *The private sector: voluntary hospitals*

The voluntary hospitals were established by philanthropy or by public subscription. Most were created in the eighteenth and nineteenth centuries, although some were older, having been founded in the early Middle Ages.

Many voluntary hospitals, however, were of more recent origin: of those existing in 1938 over a third had been founded after 1911 (Webster, 1988, p. 2)

Traditionally, the voluntary hospitals gave their care free of charge, reflecting the charitable motives behind their foundation. When originally founded the prestige of these hospitals was such that doctors often waived their fee for the privilege of being associated with them. The doctors would make up the shortfall in their incomes by treating the rich philanthropists whose contributions supported the hospital, who, like most wealthy people of the time, were treated at home rather than in hospital. The hospitals therefore catered mainly for the less well-off who could not afford to pay for treatment. Yet admission to these hospitals was quite selective: the very poor and those with infectious diseases were frequently denied access (Abel-Smith, 1960).

By the outbreak of Second World War in 1939, the voluntary hospitals had changed considerably. Only about a third of their income now came from charitable contributions. They began to charge patients for services to a much greater extent. Patients, in turn, took out health insurance or subscription plans to cover these payments. But voluntary hospitals continued to face financial problems, despite the development of these and other fundraising efforts. Yet by and large they retained their prestigious status, and continued to make a major contribution to health care. In 1938 one in three patients still received their treatment in a voluntary hospital.

□ General practice

Prior to the creation of the NHS, general practitioners (GPs) were private practitioners who charged a fee for their services. In Victorian times the fear of being unable to pay doctors' fees led to the development of club practice. The more affluent sections of the working class would subscribe to friendly societies, who in turn hired the services of GPs for their members.

Club practice covered around a third of the working class by the end of the nineteenth century (Honigsbaum, 1990). Such schemes tended to exclude those not in work, such as the unemployed, married women, children and the elderly. The limited coverage of these schemes became a cause for concern. The medical profession also became increasingly worried about other implications of club practice. In particular the hostile attitudes of the lay people who ran the clubs and who often dealt harshly with doctors contracted with them.

In 1911 the Liberal government introduced its own plans for general practice in the form of the National Insurance Act. This legislation came into force in 1913 and led to the provision of sickness benefits, free GP services and free drugs for the employed working class. Employers, workers and the government each contributed to the compulsory scheme. The scheme was administered by local insurance committees, which included the representatives of approved societies (friendly societies and industrial insurance offices and trade unions), local authorities and GPs (Honigsbaum, 1979).

The government's initial plans angered the British Medical Association (BMA). The BMA believed that remuneration for GPs under the new scheme was inadequate. It also feared that GPs operating under the scheme would be subject to the same kind of interference experienced under the club practice system. This fear was perhaps understandable, given that the approved societies had a majority on the insurance committees which administered the scheme. The government did make several compromises, removing the power of insurance committees over doctors' remuneration, and establishing the principle that patients would be free to choose their doctor. These concessions, coupled with the professions' fear about an alternative scenario – a state medical service employing salaried GPs – resulted in a rush to join the scheme and the BMA leadership were forced to capitulate (Brand, 1965).

By the outbreak of the Second World War, 43 per cent of the population were covered by the National Health Insurance (NHI) scheme and 90 per cent of GPs participated in it (Webster, 1988, p. 11). This scheme marked a new departure in state intervention in health care. Yet it only applied to the services of GPs, not specialist hospital services (except for the treatment of tuberculosis). Moreover, the scheme excluded the unemployed and dependants, such as married women and children. GP services for these groups still had to be paid for directly in one way or another.

☐ Other voluntary and commercial organisations

The health care system prior to the creation of the NHS also involved an array of other voluntary and commercial health care organisations. Insurance companies and friendly societies were involved in the financing of health care. Voluntary organisations were also involved in the provision of community health services, increasingly working in partnership with local authorities in fields such as child welfare, maternity, aftercare, district nursing, and mental and physical handicap.

□ *The public sector: municipal health services*

Even before the creation of the NHS the public sector had the largest share of hospital care. On the eve of the Second World War, two-thirds of patients were being treated in local authority municipal hospitals. Local government operated a considerable and diverse network of hospitals. Some had been set up in the previous century to cater for certain conditions or for particular categories of patient. These included the isolation hospitals for infectious diseases, hospitals specialising in the treatment of tuberculosis, maternity hospitals, and mental hospitals. From 1875 onwards local government also had the power to run general hospitals, but few authorities actually did so.

The local authorities also inherited a hospital service which had grown out of the nineteenth century system of relief known as the Poor Law (Hodgkinson, 1967). This notorious system, introduced by the Poor Law Amendment Act (1834), effectively institutionalised poverty. Local Poor Law authorities established workhouses where relief was given on the principle of 'less eligibility' in an attempt to discourage the poor from seeking help. This system, for all its defects and inhumanity, actually exposed a high level of illness among the workhouse inmates. This had two important consequences. First, the development of publicly-funded health services. This took the form of Poor Law infirmaries, initially part of the workhouse establishment and later as separate institutions for the 'sick poor'. In addition, the poor were eligible for free GP services, following a rigorous means test. Second, the recognition of the cost of the 'sick poor' led to a series of inquiries into the environmental (but not the economic) causes of their condition, such as Edwin Chadwick's famous report on the sanitary condition of the labouring population (Chadwick, 1842). These inquiries led in turn to the development of public health legislation, beginning with the Public Health Act of 1848 which gave localities the power to ensure a healthier environment.

Although public health legislation was introduced at national level, it was down to local government to implement the statutes, enforce the regulations and develop public health services. Local health committees were set up to administer this process. Local medical officers of health (MoHs) were also appointed to act as guardians of the public health. Gradually, the local authorities began to provide a wide range of health-related services. These included water supply, sanitation, food and hygiene inspection, and pollution control, and later housing as well as personal and community health services such as school health services, midwifery, community nursing, and child welfare clinics.

The system of public and community health administration grew up separately from the Poor Law hospital network. The latter fell under the responsibility of the Poor Law Boards until their abolition in 1929. After this date most of the former Poor Law hospitals became municipal hospitals under the control of local public health authorities. However, many chronically ill people continued to reside in institutions under the control of the Public Assistance Committees which took over the remainder of the hospitals.

Suggestions had been made on a number of occasions with regard to integrating health services and local authority hospital, community and environmental health services. In 1909 members of the Royal Commission on the Poor Laws produced a dissenting minority report which argued for a unified state health service run by local authorities (Cd 4499, 1909). The minority report, which was considered too radical for its time, also sought to establish the principle of free health care for the poor as a right, though it fell far short of recommending a comprehensive state health service, available to all and free at point of delivery, an idea widely accepted only three decades later.

The acceptance of a comprehensive state health system

Criticism of the British health care system began to accumulate after the First World War. Health care was fragmented into hospital, community and public health services. There was little co-ordination of health care to tackle the complex needs of vulnerable groups, such as children and the elderly. Moreover, access to health care was limited for many of these groups. The NHI scheme did not cover dependants, the long-term unemployed, and those needing specialist services. The growth of health insurance and charging for hospital services meant that, for many, health care depended on the ability to pay. Furthermore, access to high quality health care varied throughout the country and was apparently unrelated to the level of need (Political and Economic Planning, 1937). According to some, the mismatch between geographical need and availability has been exaggerated (Powell, 1992). Nevertheless, it was widely believed at the time that some form of national planning was required to relate the need for services more closely to availability.

A series of reports in the 1920s and 1930s exposed the problems of the health services and charted future paths for reform. The Dawson report of 1920 argued for the integration of preventive and curative medicine under a single health authority, which would co-ordinate a network of local hospitals and health centres. The report also stated that the provision of the best medical care should be available to all, but did not elaborate on the question of how such a system would be financed (Cmd, 693, 1920).

A further contribution to the debate was made by the Royal Commission on National Health Insurance. This body reported in 1926 against a background of concern about access to specialist medical services. It urged the approved societies which operated the NHI scheme to pool their surplus resources to fund such care. It also indicated that the long-term future lay in direct funding of health care by the state (Cmd 2596, 1926).

The failure of the health care system to cater for the needs of those requiring specialist care was also a concern in a report by the BMA in 1929 (BMA, 1929). This report argued that NHI should be expanded to cover specialist services provided by the hospitals. It also suggested that the scheme should be extended to the families of insured workers. But the BMA plan was not fully comprehensive: it intended to exclude the wealthier classes from the scheme. The issue of how the higher cost of the extended service would be funded was also sidestepped by the BMA report.

The inter-war period, with its high rates of unemployment, created conditions which undermined the operation of the NHI system. In 1932 alone 200 000 workers exhausted their right to the benefits of the national health insurance scheme because of unemployment. There was also growing criticism of the commercial insurance industry in relation to the system of health insurance, mainly from the trade unions and the GPs (Honigsbaum, 1989).

It is often thought that the Second World War, which led to a dramatic expansion in government intervention in health services, was a major reason behind the creation of the NHS. The government created an Emergency Hospital Service (EHS) to co-ordinate the patchwork quilt of public hospitals and voluntary hospitals. The task of organising the EHS, according to Abel-Smith (1964, p. 440) 'brought home to all concerned the failings of Britain's hospital system'. The experience of the EHS was no doubt useful in showing how the state could co-ordinate the health care system. But it is generally accepted that the irrationality and inadequacy of the British health care system was evident long before the EHS was created. There was a general consensus about the need for some form of national health service well before hostilities began.

■ The creation of a National Health Service

□ *Towards a comprehensive health system*

In the years before the Second World War, the government actively considered the integration of existing health services. In 1936 the Minister of Health asked his Chief Medical Officer (CMO) to report on the feasibility of a comprehensive health care system. The CMO recommended that the local authorities should provide the basis for any comprehensive scheme. From then on the Ministry of Health began to develop policy ideas along these lines. These plans included transferring the responsibility for NHI to the local authorities and extending the coverage of this scheme to cover dependants.

Such long-term plans were, however, stopped by the need to address short-term emergencies. The first emergency was the financial crisis which hit many voluntary hospitals, including the London teaching hospitals, in 1938. The second was the prospect, followed by the certainty, of war, which led to the creation of the EHS, discussed above.

During the war, the idea of a comprehensive health service became bound up with the broader aim of reconstructing Britain when hostilities ceased. A major landmark was the ministerial announcement of October 1941, which set out the government's intention to create a comprehensive hospital service after the war. It was not clear at this stage that the service would be free. Moreover, there was no question of the voluntary hospitals being taken into public ownership, though it was expected that they would co-operate closely with local authorities to produce a more coherent pattern of hospital provision.

Meanwhile, the medical profession was busy formulating its own plans for a new health service. In 1940 the BMA established a Medical Planning Commission to consider the future development of medical services. The Commission produced an interim report two years later which set out many features which were eventually incorporated in the NHS (BMA, 1942). These included the regionalisation of hospital administration; a prohibition of full-time salaried service for GPs; and the remuneration of GPs, mainly by capitation fee (a fixed payment for every patient registered with them). The Commission supported an extension of NHI to pay for hospital and community health services, but did not pronounce unequivocally on the coverage of the new scheme. Later the BMA came out in favour of a scheme which provided for the whole community rather than just sections of it (Grey-Turner and Sutherland, 1982, p. 38).

Then came the Beveridge report (Cmd 6404, 1942). In setting out a broad framework for the post-war welfare state, Beveridge supported the idea of a comprehensive health service, available to all. Yet the final version of the Beveridge report left open the precise financial and organisational details of the service. In the event, it was these detailed matters which produced most of the controversy surrounding the proposed scheme.

□ *The shape of the new health system*

In contrast with the broad agreement on the need for a comprehensive health service, there were widely differing opinions surrounding the organisational and financial principles on which such a service should be based. The Ministry of Health favoured a municipally-controlled health service, as set out in a confidential memorandum of 1943 named (after the then Minister of Health) the Brown Plan. This plan gave local government the responsibility of organising services and sought to bring general practitioners and the voluntary hospitals under the wing of local government. The GPs were not happy with this kind of arrangement and were haunted by the spectre of a municipally-run, salaried health service. Their discontent was shared by a number of local authorities which were not overjoyed by the prospect of running such a service in view of the likely financial burden. The voluntary hospitals were also unhappy, fearing the loss of independence implied by the prospect of central government funding being channelled through the local authorities. In short, the Brown Plan pleased no one.

The government offered a compromise. A White Paper containing revised proposals was eventually published in 1944 (Cmd 6502, 1944). Under this scheme, health services would be comprehensive and free at the point of delivery and GPs would come under the control of a Central Medical Board. They would not be directly under the influence of local government except where they worked in health centres run by local authorities. GPs working in such health centres would be salaried, as would new entrants to the profession (for an unspecified period), and other GPs could be salaried if they wished. Private practice was permissible and the right to buy and sell practices was retained, though some restrictions would be imposed on these activities. Finally, the hospital service was to be operated by joint local authority boards responsible for controlling municipal hospitals and co-ordinating the activities of the entire hospital network in the area.

The doctors, fearing a loss of autonomy, rejected the White Paper. Their lobbying was effective in that all the major proposals were dropped, including the establishment of the Central Medical Board. The government agreed that the responsibility for GP services would remain with local committees on which the GPs would have a majority. The local authorities' control over doctors working in health centres was eroded to the point that their function was to be little more than that of a landlord. The provision that doctors working in health centres would be salaried was also dropped.

The local authorities also obtained concessions. The joint boards that would have taken control of municipal hospitals were subsequently confined to a local planning role, leaving control in the hands of individual local authorities. This made it politically possible to allow medical representation on these boards, a move which had been resisted strongly by local authorities as long as the boards had control over municipal hospitals. In addition, expert regional planning bodies were also proposed. This was mainly to satisfy the demands of the voluntary hospitals, in particular the more prestigious teaching hospitals, which had lobbied for a regional tier to advise on planning and developing specialised medical services.

A further White Paper embodying the revised proposals was planned, but meanwhile Labour had left the war coalition government. This second White Paper was suppressed before the 1945 election and, as a result of the Conservative Party's defeat at the polls, was never published. Even so, some of the proposals it contained reappeared in the Labour government's plans, namely the regional structure and the separate local administration of GP and hospital services, discussed below.

☐ *Bevan's plan*

The 1945 General Election produced a clear victory for the Labour Party. Clement Attlee, the new Prime Minister, appointed Aneurin Bevan as Minister for Health, giving him the task of rescuing the plans for a new health service (see Foot, 1975). Despite the support within his own party for a comprehensive health service based on local authority control, Bevan opted for nationalisation of the entire hospital sector within a tripartite system of health care provision.

This option was chosen, not on ideological but on practical grounds. As Honigsbaum (1989, p. 95) correctly notes, 'far from being a dogmatic socialist, Bevan proved to be a pragmatic reformer'. Yet there was considerable opposition to his plan. Bevan was challenged by his Cabinet colleague Herbert Morrison, a staunch defender of local government interests, who argued against the nationalisation of the municipal hospitals. Bevan won this battle, but local authorities continued for the time being at least to have a significant role in health care through their provision of community services, personal social services and public health functions.

The other main source of opposition to Bevan's plan came from the medical profession, particularly the GPs, whose views were forcefully put by the BMA. Many GPs were alarmed, not only about the principle of nationalisation, but also about proposals to ban the sale of practices and to control the geographical distribution of new entrants to general practice. Their biggest fear, however, was the prospect of a salaried medical service. In an attempt to attract their support Bevan allowed GPs to remain as independent contractors. They would be allowed to provide services to NHS patients on the basis of a contract negotiated between the Ministry of Health and the profession's representatives, and would be paid mainly by capitation payments. A part-time salary element for all GPs was included in Bevan's original plan, though this was later restricted to new GPs for a limited period only. As a further concession, which was instrumental in securing the co-operation of the profession, Bevan agreed to a ban on full-time salaried medical services.

The interests of the GPs as independent contractors were also protected by the creation of a separate administrative branch. It was agreed that GP contracts, and those of dentists, pharmacists and opticians, would be administered by executive councils. These bodies would consist of part-time appointees nominated by the Minister of Health, the local authorities, and by the independent contractor professions themselves, with the last of these groups providing half the members.

The local authorities and the executive councils formed two parts of the tripartite structure (see Figure 4.1). The third was the hospital service which, with the exception of the teaching hospitals (see below), was to be operated on a two-tier structure. The top tier consisted of Regional

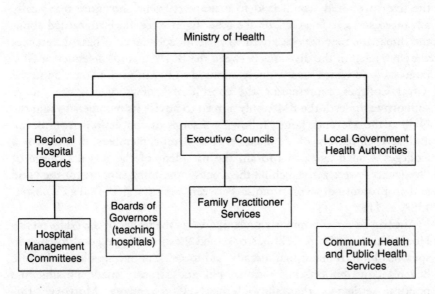

Figure 4.1   *The original National Health Service structure (England and Wales), 1948–74*

Hospital Boards (RHBs) responsible for the overall planning, co-ordination and supervision of hospital services within a large area. The RHBs were appointed by the Minister of Health after consultation with local authorities and the medical profession. The second tier, responsible for the actual running of the local hospital service, consisted of Hospital Management Committees (HMCs). The HMC members were appointed by the RHB, following consultation with local authorities, the medical profession, and voluntary associations.

The prestigious teaching hospitals were now to be administered by a separate board of governors appointed by and accountable to the Minister of Health. Though the hospitals themselves did not regard their position as being privileged, the treatment given to the élite hospitals was seen by the rest of the hospital sector as favourable. This appears to have been part of a strategy by Bevan to buy off the medical élite – the consultants – who worked in these hospitals. The consultants were also courted with promises of generous salaries, a system of merit awards, the retention of pay beds within the new NHS hospitals, and the option of combining private practice with NHS work. The strategy was apparently successful in promoting the support of the consultants. Hence the famous comment attributed to Bevan that he 'stuffed their mouths with gold'.

Aside from these concessions, the consultants tended to take a more favourable view of the NHS than did their colleagues in general practice. Many consultants believed that a comprehensive state health system along the lines proposed would lead to a more efficient and more technically advanced service. The GPs, on the other hand were more concerned about the threat the new service posed to their independence. These differences were reflected in the divisions between the BMA, a stout defender of GPs' interests (and which was strongly opposed to Bevan's initial plan), and the Royal Colleges, representing the consultants' views, which were more supportive. Indeed, the BMA only agreed to advise its members to join the NHS at the 'eleventh hour', following a series of concessions from Bevan and several ballots of its membership. Senior members of the Royal Colleges – such as Lord Moran, the president of the Royal College of Physicians – were active behind the scenes in building support for the NHS and in promoting a compromise between Bevan and the GPs (Webster, 1988, p. 116).

Aneurin Bevan is popularly remembered as the father of the NHS. Yet as Honigsbaum (1989, p. 217) has observed 'Bevan had the good fortune to spearhead a movement that already had force'. Yet one should not belittle Bevan's contribution. His vision, skill and strategy made possible the political settlement that allowed the NHS to emerge. Moreover, this political settlement forged an organisational structure, which, though in many respects flawed, was to last almost thirty years.

■ The experience of the NHS: 1948–79

The creation of the NHS brought considerable benefits. It provided for the first time a comprehensive system of health care, open to all, which was not based on the ability to pay at the point of delivery. There were other potential benefits too. The fact that the service was national raised the possibility that a high standard of health care could become universal. The bringing together of a range of services under the direct responsibility of the Ministry of Health created the potential for a more coherent, planned and integrated health care system. Finally, the funding mechanism for the new service – based on taxation (with a contribution from National Insurance funds) – meant that spending on the NHS would be under the watchful eye of the Treasury. This arrangement ensured that the NHS was one of the most cost-effective health care systems in the world.

The NHS proved also to be a popular institution. For the generation that had to live under the system which preceded it, it was a major achievement. It has also proved to be popular for the generation that grew up with the welfare state. However, despite its popularity, the NHS has faced a number of serious problems during its lifetime and has not always tackled these successfully. By the late 1970s the situation was becoming so serious that even the considerable achievements of the NHS appeared to be under threat. The NHS came to be widely perceived as in a constant state of crisis (Haywood and Alaszewski, 1980). This impression remained as the service moved into the 1980s.

Some of the difficulties facing the NHS had plagued it from its earliest days. Some arose from its original structure, which resulted from political compromise rather than administrative rationality. Other problems were new, reflecting the fact that the challenges facing the NHS, and indeed the expectations of the service, had changed since its creation. Another set of problems was caused, at least in part, by botched attempts to reform and reorganise the service, while others were caused by the wider political and economic environment which lay largely outside the control of the NHS.

□ *Problems with the structure of the NHS*

As noted earlier, the original structure of the NHS was tripartite, comprising the family practitioner services (GPs, dentists, pharmacists and opticians) administered by executive councils; local authority community health services (such as midwifery and community nursing), personal social services and public health; and the nationalised hospital service.

As time passed it became evident that the original NHS structure was flawed. The major problems were overlap, duplication and lack of co-ordination between the three parts of the structure (Ministry of Health, 1959; 1963; BMA, 1962). During the 1960s the structure came under increasing pressure, leading ultimately to government proposals to reorganise the service (Ministry of Health, 1968; DHSS, 1970). After some deliberation, and two changes of government, new proposals were brought forward (DHSS, 1971; and Cmnd 5055, 1972) and a reorganisation was eventually implemented in 1974.

The new structure created three tiers of health service management below the Department of Health and Social Security (DHSS) (which had succeeded the Ministry of Health in 1968): at regional, area and district level. New health authorities, responsible for planning and development of services were established at regional and area level. Like the RHBs and HMCs which preceded them, these bodies were accountable to, and appointed by, ministerial authority.

The reorganisation did not, however, solve the structural problems of the service. The family practitioner services supplied by GPs, dentists, pharmacists and opticians were not fully integrated. They remained separate, under new family practitioner committees (FPCs) which replaced the former executive councils. The NHS became responsible for community health services, transferred from local government. But the latter retained responsibility for environmental health services and social care. So there remained three separate agencies involved in the provision of state health care. Tripartism had proved remarkably resilient.

The new NHS structure was criticised on other grounds. It was seen as being bureaucratic, having too many tiers of management and requiring too many administrators. New systems of planning and management which accompanied these organisational changes were also criticised. These were held to be responsible for slow decision-making and a lack of accountability. Yet the search for an 'organisational fix' (Klein, 1983, p. 90) continued. Despite the problems associated with the reorganisation, policy-makers still placed their faith in structural reform (McLachlan, 1990) giving rise to a further reorganisation in 1982.

☐ *Accountability, control and planning*

The problems of the NHS went beyond the original structure. It became clear that there was a fundamental contradiction at the heart of the NHS with respect to the powers and responsibilities of Health Ministers. Health Ministers had full responsibility for health policy, but had little direct control over the activities of the NHS. It was well known that power over service developments was concentrated at local level, in the hands of doctors, who were not accountable to ministers for their actions or for the resources they used. At the end of the day the medical profession had an effective veto power over the implementation of policies. But health authorities, responsible to and appointed by ministerial authority (yet drawn in part from local government and the health professions) could not be relied upon to impose policies designed by central government. (Haywood and Alaszeskwi, 1980; Elcock and Haywood, 1980).

Ministers nevertheless attempted to influence service developments through the health authorities. Instead of clarifying the goals of the service, ministers preferred to emphasise the importance of specific service developments. They began with the Hospital Plan of 1962 (Cmnd 1604, 1962). This was essentially a plan for capital expenditure in the hospital sector, though it did set out norms for the provision of beds for various medical specialities. In the following year a similar plan was introduced for the community health services (Cmnd 1973, 1963).

A more elaborate planning process for the NHS was introduced in 1976. Ministers explicitly set out their priorities, emphasising the so-called 'Cinderella services' (the services for the elderly, the mentally ill, and the mentally and physically handicapped), primary care, and preventive medicine (DHSS, 1976a; 1977). This guidance was filtered down to the lowest tiers of the NHS, which formulated their own plans within this framework. These plans were then passed back up the structure to enable the DHSS to monitor the consistency of the local and national plans and the overall development of services.

The planning process was persuasive rather than directive. Health authorities (and the medical profession at local level) were thus able to resist a dramatic shift in priorities. The planning process was also criticised as being too cumbersome, and involving too many advisory and planning bodies. This prolonged the planning process, confused the setting of objectives, and slowed down movement towards the achievement of new priorities.

☐ Funding, efficiency and resource allocation

Since its creation, the resourcing of the NHS has been more or less a constant issue of debate. The NHS had hardly begun its life before it was faced by a financial crisis (Webster, 1988). In the 1950s the Conservative government, worried about the resources consumed by the service, established the Guillebaud inquiry into the NHS. The report of this inquiry (Cmd 9663, 1956) was unexpectedly favourable, concluding that spending on the NHS was not as extravagant as some had suggested, and that in many respects it provided good value for money. The Guillebaud report also pointed out that there were deficiencies in some services and that this required more spending on the NHS rather than less.

The Guillebaud report strengthened the case of those who argued for greater NHS expenditure and made it more difficult for those who sought economies in this area. Health expenditure began to grow both in real terms and as a proportion of national expenditure. This continued until the late 1970s, when the government attempted to exert a much tighter control over public expenditure in view of the deepening economic crisis. The NHS, like many other public services, faced financial restraint. This in turn focused attention on the need for greater efficiency in the NHS in order to maximise the use of existing resources.

At the same time it also became evident that something had to be done about the distribution of resources. Ministers were concerned to redirect resources to 'neglected' groups, such as the elderly, in line with their priorities. Also there was an increasing emphasis on geographical inequalities in health service funding. In the 1970s the highest-spending NHS regions spent around two-thirds more per head than the lowest-spending regions (Griffiths, 1971). In an attempt to iron out these inequalities, and to ensure that health authorities received a budget more appropriate to the health needs they faced, the Labour government introduced the RAWP (Resource Allocation Working Party) formula in 1977 (Mays and Bevan, 1987).

RAWP used a funding formula which replaced the existing system of allocating resources largely on an historical basis. This formula sought to allocate resources on the basis of each region's relative health care needs. There were a number of stages to this process. First, an assessment of relative need was established, based on indicators of illness, such as regional population size and structure, standardised mortality ratios for specific conditions and so on. Second, a target level of funding for each region was calculated by dividing the resources available by the estimate of relative need. Third, in view of the likely disruption caused by changing the funding system overnight, budgets were allocated in such a way as to move the regions towards their target funding levels. Hence, over a number of years, those regions below their target would receive a greater increase in their resources than those regions over target.

Scotland, Northern Ireland and Wales had their own equivalents of RAWP which similarly sought to place the allocation of resources on a more rational basis by attempting to relate budgets to indicators of need. Yet while the case for a more rational allocation system was widely accepted, there was much concern about the operation of these schemes in practice (Goldacre and Harris, 1980; Radical Statistics Health Group, 1977). This concern centred mainly on the accuracy of the indicators of need within the redistributive formula. There was particular criticism of the use of standardised mortality ratios. Many observers regarded morbidity data as being a better indicator of the need for health services, while others argued that indicators of deprivation provided a better measure of need, given the relationship between deprivation and ill-health.

The formula was also criticised for failing to account for the different costs facing each region (and each district therein). Some modifications were made to the formula to reflect the higher costs of delivering services in London, teaching hospitals, supra-regional specialties (provided for the benefit of populations in more than one region) and cross-boundary flows (the treatment of patients from another region). Despite these changes, RAWP was still regarded by many as a rather blunt instrument which in times of financial stringency could have serious effects on services in those districts which lost out in the redistributive process.

Finally, there was the related question of health inequalities and the access to health services. The NHS had been created as a free service. Yet despite the removal of financial barriers to care, social class differences in health status persisted. It was also alleged that the provision of health services favoured the middle classes and that the working classes faced problems of access to services. The Labour government responded to increasing concern by setting up a working party under Sir Douglas Black. The Black inquiry reported in 1980 with a comprehensive analysis of the various aspects of inequality in health and health care (DHSS, 1980), though, as we shall see in a later chapter, its recommendations did not find favour with the new Conservative administration.

Industrial action, professional power and the consumer

The 1970s also saw a marked deterioration in industrial relations in the health service, reflecting a general trend in British society. The government became embroiled in pay disputes with all classes of NHS staff: nurses, doctors and ancillary workers. In addition, the government faced the threat of industrial action from hospital doctors (and some of the unions representing ancillary workers) over the issue of pay beds in the NHS.

Industrial action in the NHS was not new. In 1965 GPs had threatened to resign from the NHS in a dispute over pay and conditions. The differences between the 1970s and previous disputes were in terms of scale, regularity and intensity. The 1970s not only saw more days lost (298 000 working days were lost to the NHS through industrial action in 1973 compared with only 500 in 1966), but the ferocity of the disputes was of a different order.

Industrial action, based mainly on the protection of the interests of workers and professionals, highlighted the plight of patients. Yet the disruption to services, along with the length of waiting lists, and the occasional scandals of malpractice or ill-treatment, never seriously damaged the public's support for the NHS and it remained, almost paradoxically, a popular institution. There was, however, no room for complacency. The growth of the private sector in the late 1970s (see Chapter 7) illustrated that some people (those who could afford it) were beginning to vote with their feet. There was also a feeling that once support for the NHS began to weaken slightly, the whole edifice might cave in.

Certainly, there were signs that patients were not quite as passive as they once had been. Wider concerns about the quality of health services and their responsiveness to consumer pressures grew in the 1960s and 1970s. This was enhanced by a number of developments. The 1974 reorganisation introduced Community Health Councils to represent the patients' viewpoint. In 1973 Parliament created the office of Health Service Commissioner to investigate maladministration in the NHS. Also there were moves to improve complaints procedures at around the same time, though these efforts did not come to fruition until the early 1980s.

☐ *The Royal Commission on the NHS*

The accumulation of these various problems by the mid-1970s contributed to a growing sense of crisis in the NHS and the health care system which it dominated. The Labour government responded in May 1976 by establishing a Royal Commission to consider 'the best use and management of financial and manpower resources of the NHS' (Cmnd 7615, 1979, p. 1). It is clear that the Royal Commission was not intended as a tool of radical change. Indeed, the membership was carefully selected to avoid such an outcome. Yet ironically, when the Commission reported three years later, it did so to a radical Conservative government headed by Margaret Thatcher. Unlike the Black report on inequalities, the Royal Commission's findings did not receive an outright rejection from the new government.

The Royal Commission made a number of important observations, which are worth recalling. It noted that the NHS operated in the absence of clear objectives and sought to remedy this by setting out seven key objectives. These were:

- to encourage and assist individuals to remain healthy;
- to provide equality of entitlement to health services;
- to provide a broad range of services to a high standard;

- to provide equality of access to these services;
- to provide a service free at the time of use;
- to satisfy the reasonable expectations of its users; and
- to remain a national service responsive to local needs.

Some of these objectives did not strike a chord with the new government for reasons that will become clear later in this chapter.

The Royal Commission's assessment of the situation facing the NHS was less gloomy than most. It concluded that 'we need not be ashamed of our health service' (Cmnd, 7615, 1979, p. 356) and that in many respects the NHS represented a considerable achievement. The Commission identified social and geographical inequalities as being a particular problem, but added that this could not be tackled by the NHS alone. Nevertheless, it believed that the performance of the NHS could be improved in many areas, and that much of this improvement could be achieved through greater efficiency.

The other main points raised by the Royal Commission were as follows:

- that prevention had been relatively neglected and should be given more attention in future;
- that the shortage of funds had frustrated the implementation of the priorities identified by central government;
- that the community as a whole would have to share the responsibilities and costs of looking after the elderly;
- that better co-ordination and teamwork was needed in primary care;
- that there should be an improvement of community health services in declining urban areas;
- that there should be better control of prescription costs;
- that there should be better communication between hospital and community services;
- that there should be more sensitivity to patients' needs in hospital;
- that additional resources were needed for Community Health Councils;
- that improved complaints mechanisms for patients were required; and
- that voluntary work and voluntary organisations should be encouraged.

As will become clear later in the book, many of these points were taken up by the Conservative government during the 1980s.

The Commission's 117 recommendations contained something for everybody. Many fell on stony ground. For example, the Commission unsuccessfully urged the abolition of Family Practitioner Committees and the transfer of their functions to health authorities. Other recommendations also proved unacceptable, including the abolition of charges, and direct accountability of the regional health authorities to Parliament. But the incoming Conservative government did find some of the recommendations acceptable. The Commission's argument for the abolition of a tier of management below the regional level was enthusiastically pursued, as was the recommendation for a limited list of prescribed medicines. The passage of time has also seen the Commission's recommendations for medical audit and the extension of screening programmes taken up by the government.

The acceptance of some of the Royal Commission's conclusions and recommendations by the new government exemplifies the continuities in health policy-making. Nevertheless, change rather than continuity was the theme of the 1980s, in health care as in many other areas of public policy. These changes arose from the general attitude and approach of the Thatcher government, to be explored in the next section.

■ Thatcherism and health care

□ *The Thatcher government*

The election of a Conservative government in May 1979 was in many ways a watershed. The style and approach of this government, and particularly of its leader, Margaret Thatcher, represented a considerable break with the past, according to most observers (see Jenkins, 1987; Riddell, 1991; Young, 1991). In her eleven-year tenure, Thatcher presided over a government which attempted to transform many aspects of the welfare state and the public sector established after the Second World War. The post-war settlement, broadly supported by both Labour and Conservative governments, faced its most serious challenge. The NHS, as a cornerstone of the welfare state and as a major part of the public sector, employing over a million people and accounting for more than a tenth of public-sector expenditure, could not be immune from these wider changes in British politics.

□ *The New Right*

The Thatcher government's direction was strongly influenced by the political philosophy of the New Right. Though, as Gamble (1988) has noted, this is neither a unified movement nor a coherent doctrine, yet one can identify a number of common themes among its exponents. Generally, the New Right favours more freedom for business, more choice for individuals in the market, the removal of 'impediments' in the market (such as trade unions), a greater role for markets generally and a smaller role for the state in economic affairs. This is combined with a belief in the authority of the state in social matters, where morality, social order and individual responsibility have to be preserved. The New Right philosophy is therefore in essence a fusion of conservative and liberal thought, favouring a limited but authoritarian state and a free market economy (see also King, 1987; Green, 1987).

The Thatcher government's appetite for this brand of political philosophy predisposed it towards certain social and economic policies: the privatisation of the financing and provision of public services; public expenditure control and cuts in direct taxation; the encouragement of self-help and voluntary services; restrictions on trade unions; and the encouragement of economic efficiency and business-style management practices within the public sector. For similar reasons it was also predisposed against other policies, such as restrictions and regulations on business activity and policies aimed at reducing social inequalities and deprivation. As we shall see in later chapters, this predisposition had important implications for the adoption of health policies.

Superficially, and in retrospect, the Thatcher government's programme appears to be a well-planned assault on British post-war society, and in particular on 'socialist' institutions: the trade unions, the welfare state and the nationalised industries. But although some of the elements listed above could be found in the Conservative manifesto of 1979, 'Thatcherism', as Gamble (1988, p. 222) notes, has lacked symmetry, coherence and purpose. The Thatcher government, in many ways like its predecessors, tended to react pragmatically to events rather than responding according to some master plan. Young observes that Thatcher herself was not an ideologist nor a long-term thinker, but 'a pragmatist and a problem solver' (Young, 1991, p. 603). Her government was prepared to tread carefully, particularly as the elections drew near. Indeed, as Kavanagh (1990, p. 97) has noted, some of the more hard-line adherents of the New Right philosophy believe that the Thatcher government was not radical enough. Furthermore, in practice there was often a gap between the radical intention of the government and the outcome of the policies once implemented (Marsh and Rhodes, 1992).

Nevertheless, the Thatcher government was unusual in the degree to which it did adhere to a particular vision of the world while in office. The post-war history of Britain is filled with government 'U-turns' and party political rhetoric operating within a broad consensus. The Thatcher government was, by contrast, a conviction government, not afraid of offending established interests. It also had the benefit of an environment conducive to the pursuit of these convictions, namely a long period in office, a passive (and where it mattered, a supportive) electorate, and a feeble political opposition. This enabled it not only to promote radical change in many areas of public policy, but also to change the political agenda and the terms of debate. Although Margaret Thatcher has now departed, the Conservatives have continued in office. Moreover, her legacy has been to change the landscape of British politics and policy-making in ways which will persist into the future.

☐ *Thatcherism and the health care system*

The Thatcher government's approach to health and health care was, as will become clear, typical of its overall approach to public policy: a vision in harmony with the New Right ideology, yet tempered with short-term expediency and pragmatism. The Thatcher government inherited a health care system faced with a number of internal problems and external challenges. In attempting to deal with these issues it often fell back on its own ideological predisposition. But it also drew on existing ideas, and in addition developed its own ideas in the light of experience. There were continuities, as the response to the Royal Commission on the NHS revealed, but there have also been significant changes.

In the remainder of this book these continuities and changes will be explored in an attempt to assess the extent to which the Thatcher government – and its successor under John Major – have resolved the fundamental challenges and problems facing the British health care system identified so far. The chapters in the second half of this book analyse key areas of health policy touched by the Thatcher programme. The structural and management reforms of the NHS; privatisation and public expenditure on health care; the introduction of market mechanisms into the NHS; primary care; community care; and finally, public health. Before embarking on this analysis, however, it is important that we bring ourselves right up to date by setting out the main features of the British health care system today.

■ *Chapter 5* ■

The British Health Care System Today

The main purpose of this chapter is to outline the major features of the British health care system today. Before doing so, however, it is important to place these features in a broader context, by looking at the variety of contemporary health care systems to be found in advanced industrial societies.

■ Health care systems

In practice it is difficult to pin down the meaning of the term 'health care system'. Field (1989, p. 10) uses the general term 'health system' to identify 'the totality of formal efforts, commitments, personnel, institutions, economic resources, research efforts (both basic and applied) that a nation state or a society earmarks or devotes to illness, premature mortality, incapacitation, prevention, rehabilitation and other health-related problems'. In one respect this broad definition is useful as it focuses attention upon the range of factors and agents which may significantly affect health, such as poverty, environmental factors and individual lifestyles.

Health impinges upon almost every aspect of life in some way. Ultimately, the health system is boundless. But, as Field himself recognises, for analytical purposes, boundaries have to be set. One way forward is to focus purely on the delivery of a more narrowly defined set of health care services, such as hospitals, primary care services, and community care facilities.

Another attempt to set boundaries has been undertaken by Moran (1991, p. 3) who defines the term 'health care state' as 'that part of any state concerned with regulating access to, financing, and organising the delivery of, health care to the population'. This is a helpful concept because it focuses attention upon key features of modern health care systems: the extent to which the state intervenes, and the different forms of intervention adopted, though this focus should not (and indeed is not intended to) divert our attention away from the significant and increasing role undertaken by voluntary and commercial organisations in relation to health care.

Most classifications of health care systems are, in fact, based on characteristics related in some way to the nature and extent of state involvement and the scope for independent provision. Field's (1989) typology of health care systems shown in Figure 5.1 is one such example.

The focus of Field's classification is mainly, though not exclusively, based upon allocative mechanisms. Health care systems allocate resources mainly or wholly through the market (for example, emergent and pluralistic systems), or mainly or wholly through the state (state insurance, national health service and socialised systems). State involvement takes a number of forms, ranging from direct ownership of health care facilities and the direct employment of health care workers (as in the NHS) through to the provision of funding schemes to reimburse the population's health care expenses (see Exhibit 5.1). The relationship between state and market is, however, increasingly complex, as countries adapt their systems both in the light of common problems and in view of other countries' experiences.

☐ *Different systems: common problems*

Increasingly, it seems that different health care systems around the world are facing the same kinds of problem. Countries such as the USA, France, Holland and Italy, like the UK, face growing dissatisfaction with their health systems. The majority of OECD (Organisation for Economic Co-operation and Development) member countries have, in fact, under-taken significant reforms in their health care systems in recent years. The UK is far from alone in considering radical reform (see Ham *et al.*, 1990).

The industrialised countries have similar problems, in two respects (OECD, 1987). They face the same kind of health trends, as outlined in Chapter 1, such as lifestyle and environmental factors in ill-health, new infectious diseases, the burden of chronic illness, growing numbers of elderly people and so on. Second, these countries are experiencing similar problems in terms of the organisation and funding of health care, such as the need to control costs, improve accountability and efficiency, monitor the effectiveness of care, establish priorities, and ensure that health care is accessible to those who are in need. In the light of these common problems, it is not surprising that similar solutions are being sought.

Policy imitation is a recognised feature of health planning, with countries borrowing ideas from each other (Leichter, 1979). It has been suggested that there is a kind of convergence at work, with health care systems becoming increasingly similar (Jönsson, 1990). One writer, for

Type 1:   EMERGENT
Health care viewed as item of personal consumption
Physician operates as solo entrepreneur
Professional associations powerful
Private ownership of facilities
Direct payment to physicians
Minimal role in health care for the state

Type 2:   PLURALISTIC
Health care viewed mainly as consumer good
Physician operates as solo entrepreneur and in
    organised groups
Professional organisations very powerful
Private and public ownership of facilities
Payments for services direct and indirect
State's role in health care minimal and indirect
Example: USA

Type 3:   INSURANCE/SOCIAL SECURITY
Health care as an insured/guaranteed consumer good or
    service
Physicians operate as solo entrepreneurs and members
    of medical organisations
Professional organisations strong
Private and public ownership of facilities
Payments for services mostly indirect
State's role in health care central but indirect
Example: France

Type 4:   NATIONAL HEALTH SERVICE
Health care as a state-supported service
Physicians solo entrepreneurs and members of medical
    organisations
Professional organisations fairly strong
Facilities mainly publicly owned
Payments for services indirect
State's role in health care central and direct
Example: UK

Type 5:   SOCIALISED
Health care a state provided public service
Physicians are state employees
Professional organisations weak or non-existent
Facilities wholly publicly owned
Payments for services entirely indirect
State's role in health care is total
Example: Former Soviet Union

Source: M. G. Field (ed.) *Success and Crisis in National Health Systems* (London:
          Routledge, 1989) p. 7.

Figure 5.1   *Health care systems*

Exhibit 5.1   *The health care systems of France and the USA*

France

Finance   70 per cent of health care costs funded by the state from the social security fund. The fund is raised by levies upon employers and employees. The poor do not pay a contribution. For certain illnesses (for example, cancer) the state funds 100 per cent of the cost.

For other conditions, individuals have to pay the balance of the cost of care (30 per cent). This is usually financed by subscribing to non-profit-making insurance societies.

The scale of medical fees is negotiated between the profession and the health ministry.

Ownership of facilities/employment   Approximately 80 per cent of the hospitals are publicly owned and are the responsibility of the health ministry. The rest are operated for profit, and mainly cater for the upper classes, though patients can get some reimbursement from the social security scheme.

Most hospital physicians are salaried, but family doctors are independent. In all, over half the doctors in France are private practitioners.

Patients are not assigned to a specific list as in the UK, but can consult any (and any number of) doctors (though the government is currently attempting to restrict choice).

United States of America

Finance   The state operates two schemes: Medicaid for the poor, and Medicare for the elderly and disabled, which reimburse the medical fees of these groups. The schemes are far from comprehensive. Medicare patients often have to make top-up payments for care, and long-term care is not covered. Medicaid does not apply to single people, the childless, or the low-paid. The remainder of the population (two-thirds) are insured privately, often as part of their employment package. A fifth of the population subscribe to Health Maintenance Organisations (HMOs – see Chapter 8). A limited amount of free care is provided by the public hospitals. Some private hospitals have in the past cross-subsidised patients who are unable to pay.

Ownership of facilities/employment   Three-quarters of hospitals are privately owned, of which a minority (a fifth) are operated for profit. The remainder are public hospitals run by local or state authorities.

The bulk of the medical profession has traditionally consisted of independent private practitioners who charge a fee for services as they are provided. But increasing numbers are employed directly by hospitals and by third-party organisations such as HMOs.

Note With the election of President Bill Clinton in 1992, amid growing dissatisfaction with the US system of health care, reform has moved up the political agenda. At the time of writing, no national health scheme has been introduced, although individual states are experimenting with various schemes.

example, has likened the US and British health care systems to two ships moving across the Atlantic towards each other (Roberts, 1991a). While the British government has appreciated the benefits of market forces in the American system of health care, the Americans themselves are considering a more universal health scheme.

Yet it should be stressed that considerable differences continue to exist between health care systems. While there may be a long term trend towards convergence in some aspects of health care finance and organisation, considerable differences are likely to remain as systems retain their own particular cultural identities.

■ The British health care system

□ *Organisation*

Having placed the British health care system in context, it is now possible to take a look at some of its main features. Essentially, there are four main parts to the health care system in Britain: central government; the NHS; local government; and the independent sector. The picture is complicated somewhat by the fact that each part of the UK has its own separate structure. In this section the focus is mainly upon the health care system in England, though important differences with Wales, Scotland and Northern Ireland will be noted.

□ *Central government*

Central government provides few health services directly. Most services are, in fact, delivered through the NHS. Even so, central government bears the burden of political responsibility for health service delivery. In England the Department of Health (formerly the Department of Health and Social Security) is responsible for overseeing health services. The specific functions of the Department of Health are to determine policy and priorities, circulate advice to NHS authorities, to review their performance, and to allocates resources to them. The department also advises, inspects and provides some resources for the personal social services operated by the local authorities.

Political responsibility for health and personal social services lies with the Secretary of State for Health, the senior minister and constitutional head of the department. The minister is accountable and responsible to Parliament for a range of matters. This involves explaining and justifying the department's policies to individual MPs and Parliamentary commit- tees. The Secretary of State is also accountable for the financial resources spent by the department and the NHS. Furthermore s/he has a general responsibility to promote the health of the people.

The Secretary of State for Health is also responsible to Parliament for the detailed operation of NHS services, though not for local authority personal social services. However, the Secretary of State does have some specific responsibilities for approving arrangements made by local authorities for the care of the elderly, for child welfare, for the mentally and physically handicapped, and for the mentally ill. The growing importance of issues such as child abuse and community care, and criticism of current arrangements in these areas, have led ministers to take a much closer interest in the details of local authority personal social services in recent years.

The extent of ministerial responsibility for the NHS was captured in Aneurin Bevan's phrase: 'when a bedpan is dropped on a hospital floor its noise should resound in the Palace of Westminster' (quoted in Nairne, 1984). Maxwell (1981) has described the responsibilities of the Secretary of State for Health as being unique in terms of the numbers of staff, organisational complexity, the degree of discretion involved in individual cases, and the amount of expenditure. In practice, detailed ministerial responsibility for health services is, as the Royal Commission on the NHS noted, largely a constitutional fiction. Yet the Department of Health has been a political hot-seat for a number of years. Ministers themselves have been well aware of the extent to which they have been held personally and publicly responsible for policies and services (Castle, 1990; Crossman, 1977; Fowler, 1991).

The Secretary of State for Health is assisted by a number of junior ministers. Currently, the Department of Health has four junior ministers. Three are responsible for specific areas of policy (such as preventive medicine and community care for example) and operate with the delegated authority of the Secretary of State. A further minister is drawn from the House of Lords and acts as the department's spokesperson in this chamber.

The Department of Health also employs over 4500 civil servants who have the task of advising ministers and implementing policy decisions. In practice civil servants can have considerable influence over policy in view of their permanence (the civil service is a career, but ministerial tenure is short, lasting on average only thirty months), their knowledge of departmental issues, and their familiarity and experience with the procedures of departmental policy-making (Hennessy, 1988). Civil service influence is at its greatest where ministers are not committed to a particular policy response. In general, technically-complex issues, matters currently attracting little attention from the public or from major pressure groups, and issues of little party-political significance, are those decisions which tend to be dominated by the civil servants, in view of the low levels of ministerial interest in these matters.

There are two types of civil servant within the Department of Health: the generalists, who have a general administrative background; and the specialists, who have specific professional qualifications. A similar dichotomy is found in other departments, though in the Department of Health the key feature is that many of these specialists, as one might expect, have a professional background in health care. The department employs civil servants drawn from medicine, nursing, social work and a range of other caring professions, who are able to contribute to policy-making and implementation on the basis of their specialist training and knowledge.

The structure of the Department of Health reflects the need to combine generalist administrative skills and specialist advice. Although the department is headed by a generalist permanent secretary, professional advice is incorporated at every level. At the top there is the Chief Medical Officer (CMO), who has direct access to ministers and who is also the chief medical adviser to the government as a whole. Although the CMO is in effect the professional head of the department and stands at the apex of the medical advisory structure, each professional group has its own chief officer (such as the Chief Nursing Officer, for example) to whom it is professionally accountable. Professional advice is not, however, confined to 'big issues'. Highly specific contributions are made by the professional officers within the various groups and divisions which make up the bulk of the department. These smaller units, which either focus on specific functions or particular policy areas, frequently require specialist input from the professions on a range of technical matters.

Given the complexity of health care policy and its increasingly controversial nature, there have been moves in recent years to reduce the burden on health ministers through reorganisation of the department's functions. From 1968 to 1988 the responsibility for health and social security was combined within the Department of Health and Social Security (DHSS). The original merger between the health and social security ministries had been devised partly in an attempt to co-ordinate these two areas of policy and partly (so the story goes) to provide a suitably prestigious job for one of the ministers in the then Labour government, Richard Crossman. Twenty years later there were both political and rational grounds for dividing the department. This enabled the government to appoint a new health minister without having to remove the incumbent, Jon Moore, who was subjected to enormous political pressure during the NHS crisis of 1987/8 (Moore became Minister of the Department of Social Security after the split). Yet it was also apparent that the DHSS was simply too large to be able to formulate and co-ordinate such a wide range of policies in an effective manner.

Attempts have also been made to devolve many of the management responsibilities for the day-to-day running of health services to the NHS, in an effort to limit ministerial responsibility and to distance them from some of the more detailed matters relating to the service. Though this has been part of a general reform of central government undertaken since the late 1980s, the attempt to devolve management responsibilities within the Department of Health began much earlier. Following the Griffiths report (DHSS, 1983), separate policy and management boards were established for the NHS. For reasons that will be discussed in Chapter 6 this arrangement was not initially successful. The attempt to divide policy and management was revived again in a slightly different form in 1989 with the creation of a new Policy Board and the NHS Management Executive (NHSME).

The Policy Board, which is responsible for the overall policy and strategy of the NHS, is chaired by the Secretary of State for Health, and consists of ministers, senior civil servants from the Department of Health, the Chief Executive of the NHS, special advisers and others appointed for their knowledge of business and public-sector management.

The NHSME is chaired by the Chief Executive of the NHS and consists of senior managers, each of whom takes responsibility for a particular area of management, such as finance, personnel and so on. The NHSME is charged with implementing the policies and strategies formulated by the policy board and is responsible for day-to-day management of the NHS. In 1992, the theoretical division between policy and management in the Department of Health became a physical separation when the NHSME moved to Leeds. Figure 5.2 shows the current structure of the Department of Health, the NHSME, and their various functions.

☐ *Other departments and agencies*

Other government departments and agencies have some responsibility for health services and policies. The Secretaries of State for Scotland, Wales and Northern Ireland are responsible for health policy and services in the

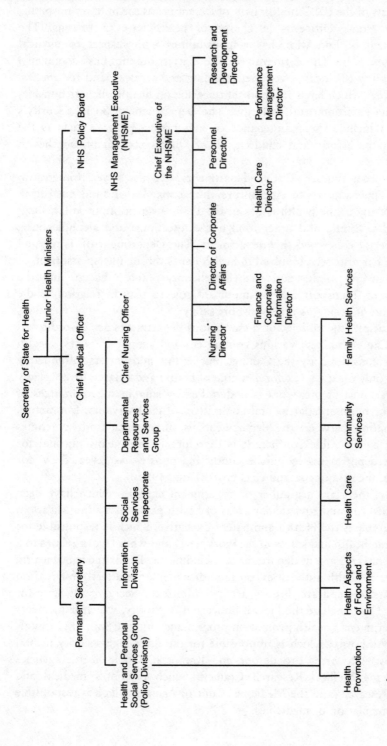

Note: *The Chief Nursing Officer is also the Director of Nursing in the NHSME.

Figure 5.2 *The Department of Health*

other parts of the UK. The Ministry of Defence runs the military hospitals, and the Home Office is in charge of health care in prisons. The Department of Education has responsibilities with respect to medical education. The Department of the Environment has a general responsibility for local government funding and services, and for specific policy areas which have an important bearing on health, such as housing, water and environmental pollution. The Department of Social Security's functions include the maintenance of low-income groups, such as the disabled, the elderly and children, all of whom have significant health needs.

There are a number of other departments who also have an interest in health. The Ministry of Agriculture is responsible for food and drink policy. Many of the health issues of the 1980s – nutrition; food labelling; salmonella, listeria and other food borne infections; and alcohol abuse; have directly concerned this department. The Department of Trade and Industry has also been involved in health issues through its sponsorship of health-damaging industries, such as chemicals and tobacco, and the Ministry of Transport has an important role to play in relation to the prevention of accidents and transport safety.

In principle, the policies of these various departments are co-ordinated by the Cabinet and its various committees and support services. Health policy is considered by the Cabinet, but as this body meets infrequently (usually only once a week for a couple of hours) and is large (over twenty members) most of this work is undertaken by smaller subcommittees of cabinet or by interdepartmental committees of civil servants. In practice, co-ordination between the departments is often weak and sometimes involves considerable conflict. It is therefore by no means unusual for different departments to pursue conflicting policies, as revealed by, for example, the salmonella and eggs crisis (Doig, 1990).

Finally, there are a number of government agencies which have been established to handle particular areas of health policy and administration. One example is the Health and Safety Executive, which is responsible for promoting health and safety in the workplace, and whose work relates to a number of government departments, including the Department of Health. The special health authorities, on the other hand, are directly focused on health matters and are directly accountable to the Secretary of State for Health. These include the Health Education Authority, which implements the government's health promotion programme; and the Special Hospitals Service Authority, which is responsible for the three high-security mental hospitals: Ashworth, Broadmoor and Rampton. Other health agencies include the Medical Research Council, which promotes medical and related research; and the Medicines Control Agency, which is responsible for the regulation of medicines.

□ *The National Health Service*

The provision of hospital and community health services in the UK is dominated by the NHS. Later chapters explore the evolution of the NHS and how it has changed over the past decade. The purpose here is to set out in a very basic way its present structure and organisation.

The main organisational components of the NHS are shown in Figure 5.3. The roles of the Policy Board and the NHSME have already been mentioned. The remainder of this section briefly explains the roles of the Regional Health Authorities, the District Health Authorities, the Family Health Services Authorities, the GP fundholders, the self-governing trusts, the directly managed units, and the Community Health Councils.

□ *Regional Health Authorities*

There are fourteen Regional Health Authorities (RHA) in England, accountable to the Secretary of State for Health. Each RHA is controlled by a board which consists of a chairman and five non-executive members, appointed by the Secretary of State. Of the non-executives, one must be a chairman of one of the Family Health Service Authorities within the region. The RHA board also includes a further five executive members, including the general manager and the finance officer.

The RHA's role is essentially strategic. First, it is responsible for planning services within its boundaries, within the guidelines set by the Department of Health. Second, it allocates resources to purchasers of health care (the District Health Authorities – DHAs – and GP fundholders – GPFs) and Family Health Service Authorities (FHSAs). Third, the RHA oversees the work of lower-tier authorities such as the FHSAs and the DHAs, monitors their performance and holds them to account. Fourth, the RHAs are responsible for managing the internal market. This involves sorting out any disputes that might arise between the purchasers of health care (DHAs, GPFs) and the providers of health care (the trusts and the directly managed units). Finally, RHAs have in the past provided services that are too large-scale to be managed at district level, such as the blood transfusion service and, in some areas, the ambulance service. However, following pressure from the Department of Health, RHAs have mostly divested themselves of such functions in order to concentrate on a strategic management role.

Furthermore, it should be noted that the very existence of the RHAs has been threatened in recent years. Those who support a more flexible internal market in health care have argued that RHAs represent an

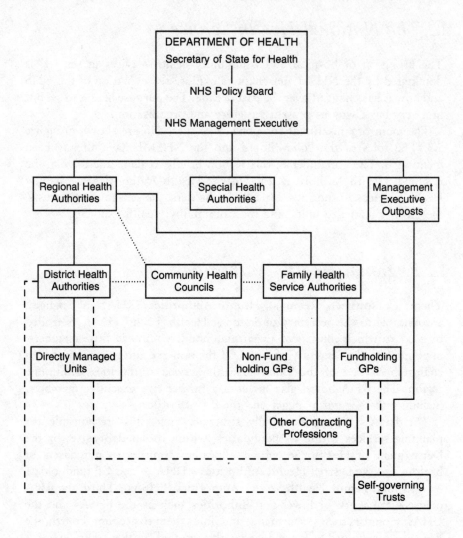

Figure 5.3   *The National Health Service*

unnecessary tier of bureaucracy and should therefore be abolished. In 1993 the Department of Health responded by proposing that the RHAs would be 'slimmed down', reduced in number, and eventually abolished.

One of the reasons why the RHAs have come under pressure is the growth of a parallel regional structure under the auspices of the NHSME. In April 1992, the NHSME established six regional outposts to deal directly with the growing number of NHS self-governing trusts (which are directly accountable to the Secretary of State for Health). The number of outposts will rise to at least eight as trust status becomes widespread. The growth of the NHSME regional structure will be at the expense of the existing RHAs.

☐ *District Health Authorities*

The DHAs are responsible for assessing the health needs of those living within their boundaries. They are also major players in the NHS internal market. They are the purchasing agencies for those health needs not covered by the GP fundholding scheme. In this capacity they agree contracts with providers for a particular level and standard of services. The precise nature of this contracting process is discussed in Chapter 8. Finally, DHAs have overall management responsibility for services that are not provided by self-governing trusts, including the remaining directly managed units (DMUs).

DHAs are accountable to the RHA, which in turn monitors their performance. They are expected also to work closely with other health agencies, such as the GP fundholders and Family Health Service Authorities in drawing up purchasing plans. These plans include a statement of priorities, statements about how improvements in services are to be secured and monitored, and the pattern and range of services to be funded.

The composition of the DHA is as follows. The chairperson is appointed by the Secretary of State for Health. The remaining members include five non-executives (appointed by the RHA) and five executive members (including the general manager and finance officer). Where a district contains a teaching hospital, one of the non-executive members must be drawn from the medical school.

In 1991 there were 190 DHAs. But since this time there have been a number of mergers, as districts have sought to combine their purchasing power in the NHS internal market. At the time of writing the number of DHAs has fallen to 140. It is believed that this figure could fall below a hundred by the end of the 1990s. In addition to the mergers of DHAs, there have in recent years been examples of closer working arrangements between DHAs and Family Health Services Authorities. In the future it is likely that these arrangements will also lead to mergers (p. 196).

□ *Family Health Services Authorities*

In England there are currently ninety Family Health Service Authorities (formerly known as Family Practitioner Committees). Each FHSA is responsible for managing the family practitioner services within their boundaries. These services include those provided by the four independent contractor professions – GPs, dentists, pharmacists and opticians. Although the contracts under which these professions operate are determined nationally, the FHSAs are responsible for implementing them at a local level. This involves paying the contractor professions, and monitoring the quality and availability of their services.

The FHSA deals with the public in a number of ways. It provides information about services and manages the process of complaints against family practitioners. It is also responsible for assessing the public's attitudes and needs with respect to these services. The FHSA also has a role in developing and improving such services. For example, practice development funds can be used to direct resources towards the priorities the FHSA has identified.

Each FHSA, which like the DHA is accountable to the Regional Health Authority, is chaired by an appointee of the Secretary of State for Health. The rest of the authority consists of five non-executive members from a lay background, and four drawn from the professions (a GP, a dentist, a pharmacist and a community nurse).

□ *GP fundholders*

By the mid-1990s, almost half the population will be covered by 'fundholding' general practitioners. Under the GP fundholding scheme, each practice receives a budget which covers the cost of running the practice, buying drugs, the use of selected non-emergency hospital services and some community health services. When first introduced, the scheme was confined to larger practices with over 9000 patients. This was later extended to those with practice lists of 7000 and over. In future it is likely that smaller practices will be eligible to become fundholders, implying that an even greater proportion of the population will be covered by the scheme.

GP fundholders (GPFs) are, in effect small purchasing authorities. They contract with self-governing trusts, directly managed units and independent hospitals, who will then provide services for the patients on the GPs' list. This scheme, and indeed operation of the internal market as a whole, will be discussed in more detail in a later chapter.

Self-governing trusts and directly managed units

In the NHS internal market there are two main types of organisation providing services. The trusts (or more correctly self-governing trusts – SGTs) and the directly managed units (DMUs). These provide hospital and community health services for the purchasers of health care, namely the GPFs and the DHAs.

DMUs, as noted earlier, are accountable to the District Health Authority. However, these providers have been given a greater degree of delegated management, partly in preparation for trust status. The majority of providers are now SGTs. It is envisaged that by the mid-1990s these units will be providing 95 per cent of NHS hospital and community health services in England.

SGTs are directly accountable to the Secretary of State for Health, through the NHSME outposts mentioned earlier. SGTs have, in principle, considerable freedom to determine their own management arrangements, although the Department of Health has stipulated that at least two of the non-executive members sitting on a trust board must be drawn from the local community. SGTs also have considerable discretion in principle over the employment terms and conditions of service of their staff, and over their own investments, borrowings and assets.

SGTs remain part of the NHS. The government has stressed that SGTs will continue to provide essential health services at a local level. It has also made it clear that their services will be still be free to NHS patients. Furthermore, the government has reserve powers to control the activities of SGTs if the need for this should arise.

Community Health Councils

Community Health Councils (CHCs) were established in England and Wales in 1974 as a means of establishing a consumer voice in the NHS. CHCs are statutory bodies funded by the Regional Health Authorities

(RHA). Normally there is one CHC for each district. Similar bodies are found in Scotland and Northern Ireland.

CHC members are nominated by voluntary organisations, local authorities and the RHA. They have no specific powers but they do have a number of specific rights to enable them to perform their function of presenting the patients' views. These include a right to information, consultation and to observe proceedings at health authority meetings.

Deprived of formal powers and financially constrained (on average CHCs have a budget of £35 000 and two full time staff), the CHCs nevertheless play a useful role in informing patients, assisting them with complaints and representing the views of the community. In recent times the CHCs have faced a number of serious problems, including in some cases exclusion from health authority meetings and consultative processes. Despite the new emphasis on consumerism, their future in the new NHS market-place looks rather uncertain.

☐ *The NHS in other parts of the UK*

There are important differences in the structure of the NHS in Scotland, Wales and Northern Ireland.

In Wales there is no regional tier of health authorities, only districts. There is, however, a common services agency, the Welsh Health Technical Services Organisation, which provides most of the services that the English RHAs provide for their districts. Wales also has eight Family Health Service Authorities.

Scotland has a Common Services Agency instead of regional authorities. The Scottish Health Boards also have responsibilities, not only for hospital and community services, but also for the family practitioner services. There is no counterpart to the Family Health Service Authorities of England and Wales.

In Northern Ireland there is also a Common Services Agency, but perhaps the most important features of health administration in Northern Ireland are the Health and Social Services Boards. These are responsible for social services as well as hospital, community and family health services.

Finally, the introduction of the internal market in health care in the other parts of the UK has led to the creation of similar structures and institutions, such as trusts and GP fundholders. However, it should be noted that the implementation of the internal market has generally proceeded at a much slower pace in Scotland and especially in Northern Ireland, compared with England and Wales.

□ *Local authorities*

Although the NHS provides the bulk of public sector health care, one should not forget the role of local authorities in the provision of health and health-related services. As Chapter 4 showed, local government has had a long history of involvement in health service provision. While over the years most of these responsibilities have been removed, local authorities have retained two important health responsibilities: personal social services and environmental health services.

Personal social services cover a range of caring, protective and support services for children, the family, the elderly, the mentally ill, and the mentally and physically handicapped. Local authorities provide residential and community-based care and support services. In some cases these services have been jointly provided in collaboration with the NHS and the independent sector.

Local authorities have a particularly important role to play in the development of community care. Indeed, central government has recently decided that local authorities should be the lead agency in this field. These authorities will in future bear the burden of responsibility for arranging community care for those who need it.

The second major area of local authority activity is the environmental health service. This incorporates a variety of services aimed at the protection of public health. Local authority environmental health services are responsible for a variety of matters which affect health, ranging from pest control and noise pollution to the inspection and registration of food premises.

In addition to these health services, local authorities are also responsible for other services which have an important health dimension. These include housing, education, cleansing, waste disposal, and the provision of sport and leisure facilities. Such services, if adequately provided, contribute to a healthy environment and a healthy society.

At the time of writing the structure of local government is being reorganised, and it is unclear where the responsibilities for these services will lie in the new structure. There are strong arguments in favour of unitary authorities, which may be better placed to co-ordinate the various functions in the interests of health. There are also similarly strong arguments for bringing health services under some form of local authority control (Hunter and Webster, 1992; Regan and Stewart, 1982). Proponents argue that this would, for example, lead to more local accountability and would improve the prospects for co-ordinating health, social and environmental services. Such a scheme does not, however, have the support of government at the present time.

□ *The independent sector*

The independent (or private) sector consists of the commercial provision of health care (the commercial sector), that provided by charitable and voluntary organisations (the voluntary sector), and the care provided by friends, neighbours and families (the informal sector). At the margins, however, a clear-cut distinction between these categories is not always easy to maintain. The main distinction between commercial providers and the rest of the independent sector is that the former expects to make a profit from its involvement, though charitable organisations often make a surplus which many see as the equivalent of profit in a commercial organisation.

The three parts of the independent sector frequently intertwine during the delivery of care, not only with each other but with services provided by the public sector. For instance, the NHS is involved in selling its services to the private sector. This takes the form of hiring out equipment to private hospitals, and treating private patients. Another feature of the interdependence between the private and public sectors, as will become clear in the next section, is the extent to which funding for commercial, voluntary and informal care is provided by national and local government and the NHS.

The independent sector provides a considerable proportion of Britain's health care. Moreover, the contribution of this sector has grown substantially over the past decade or so. In 1984, private and voluntary hospitals and nursing homes supplied only 7.5 per cent of UK hospital based treatment and care. By the end of the decade this had grown to 15 per cent (Laing, 1990).

□ *The commercial sector*

Commercial providers are involved in many aspects of health care: in particular, acute hospitals, nursing homes, and the provision of health insurance. With the advent of competitive tendering for NHS ancillary services, commercial firms have secured a considerable role in the provision of NHS cleaning, catering and laundry services.

Commercial health care is more common in some sectors than others. This is because some treatments and forms of care are more profitable than others, and some are not profitable at all. The involvement of the commercial sector traditionally has been highest in the area of routine, non-emergency surgery, and abortions. In recent years the commercial sector has also increasingly been involved in long-term care, particularly the care of the elderly, and in primary care, for example the provision of health screening facilities. Furthermore, it should be remembered that the provision of medical equipment, medicines and appliances is in the hands of commercial suppliers.

All forms of independent provision of health care have been actively encouraged by the Conservative government since it came to power in 1979 (see Chapter 7), but within the independent sector it is the commercial providers that have shown the most significant growth (Higgins, 1988). For example, 'for profit' organisations now control over half the beds in private hospitals and over three quarters of the places in private residential homes.

☐ *The voluntary and informal sectors*

The voluntary and informal sectors have also been actively encouraged by the government over the past decade or so. The term 'voluntary sector' covers a diverse range of activities (Brenton, 1985). These activities can range from the rather small-scale activities of local volunteer groups to large national charities and non-profit-making bodies.

The voluntary sector has a long history of involvement with the provision of health services. As noted in Chapter 4, many hospitals were, in fact, created and financed by philanthropists. Today, voluntary organisations supplement NHS provision in both the hospital and the community health sectors. An example is the Womens' Royal Voluntary Service (WRVS) which assists with patient services in hospital, meals on wheels, old peoples' clubs and so on. The fact that the WRVS provides 15 million meals every year gives a guide to the scale of this voluntary effort. Other examples of voluntary organisations at work in the health field include the London Lighthouse which provides advice and support for those suffering from HIV and AIDS, and the National Childbirth Trust (NCT) which provides help and advice for parents-to-be.

Although voluntary bodies, particularly at a national level, are increasingly large-scale and professional in their organisation, they nevertheless continue to depend on unpaid volunteers to raise funds and to deliver services. According to the latest figures, around 25 per cent of women and 21 per cent of men participate in various forms of voluntary work (Central Statistical Office, 1992).

Voluntary work is generally regarded as being a good thing. It is a relatively cheap (though not cost free) and flexible way of delivering services. Yet there are worries about an over-reliance on voluntary services. Some believe that voluntary organisations could be led into performing a role for which they are unsuitable, and replacing rather than complementing services currently provided directly by the NHS and local authorities.

Informal care refers to the care undertaken by friends, relatives and neighbours. This is not necessarily a bad thing. If adequate support from statutory and other services is provided, such care may well be far more humane and effective than institutional care, though it is argued, with some foundation, that the informal sector is being used as a dumping ground for long-term patients in order to save public money, and that support for carers is patchy and in some cases non-existent.

There has also been a movement in the past decade towards self-help and greater personal responsibility regarding health. This is a favourable trend. Given the growing importance of lifestyle factors in producing ill-health it is, of course, important that individuals take some responsibility for their own well-being. However, there also has to be a role for the government, both in the prevention of ill-health and in the provision of an adequate level of caring services when individuals are unable to help themselves.

■ Funding the health care system

The organisational structure of the health services, sketched out above, is, of course, an important aspect of the health care system. But equally important is the way in which the health services are funded, and how these resources are spent.

☐ *Private funding*

Services provided by the independent sector are not necessarily privately funded. Private health care may be purchased out of public funds. For example, a health authority may try to reduce its waiting lists by buying services from a private clinic. Conversely, health care can be provided by the public sector and funded by the private sector. For example, a private clinic may hire equipment from the NHS. These various combinations are explored in more detail in Chapter 7, but at this stage they serve as useful illustrations that the private provision of health services is not the same as private expenditure on health services.

Approximately 14 per cent of health care in the UK is privately funded. This is a low proportion relative to most other developed countries (see Figure 5.4). But, as with the provision of services, there are wide differences in the levels of private funding for various types of care. Private

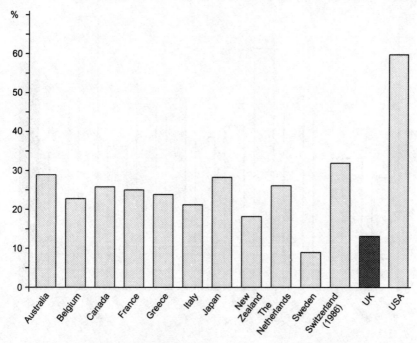

Figure 5.4 *Proportion of health care privately funded (selected OECD countries), 1987 (private expenditure as a percentage of total health care spending)*

funding is higher than the UK average for all services, in the following areas: long term care of the elderly, abortions, non-emergency surgery, medicines and opthalmics (see Table 7.1).

Private financing takes two forms. In the first, people can subscribe to an insurance scheme. The scheme then pays for health care when the subscriber requires treatment. Or they can pay directly for health care as they receive it. The second method is obviously more popular for low-cost health care items such as medicines, and for long-term care where the payments are, in effect, spread over a period of time. The first is used mainly for medical care where the cost is high and indivisible.

☐ *The public sector: income*

The majority of health care in Britain is publicly funded. But how is this money raised? Since the NHS began in 1948, the vast majority of funding has been in the form of general taxation (81 per cent in the 1992/3 financial year). This is supplemented by a contribution from the National Insurance

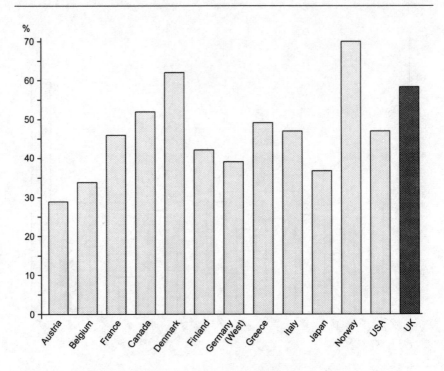

Figure 5.5 *Spending on in-patient care as a percentage of total health care spending (selected OECD countries), 1987*

Fund (14 per cent). Most of the remaining (5 per cent) is raised from patient charges for dental treatment, prescriptions and so on, and other receipts, such as the sale of land and other assets.

Local authority spending on health and social services is funded in several ways: through central government grants; the council tax; business rates; and charges for specific services. Only a small amount of income (representing only 2 per cent of the total expenditure on personal social services) is raised in fees and charges. The majority of the funds (around two-thirds of the total) takes the form of central government grants.

□ *Public expenditure*

Having explored the sources of public finance for health care, it is now possible to look briefly at the broad categories of expenditure. The majority of public expenditure on health care has in the past been allocated to the hospital sector, and within this category, in-patient care. Figure 5.5 illustrates that the UK appears to spend a large proportion of health expenditure on in-patient care. Yet, taking into account the difficulties of international comparison of such expenditures, the UK is perhaps not significantly out of step with others in terms of the balance between hospital and community care spending.

However, the picture is definitely changing and there are signs that the dominance of the hospital sector is being challenged. Figure 5.6 illustrates that if personal social services spending and social security funding are taken into account, community-based care has consumed a growing share of resources compared with the hospital sector over the past decade.

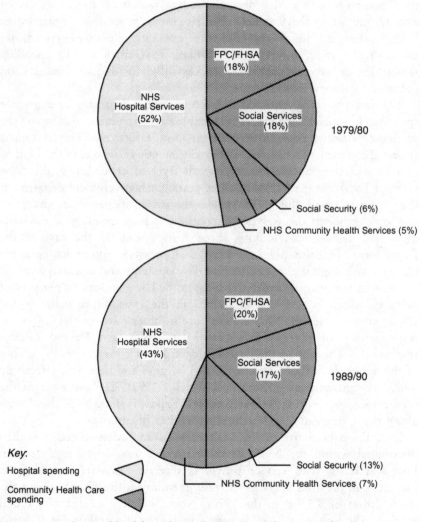

Figure 5.6 *Share of health and social care expenditure, England*

□ *The public expenditure process*

The NHS (and central government financial support for local authority personal social services) has to compete for resources at a national level with other priorities such as defence, education, housing, social security and so on. The budgets for these services are determined through the annual process known as the Public Expenditure Survey.

The machinery of the public expenditure survey has recently been altered (Cm 1867, 1992). Under the previous system, departments would bid for funds for their various programmes. They would then bargain with the Treasury over the size of their budget within an overall target of expenditure set by the Cabinet. The bargaining process was regarded as being rather irrational and did not explicitly identify expenditure priorities. In addition, it proved difficult to control overall spending when the departments lobbied successfully for higher budgets on politically sensitive issues.

The new system is expected to exert a tighter control over aggregate spending. It is also hoped that it will enable the government to compare the spending priorities of each department more effectively. This system is expected to operate as follows. The government as a whole, in the light of economic circumstances, sets an overall level of expenditure (the New Control Total) for the following three years. Each government department then negotiates with the Treasury over the size of its particular share.

The departments themselves will continue to plan spending on the basis of annual assessments, looking three years ahead. In the case of the Department of Health, plans are based on forecasts of future demographic trends, technological changes, service developments and disease patterns.

The vast majority of health spending in the UK – around 80 per cent of NHS spending, in fact – is contained in the expenditure plans of the Department of Health. NHS expenditure in other parts of the UK is the responsibility of the Welsh, Scottish and Northern Ireland Offices respectively. The size of the health budget depends largely on the ability of the ministers in these departments to bargain and negotiate effectively within the government (Thain and Wright, 1992). The outcome of the public spending process is examined in Chapter 7 along with the debate about the appropriate level of funding for health care.

Once the overall size of the health allocation is determined it is then distributed within the NHS. In the past this was done largely on an historical basis, with service providers receiving similar shares of the budget as in previous years. As already mentioned, this changed with the introduction of RAWP in the 1970s. Now, with the advent of internal markets, the bulk of the funds passes to purchasing authorities (District

Health Authorities and GP fundholders). These in turn negotiate contracts with provider units (hospitals and community health service units), to which the funds are then allocated.

☐ *The British health care system in transition*

To recap, the British system of health care is still predominantly a state-dominated one. The vast majority of non-informal care is given by public-sector organisations. The public sector of health care is, in turn, dominated by the NHS, though local authorities play an increasingly important role through their responsibilities for environmental health and community care. The vast majority of health expenditure is also public expenditure, raised mainly through general taxation.

The expansion in the private sector of health care, to be discussed in more detail in later chapters, has been considerable and may continue in the future, but this expansion has to be put in context. The private health sector is at present dwarfed by the public sector. The British system of health care therefore remains, for the time being at least, in the category of 'national health service' in Field's typology, outlined earlier in this chapter.

Nevertheless, there have been significant changes in the British system of health care over the past decade or so. These changes require a much more detailed analysis than has been provided by this outline. Each of the remaining chapters explores an area of health policy and service development, identifies the key reforms, explains their origins, and draws out the implications for the future of health care in Britain.

■ *Chapter 6* ■

The Management of Health Care

The shortcomings of the NHS have largely been attributed to the fragmentation of responsibility for various services between a number of different authorities, and a failure to establish an appropriate balance of responsibility between the various 'tiers' of the service, from central government down to local service providers. Previous governments sought to address these organisational problems mainly by structural reorganisation, accompanied by management reform and the development of new planning procedures. On taking office in 1979, the Conservative government adopted a similar approach, but these initial changes were overtaken to a considerable extent by further management reforms, which represented an attempt to change the style of decision-making in the NHS, to make it more 'business-like'.

■ The 1982 reorganisation

The Conservative government came to office with a manifesto commitment to simplify, decentralise and cut back the NHS bureaucracy. It seized immediately on a recommendation of the Royal Commission on the NHS that there should be only one tier of management below regional level carrying responsibility for the operation of services.

In December 1979 the government published its proposals for reform in a document entitled *Patients First*, which included plans to abolish the middle tier of the NHS – the Area Health Authorities (AHAs) (DHSS, 1979). New authorities were to be established at district level. A greater delegation of management responsibility to those providing hospital and community services at unit level (the basic administrative unit of the NHS, such as a single large hospital, a group of smaller hospitals, or a collection of community health services) was proposed. No major management changes were envisaged at this stage. Indeed, *Patients First* opposed a management system based on the appointment of a 'chief executive', which had been advocated as means of focusing responsibility and accountability within the NHS, and which was to become government policy only a few years later.

The reorganisation heralded by *Patients First,* which came into force in 1982, also simplified the planning and professional advisory systems established following the 1974 reorganisation (Barnard *et al.,* 1979; Hambleton, 1983). Extensive consultation over plans was to be reduced. In addition, the DHSS replaced the previous practice of giving detailed guidelines to NHS authorities with rather more general statements about the department's priorities.

These priorities were outlined by the DHSS in the policy document, *Care in Action,* published in 1981 (DHSS, 1981c). Some of the priorities were similar to those of the previous Labour government. The emphasis upon preventive medicine, community care, and services for priority groups (the elderly, children, the mentally ill and the mentally and physically handicapped) remained. On the other hand, there was a new emphasis on the importance of the commercial and voluntary health care sectors and upon the quality and efficiency of services.

Care in Action continued the theme set out in *Patients First,* that management responsibility would be delegated downwards to localities. This idea was popular with ministers, who saw it as a way of shifting at least some of the burden of responsibility for the NHS. It was also welcomed by those within the service who relished the prospect of reduced political interference. Others were more critical, seeing the new policy as an attempt on the part of central government to evade responsibility for the shortcomings of the service (Chaplin, 1982).

☐ Planning and review

The attempt to decentralise responsibility within the NHS was in fact relatively short-lived. There was increasing pressure from Parliament to abandon the 'arm's length' approach adopted by the government and to improve the central monitoring of the NHS. A new planning process, foreshadowed in *Patients First* and introduced in 1982, addressed some of these concerns (DHSS, 1982). Strategic plans, looking ten years ahead, would now set out the existing state of services, perceived needs and future priorities. These plans were drawn up by both the Regional Health Authorities (RHAs) and District Health Authorities (DHAs) every five years. Second, within this framework annual programmes produced by the DHAs (and by RHAs for services which at this time were managed directly at this level) would set out the implementation of policies and service developments over the following two years. Third, annual performance review meetings, held between the districts and the regions, and also in turn between the regions and the DHSS, were established. These meetings enabled the higher authorities to monitor the performance of the lower tiers, and in particular their progress in moving towards certain objectives or targets set previously.

The Griffiths Inquiry: towards a new model of management

A further move away from the decentralist approach occurred with the appointment of the Griffiths management inquiry in 1983. This reflected a change of leadership at the DHSS. Norman Fowler, who had succeeded Patrick Jenkin as Secretary of State in the autumn of 1981, had become convinced that the real problem of the NHS was one of management (Fowler, 1991). Fowler asked four businessmen under the chairmanship of Sir Roy Griffiths (Deputy Chairman and Managing Director of Sainsbury's, the supermarket chain) to look at the management arrangements in the NHS in England. The inquiry's remit did not cover Scotland, Wales or Northern Ireland. Nevertheless, the main recommendations of the inquiry were gradually applied to these parts of the UK as well.

The use of business advisers to inquire into the workings of the NHS was not unprecedented. Business advice was previously sought during the reorganisation process of the early 1970s when Sir Keith Joseph commissioned a report from McKinsey and Company, the management consultants. However, in the new climate of the 1980s the business viewpoint was to dominate rather than simply to be one of several perspectives taken into account by policy-makers. In appointing businessmen, the government already knew what it wanted to hear from the inquiry team (Black, 1987, p. 82). The politicians at the top, who were being held responsible for the NHS, sought a management structure which facilitated greater control, particularly over the costs of the service.

☐ The Griffiths report

The Griffiths report (DHSS, 1983) focused on the absence of a clear line of management responsibility in the NHS, summed up in the cutting observation that 'if Florence Nightingale were carrying her lamp through the corridors of the NHS today, she would almost certainly be searching for the people in charge'. Much of the blame was laid at the door of consensus management, the existing method of decision-making which had been introduced following the 1974 reorganisation.

Consensus management operated at each level of the NHS. Management teams, responsible for day-to-day management of health authority business, were drawn from a variety of professional and management backgrounds including administration, finance, nursing and medicine. In principle, no member of the management team had superior status and each had the power to veto decisions. Ultimately, decisions emerged through bargaining, negotiation and agreement between the various managers and professions involved.

This style of decision-making had its advantages. By involving managers from different backgrounds it enabled the management team to consider a wide range of perspectives before arriving at a decision. Also as the importance of securing agreement was emphasised, it was widely believed that the decisions made stood a greater chance of being accepted and implemented by all the staff.

On the negative side, consensus management was also held to be responsible for delays in decision-making, the avoidance of tough decisions, and the blurring of responsibility. This was certainly the view of the Griffiths inquiry. It was not alone in this regard: the Royal Commission on the NHS had also found problems with consensus management. Griffiths went further and actually recommended a new management system to replace it.

The Griffiths inquiry also found a blurring of responsibilities between the DHSS and the NHS. As a remedy it sought to prune the existing activities of the DHSS. The DHSS had continued to intervene directly in the detailed affairs of health authorities, contrary to the declared policy of decentralisation and delegation. Moreover, this intervention was undertaken in a haphazard and inconsistent way. These findings echoed an earlier inquiry into the workings of the DHSS by three regional chairmen (DHSS, 1976b).

Finally, the inquiry team was highly critical of the way in which the service failed both to address the needs of the consumer and to achieve explicit national policy objectives. Griffiths saw an absence of clear objectives for the NHS, and a failure to monitor the performance of the service. The inquiry did, however, recognise that the recent adoption of regional and district annual performance reviews, mentioned earlier, could improve this situation.

☐ The Griffiths inquiry recommendations

The Griffiths inquiry made a number of specific recommendations. First, at the national level, the creation of two new boards within the DHSS itself. The Health Services Supervisory Board (HSSB), chaired by the

Secretary of State, would be responsible for determining the strategy and direction of the NHS, reviewing the general performance of the NHS and approving the overall level of resource allocation to the service. Beneath the HSSB and responsible to it would be the NHS Management Board. This board would take over existing DHSS responsibilities for the management of the NHS. It would be chaired by a general manager from outside the NHS and the civil service, and would include the managers of other functions such as personnel, finance, procurement, property and service planning.

This first set of recommendations was intended to achieve two things: to separate and distinguish policy (and by implication politics) from management; and to rationalise and make explicit the links between the central department and the NHS. This experiment was a failure, at least initially, for reasons discussed later.

Second, Griffiths recommended the replacement of the system of consensus management with one of general management, defined as 'the responsibility drawn together in one person, at different levels of the organisation, for planning, implementation and control of performance'. It was intended that general managers would be appointed to take overall responsibility for service performance and management at each level in the NHS: region, district and unit. At regional and district level the managers would be responsible to their respective health authorities for the achievement of policy objectives. General management was also to be established at unit level, where it was envisaged that a greater number of decisions would be taken in the future.

The rationale for introducing general management was rooted in the belief that it would clarify responsibility for carrying out policies. In particular, it was seen as being crucial to the attainment of greater cost-efficiency and better use of resources. Griffiths argued that general management would also provide better leadership, producing an improvement in the motivation of staff working in the NHS.

The idea of general management was not entirely new to the NHS reform agenda. Proposals aimed at focusing day-to-day management responsibility on one individual had surfaced on a number of occasions in the past. The Farquharson–Lang report of 1966, which considered the administrative practice of the Scottish Hospital Boards, recommended the appointment of a chief executive at each board level (Scottish Health Services Council, 1966). The chief executive would take prime responsibility for day-to-day management and would be expected to take a leading role in the organisation of the board's work. A similar proposal was floated in the Labour government's consultative paper on NHS reorganisation in 1968. It will also be recalled that the idea of a chief executive was rejected in the Conservative reorganisation plans of 1979.

The third set of recommendations put forward by the Griffiths inquiry concerned accountability. It was argued that accountability would be further strengthened by including the units within the annual review process, as discussed earlier. Districts would therefore become directly involved in monitoring the performance of the units at the level of service delivery. This, in theory, would create a line of accountable management from the unit through the regions and districts up to the new Management Board.

Fourth, Griffiths focused on the health authority chairpersons at regional and district level. The chairpersons were to have a special role in relation to the introduction and operation of general management. At each level they would be expected to take a leading role in the identification of the general manager, the review of the general manager's performance, the organisation of health authority business, and the introduction of efficiency initiatives.

The report also made a number of specific recommendations concerning efficiency and the management of resources. The introduction of cost improvement programmes (CIPs), to achieve savings in budgets, for example. A further recommendation was the development of management budgeting at unit level, relating clinical workload directly to financial budgets and manpower allocations. More generally, Griffiths urged that doctors should become more closely involved in processes of management and budgeting.

Finally, the report concentrated on improvements in the quality of service by recommending that managers take steps to evaluate performance, particularly from the patients' perspective. It also urged that this be incorporated in the planning and management of services, along with improved information about the effectiveness and efficiency of services.

☐ *Implementing Griffiths*

The government accepted the recommendations of the Griffiths report and set in motion a fairly tight timetable for the introduction of the changes. This haste was criticised in many quarters, notably by the medical and nursing professions. Despite this, the government continued to press ahead, and within two years the new management arrangements were largely in place.

By 1986, most of the new general managers had been appointed at each level. Although the individual health authorities, and in particular their chairpersons, were responsible for these appointments, their decisions were subject to DHSS approval. A number of internal candidates were, in fact, vetoed by the department. In the South Western Regional Health Authority, for example, two DHAs had their chosen candidate for the general manager's post rejected. In another case, the West Midlands Regional Health Authority had to battle strongly to win DHSS approval for their chosen candidate.

Health ministers were keen that a substantial proportion of candidates should be appointed from outside the NHS, and in particular from the world of business. But the attractions of NHS management were limited. Salaries were lower than those in the business sector. Fringe benefits and perks were virtually non-existent. Moreover, the general managers were appointed on three-year contracts (in some cases, five years) and therefore had limited security of tenure. Despite the interference of the DHSS, as Figure 6.1 clearly shows, the majority of general managers came from the ranks of former NHS administrators.

☐ The impact of Griffiths

In the remainder of this chapter, the impact of Griffiths, and of other management reforms that have followed in its wake, are examined in relation to three key relationships within the NHS. The internal operation of health authorities; the relationship between managers and professionals; and relationships between the DHSS (and subsequently the Department of Health) and local health authorities.

▌ Management in Health Authorities: members, officers and chairpersons

The Griffiths report appeared to suggest a greater role for health authority chairpersons and managers relative to the ordinary member. However, Roy Griffiths himself emphasised that the recommendations were not intended to undermine health authority members. Ministers also stressed that there was no threat to the role of members.

Despite these assurances it was widely felt that the decline in the influence of the health authority member would be hastened by the implementation of the Griffiths report. The Select Committee on Social Services (House of Commons, 1984) commented that the report was being interpreted by some as a blueprint for the reduction of the member's role, mainly in view of the proposed concentration of authority in the hands of the chairperson and the general manager.

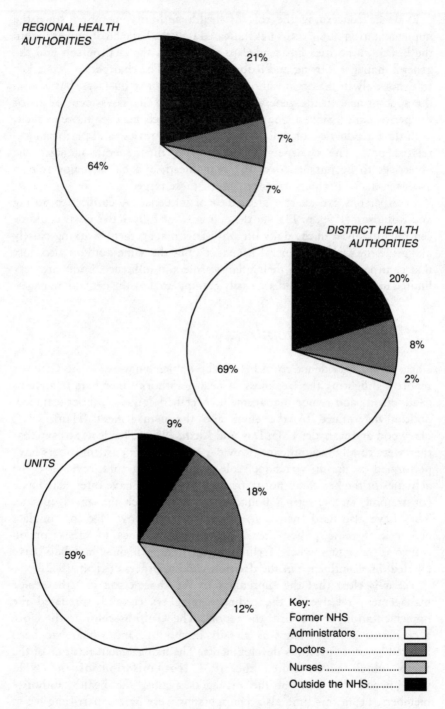

REGIONAL HEALTH AUTHORITIES

21%

7%

7%

64%

DISTRICT HEALTH AUTHORITIES

20%

8%

2%

69%

UNITS

9%

18%

12%

59%

Key:
Former NHS
Administrators ....
Doctors ....
Nurses ....
Outside the NHS............

Figure 6.1 *Backgrounds of the new general managers, 1986 (England)*

Evidence concerning the role of health authority members since the implementation of Griffiths has indicated that the balance of power within the health authorities has tended to reside with the chairperson and the general manager (Strong and Robinson, 1990). The chairperson has a key role, not only in the organisation of health authority business, but also in the appointment of the general manager, and in the assessment of his or her performance. Since 1986 this latter role has become even more explicit, with the introduction of individual performance review and performance-related pay. The chairperson agrees with the general manager the objectives to be pursued over the year ahead, and has a major role in assessing his or her performance against these targets.

Chairpersons can exert a great deal of influence. According to Strong and Robinson (1990, p. 135) 'at the extreme, the fully active chair could be centrally involved in the daily life of district management working closely alongside the District General Manager'. But the same authors also note that chairpersons vary in their quality, role and influence. Some are very limited in their abilities and are easily manipulated by the general manager.

☐ *The role of members*

There is much evidence from before the implementation of the Griffiths report highlighting the weakness of health authority members relative to chairpersons and senior management. Members largely 'rubber-stamped' policies determined by the chair and the management (Ham, 1986; Haywood and Ranade, 1985; Day and Klein, 1987). This is not to say that they were totally insignificant (Ranade, 1985). In the past, members have performed a useful watchdog role – monitoring and reviewing the activities of the health authority management. They have often acted as a constraining factor, setting boundaries within which managers operate. They have also used their own experience and knowledge to stimulate action in specific policy areas. Moreover, in times of crisis, or on controversial issues where feelings were running high – members have exerted direct influence in the decision-making process (Klein, 1982).

Yet it is clear that the supremacy of the chairperson and the senior management relative to the ordinary members certainly predated the implementation of the Griffiths report. The Griffiths reforms therefore accentuated a trend that was already in motion, and which had been assisted by other previous developments. The management reforms of the 1970s which accompanied the 1974 reorganisation of the NHS strengthened the hand of the managers against the health authority members. From this time also, chairpersons were paid a part-time fee in recognition of their workload. Even before this, during the late 1960s, there had been an attempt to reduce the role of the part-time members in day-to-day management in a number of health authorities throughout Britain following the recommendations of the Farquharson–Lang report on Scottish hospital administration (Ham, 1981).

In the early 1980s, the roles of the chairperson and senior management were further strengthened by the introduction of annual reviews of regions and districts, discussed earlier. It appears that by focusing responsibility on these individuals, the reviews ensured that the ordinary health authority member became increasingly marginalised.

The rising profile of health authority chairpersons was reflected in increasing allegations of political bias in these appointments. Haywood and Ranade (1985, p. 47) report that only four out of the ten chairmen in their study were overt supporters of the present government, while two were overt supporters of opposition parties. In 1985 the Labour party undertook a survey of health authority chairpersons and came to the conclusion that 60 per cent were Conservative supporters. Not surprisingly in view of its partisan source, the objectivity of this survey was challenged (Phillips, 1985).

There is, in fact, very little hard evidence as to the extent to which health authorities have become politically biased during the past decade. It is true that a number of chairpersons were not reappointed by ministers during the mid-1980s after criticising government policy. Certainly, ministers have been more active in vetting chairpersons, and for that matter members and senior managers. But, oddly, some of those who were removed from their posts were Conservatives. It seems fairly clear that the main reason for refusing to appoint and reappoint certain individuals was not simply their party political loyalties, but whether or not they had publicly expressed criticism of government policy. Through its power of appointment and reappointment the government made it clear that such criticism would not be tolerated.

☐ *The new health authorities*

Concern about political bias in health authorities has moved up a gear in the light of changes in the composition of health authorities. Until 1990, health authorities were drawn from a range of backgrounds. Some members were nominated by local councils, providing at least a tenuous link with the local community. Some were drawn from the ranks of NHS staff. Since then health authorities have been reconstituted. There is no longer a general obligation for health authorities to include people from the health professions or representatives of local communities. There are a few exceptions, as noted in Chapter 5. Family Health Service Authorities must include a specific number of health care professionals. Districts with a teaching hospital have to include a medical school member, while self-governing trusts (SGTs) must include at least two members drawn from the local community, and a medical school member if the trust is a teaching hospital.

The new health authorities are composed of a smaller number of people than before. The executive members are appointed to the health authority in recognition of their management responsibilities. They include the general manager and the finance manager. This is a new departure. Previously, senior management were not included on the health authority itself. The remainder of the new authorities consist of the chairperson and part-time non-executive members appointed not as representatives but for their knowledge and expertise.

Recent research has explored the backgrounds of the members of these new authorities (Pettigrew *et al.*, 1991). The main findings are as follows. First there is a surprising degree of continuity between the membership of the old and the new health authorities. At regional level, around three quarters of the non-executive members and chairpersons are continuing previous service. However, there are some important differences. The new authorities do seem to have a lower proportion of women than did their predecessors (slighly under 27 per cent of the new health authority membership). Ethnic minorities are also similarly under-represented, with less than 2 per cent of members being non-white.

The new authorities also seem to have more members with a business or self-employed background than their predecessors (see Figure 6.2) The majority of non-executives and chairpersons are either employed by the private sector or are self-employed. Nevertheless, health authorities have retained some members with experience of the public sector and voluntary organisations. Despite the removal of the obligation to include local councillors, 15 per cent of the non-executive members of the new health authorities had served in this capacity. A final point to note is that, regardless of Department of Health advice, one in eight chairpersons and non-executive members did not live or work in the health authority area which they served.

The same research programme also looked at the composition of the new self-governing trusts (SGTs). Compared with the new health authorities, a higher proportion of the non-executive directors on 'first wave' SGTs established in 1991 are new to the NHS (Ashburner and Cairncross, 1992). Only a third of these directors have had previous experience of the NHS. Figure 6.2 shows that SGTs also have a higher proportion of non-executive directors drawn from the business sector. Ethnic minorities and women are under-represented on SGT boards to a similar extent as in the health authorities.

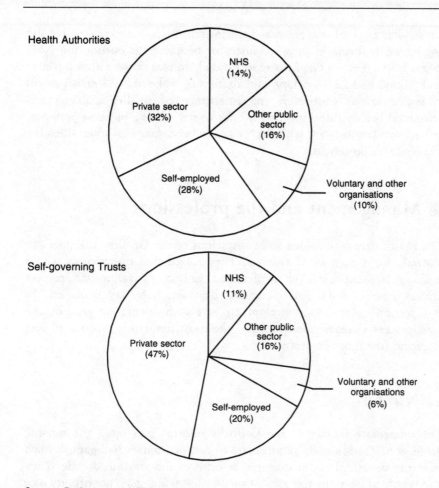

Health Authorities

NHS (14%)

Private sector (32%)

Other public sector (16%)

Self-employed (28%)

Voluntary and other organisations (10%)

Self-governing Trusts

NHS (11%)

Private sector (47%)

Other public sector (16%)

Voluntary and other organisations (6%)

Self-employed (20%)

Source: Pettigrew *et al.* (1991) pp. 11, 18.

Figure 6.2 *Backgrounds of health authority and trust members, chairpersons and non-executives (England)*

Further evidence supplied by the Labour Party adds to this picture. A survey of 67 of the 128 trusts which were to become operational in 1993 showed that 56 per cent of the chairpersons had a business background, and only half had previous experience of the NHS. Of those chairpersons which had disclosed their political background, two thirds were Conservative. This survey reports an even greater business presence among trust non-executives, with five out of six being drawn from the private sector (Labour Party, 1992a).

It should be noted that the Griffiths report did not explicitly recommend an influx of businessmen on to health authorities. Indeed, Sir Roy Griffiths himself has claimed that the management reforms his inquiry inspired did not intend to bring in large numbers of people from outside the NHS (May, 1991). Yet the Griffiths report did claim that those with a business background had an important contribution to make to NHS management at senior levels. Moroever, the emergence of smaller management-orientated health authorities, with their overwhelming business presence, seems entirely consistent with the 'businesslike' managerial style which the inquiry team promoted.

■ Management and the professions

The health care professions were suspicious of the Griffiths management reforms, for a number of reasons. They feared that the reforms would lead to the exclusion of professional advice, a failure to respect professional interests, and increasing domination by lay managers. In this section there is an attempt to assess the actual impact of the management changes upon nursing (the most numerous profession) and medicine (the most powerful).

□ *Nurses*

The immediate impact of the Griffiths reforms was upon the nursing profession. Traditionally subordinate to doctors, nurses had gained much from the structural and managerial reforms of the previous decade. They had benefited from the reorganisation of 1974, winning an important voice on the new management teams. The retention of consensus management in the 1982 reorganisation consolidated their position. The Griffiths recommendations seemed likely to have the opposite effect, threatening to diminish the role of nurses at senior levels in the management structure, and were thus seen as a direct assault on their hard-won victories in the previous decade.

The nurses' fears were to some extent justified. Few nurses were, in fact, appointed as general managers (see Figure 6.1). Moreover, under the new regime, general managers had considerable freedom to determine their own management structures. These structures often changed in ways unfavourable to nursing interests, especially at district level. The newly-created management boards contained new posts such as director of personnel, director of research, or director of information. In some districts the inclusion of such posts was at the expense of the district nursing officer, who had previously been a member of the consensus management team. Many former nursing officers were retained in the less influential role of nursing adviser. Others combined this advisory function with an additional role (such as director of quality assurance, director of personnel, or director of nursing education) and thereby retained their seat on the management board.

In the light of these changes, the nursing advisers that remained often suffered from low morale. Their role now lacked line management responsibilities, yet those who combined this post with an additional role faced workload problems. Interestingly, only three out of fourteen district nursing officers in the North West Thames health authority, who were in post before the implementation of the Griffiths report had been retained by the end of 1988 (Owens and Glennerster, 1990).

In some health authorities, changes in the management structure were successfully resisted by nurses at a local level. The nursing unions, worried that the Griffiths reforms would remove the voice of the nurse at regional, district and even unit level, had campaigned strongly against their introduction. Although this strategy failed, the DHSS was persuaded to take some action to reassure the profession. Proposed management structures in a number of districts where nursing advisers had been excluded were vetoed accordingly. Although the nursing profession was not actually guaranteed a seat on the top management boards, every district now had to have a nurse adviser. The Royal College of Nursing (RCN), supported strongly by the House of Commons Select Committee on Social Services, successfully reversed a decision to exclude the DHSS Chief Nursing Officer (CNO) from the Health Services Supervisory Board (HSSB). However, the CNO was subsequently excluded from the HSSB's replacement, the NHS Policy Board, when this was created in 1989.

The longer-term impact of Griffiths upon the nursing profession is difficult to ascertain. There are some signs that nurses may be reasserting their influence. According to Harrison (1988b), the loss of status suffered by senior nurses is temporary. He argues that such nurses will regain status in view of their new roles, particularly through quality assurance. Owens and Glennerster (1990) point out that nurses are now well-established at middle management level and so are well placed to be general managers in the future.

At grassroots level, the picture is even less clear. Nurses certainly have the potential to exert influence in the future. The devolvement of managerial responsibilities to unit or ward level post-Griffiths has often been seen in a positive light by nurses themselves, although it has also been noted that extra responsibilities have added to increased workload and stress among nurses (Owens and Glennerster, 1990, pp. 131–40). It is also debatable whether or not increased responsibility for nurses at this level equates with increased authority and managerial discretion.

☐ *The medical profession*

The medical profession reacted cautiously to the Griffiths report. Many doctors initially appeared to accept the need for clearer management responsibilities, but argued that reform should be piloted. Once it became known that most of the general managers were, in fact, likely to be former administrators (rather than doctors), medical opinion hardened. The removal of doctors from the new management structures at regional and district level confirmed the worst suspicions of the profession.

Doctors were able to reduce the impact of the Griffiths reforms in a number of ways. Like the RCN, the British Medical Association (BMA) lobbied ministers, who responded by insisting that all new management boards should include a medical officer. Yet the main weapon of the medical profession was not its lobbying power, but its ability to frustrate management initiatives at a local level.

As we saw in Chapter 2, the medical profession has a formidable power base. Most general managers, knowing they could not ride roughshod over senior doctors, adopted a consensual approach. Others simply avoided confrontation. A few did take on the local medical establishment, at their peril. These were mainly drawn from outside the NHS and had no previous experience of medical politics. For example, a former army colonel resigned as general manager of Nottingham DHA after less than two years, after facing difficulties with the profession. Other 'military' casualties occured in Central Birmingham and in Gwent.

Haywood (1987) agrees that some managers were forced out by pressure from senior doctors. He observes that the general manager's authority was not extended to the clinical domain. As a result, the authority of the general manager was less than the formal job description suggested. Indeed, it is clear that general managers made only limited progress in setting clinical targets and that the power of the medical profession in determining priorities at a local level remained formidable (National Audit Office, 1989b). Managers were largely unable to exert control over the resources for which they were held accountable because the demand for patient services was determined by clinicians.

Harrison *et al.* (1992) point out that the manager–doctor relationship remains to be renegotiated. Doctors and managers are not, however, always in conflict, and in places they work together well. But where conflict between doctors and managers has taken place, the former have usually been victorious.

It seems evident that in most health authorities, despite the demise of the formal structures of consensus management, management by consensus was not an immediate casualty of the Griffiths reforms. Most general managers realised that change could only be brought about with the consent of the professions, particularly the doctors (Davison, 1988).

Local medical power was not immediately challenged by general management. However, the reforms did lay the foundation for further attempts to bring doctors more closely into management, which perhaps had more scope for altering the balance of power between medicine and management. These reforms included the resource management initiative (RMI), medical audit, and quality management initiatives.

☐ *Resource management initiative (RMI)*

The RMI was launched in 1986, on an experimental basis. It was introduced in an atmosphere of consensus, following agreement between the DHSS and the medical profession. Four main aims of RMI have been identified (Packwood *et al.*, 1991). These are: first, to control resources, which are largely allocated as a result of clinical decisions; second, to involve clinicians in the management and budgeting process; third, to provide a way of assessing the quality of services; fourth, to provide adequate information for better decision-making.

The RMI was therefore an amalgam of ideas, none of which were particularly new (Perrin, 1988). There had been a number of experiments since the early 1970s to provide clinicians with greater information about the resource implications of their decisions. Such initiatives were clearly a step in the right direction in the view of the Griffiths report, which saw 'management budgets' relating workload to resources as a vital management tool.

There are significant differences between 'management budgets' and the resource management initiative that was actually implemented. Management budgeting was essentially a 'top-down' exercise. The main aim of this programme was to provide clinicians with some idea of their share of total costs, and to attempt to get them to accept some responsibility for their budgets. Resource management is generally depicted as a 'bottom-up' exercise, where information is generated which relates resources to activity. This information is then used by clinicians and managers to identify cost-effectiveness and to inform future resource allocation.

Resource management consists of two main components. First, the development of an information base on the cost-effectiveness of services. Second, a management structure which explicitly incorporates clinicians into the decision-making process and gives them responsibility for budgets. Neither aspect has been easy to achieve in practice. In the six pilot sites chosen for RMI, not one had a fully operating resource management system up and running within three years of the initiative's launch (Packwood *et al.*, 1991).

The development of information systems is particularly problematic. An effective system requires accurate data collection procedures; means of analysing the data; and ways of bringing the data into the decision-making process. There are large obstacles to be encountered in each of these areas, not least being the shortage of adequately trained information technology (IT) staff (Brittain, 1992).

There have also been difficulties in establishing effective management structures. A large number of hospitals – including those not participating in the original pilot RMI schemes – have now developed clinical directorates in an attempt to incorporate clinicians within the management structure. Though there is a great deal of variation in the management structures adopted by units, a clinical directorate in its pure form can be said to have a number of typical features, outlined in Exhibit 6.1.

Exhibit 6.1   *Clinical directorates*

1. Clinical work is divided into 'speciality departments' and 'diagnostic/support' departments and each is led by a clinical director appointed from among the clinicians in each department.
2. The clinical director is responsible for budget, staff and clinical activity within the department. He or she usually continues to practise, undertaking the management function on a part-time basis.
3. The clinical director is usually supported by a full-time associate manager who undertakes the day-to-day management function.
4. Each clinical department also has a senior nurse responsible for the management of the nursing staff. There may also be a paramedical staff manager.
5. The clinical directors participate in the setting of priorities and targets, and the allocation of resources.

It has proved easier in practice to create these structures than to make them work as part of a system of resource management. The main difficulty faced has been in making clinical directors fully responsible and accountable for the activities of their colleagues. Doctors are particularly suspicious of anything resembling line management, and may ultimately refuse to co-operate with the plans agreed by the clinical director at unit level.

Confidence in the benefits of RMI were shaken further following the final report of an evaluation study by researchers at Brunel University

(Packwood *et al.*, 1991). The study confirmed that the process of introducing resource management into the six pilot sites had been subject to delays. No conclusive evidence of benefits in terms of patient care were found by the researchers. But the cost of implementing the resource management system was twice as high as originally expected.

Given these difficulties, it is not surprising that RMI made slow progress. The tempo – and the temperature – was increased by the government's White Paper, *Working for Patients*, published in 1989, before the evaluation of the RMI 'experiment' was complete. Not only was resource management to be extended – to 260 acute units by 1992 – but its purpose also seemed to have become clearer. Resource management was no longer simply seen as a way of improving the management of resources, or creating cost-awareness among clinicians. Instead, it had become a cornerstone of the internal market, providing information on the costs of clinical activity. What had begun as a fairly innocuous experiment, introduced with the consent of the profession, now appeared quite threatening in the eyes of many clinicians. Talk of doctors 'seeing off' the threat to their autonomy posed by general management was perhaps premature.

☐ *Contracts and markets*

In addition to the widespread introduction of RMI there are one or two other developments which may perhaps give managers more leverage over doctors in the future. The first of these concerns a range of proposals in *Working for Patients* regarding consultants' contracts. Following the implementation of these proposals, consultants' contracts are now more tightly drawn than before. Consultants have to agree specific job descriptions with managers. Managers are also likely to have a greater role in relation to the appointment of consultants, and in the recommendation of merit awards for existing consultants.

In addition, the government stated its intention to manage consultants at a local level (that is, at district or trust level rather than at regional level). The new self-governing trusts (SGTs) will be able to take this further in view of their discretion to set pay and conditions for all staff, including medical staff. The operation of a competitive internal market may also give hospital managers considerable influence over the medical profession. Ultimately they may be able to use 'market forces' as a means of persuading doctors to alter their practices and to participate to a greater extent in management processes.

The other main branch of the medical profession – the GPs – have also been subject to contractual changes. The new GP contract defines the doctors' responsibilities more closely and ties remuneration more closely to specific performance targets. At the same time, the Family Health Service Authorities have adopted a similarly managerialist role in relation to the contractor professions. These issues are discussed in further detail in Chapter 9.

☐ *Medical audit and quality management*

A further development in recent years has been the introduction of medical audit. The assessment of medical procedures and practices has been accepted by the profession on condition that the process of audit remains under its control.

The first report of the National Confidential Enquiry into Perioperative Deaths (NCEPOD) (Buck *et al.*, 1987) (the main results of which were discussed in Chapter 3) was not the first attempt at medical audit, but it was certainly by far the most significant attempt to date. It was, moreover, a voluntary exercise, promoted mainly by the medical profession itself. In *Working for Patients*, however, the government sought to institutionalise medical audit procedures by establishing advisory committees at district and regional level. Similar committees were established by the Family Health Service Authorities. Although managers were given a role in the establishment of these committees and have some influence over their general direction, the Department of Health agreed that the process of medical audit should be managed by the doctors themselves.

Medical audit has not really challenged the autonomy of the medical profession to date. Pollitt (1992) argues that medical audit has been set up in such a way that management and patients are excluded, so that in the short term at least, it has not offended medical interests. Indeed, medical audit may well be used to further these interests. Notably, a second report of the National Confidential Enquiry into Perioperative Deaths in 1992 attributed a significant proportion of deaths to factors outside doctors' control (Camplin *et al.*, 1992). For example, it was pointed out that around a quarter of deaths in orthopaedic and trauma surgery occurred at weekends and on public holidays. Personnel and resource shortages were associated with 5 per cent and 4 per cent of deaths respectively. By drawing attention to the inadequacy of facilities, medical audit may deflect the burden of responsibility back on to managers, and may even be used to make a case for more resources.

So far, medical audit has not been a managerial stick with which to beat the doctors. However, once again, the internal market may have an impact upon this relationship. As the purchasers of care begin to specify a certain quality of service they expect from providers, medical audit will probably be used by managers to improve to some extent the quality of medical practice. In such circumstances medical audit ceases to be simply a measure of the effectiveness of care and becomes part of the 'discipline' of the market.

Increasingly, doctors and other health care professionals are being forced to acknowledge the issue of quality. There has been a greater emphasis on quality assurance and the management of quality in recent years, across all levels of clinical competence and health service provision. One concept which is receiving considerable attention at the moment is 'total quality management' (TQM). Essentially, this concept is rooted in four principles: that organisational success depends on meeting customer needs; that quality (defined by the customer) is achieved by the production process; that most employees are motivated to work hard and perform well; and that simple statistical methods can assist the discovery of faults in the production process and thereby lead to continuous improvements in quality (Berwick *et al.*, 1992).

Despite the interest in this approach, which originated in the management and production processes of successful Japanese companies, it has nevertheless been criticised on several grounds (Freemantle, 1992). Two main dangers have been identified. First, it is argued that health care is a complex personal service not suitable for 'production line' quality evaluation techniques developed for manufacturing industries. Second, it is likely that the measurement of quality under TQM may respond to superficial consumer reaction rather than the real need to improve efficiency of service provision.

It seems likely that the application of quality assurance techniques, underpinned by the pressure of market forces, will strengthen the hands of managers. The weaker professions are increasingly succumbing to this process. It is also a further tool which could be used to assess the work of the medical profession, and reduce its autonomy in the future.

■ Central–local relations

The Griffiths reforms and the other management initiatives mentioned so far in this chapter are often depicted as centralist: increasing the power of the centre relative to the locality (Paton, 1992). According to this view, the Griffiths reforms have created a system of line management, a 'mechanistic management hierarchy' (House of Commons, 1984), or a 'professionalised management hierarchy' (Loveridge and Starkey, 1992). Some argue that this has enabled the politicians and civil servants in the Department of Health to direct the service from the top down (Best *et al.*, 1988; Thwaites, 1988).

□ *Politics and management*

One of the themes central to the Griffiths report was devolution of management responsibility. In theory, ministers and their senior advisers would set policy objectives, while the NHS managers would be responsible for implementing policies in the most efficient and effective manner. According to Griffiths 'the requirement for central isolated initiatives should disappear once a coherent management process is established' (DHSS, 1983, p. 16).

The division between policy and management was, as we have seen, institutionalised in the form of separate management and supervisory boards. The Department of Health's role was to be drastically pruned. According to the Select Committee on Social Services, for example, the Griffiths report had 'quietly proposed the decimation of what used to be the Ministry of Health' (House of Commons, 1984). This did not happen. As Klein (1990b) has pointed out, the Department's officials fought a successful rearguard action against moves to limit their power, while ministers, in view of the political sensitivity of health issues, were not content to leave health authorities to manage their own affairs (Stowe, 1989).

The tensions created within the Department of Health by the attempt to divide policy and management were clearly illustrated by the resignation of the first chairman of the NHS management board. The Griffiths inquiry had urged that the new chairman be an outsider with experience of general management. The government appointed Victor Paige, an industrialist, to the £70 000 a year post. Paige resigned from the job in 1986 after only sixteen months following alleged disagreements with ministers. He later claimed in a statement to MPs that 'Ministers took all the important decisions: political, strategic and managerial' (House of Commons, 1988c, p. 94).

Paige's resignation led to the return of explicit ministerial control over management. His replacement, the management board's director of personnel, was confirmed as NHS chief executive, but only as acting chairman of the management board. He was succeeded in this latter capacity by the Minister of State for Health, and subsequently by the Secretary of State himself. This move was a fundamental contradiction of the Griffiths principle of separating policy from management. An attempt to re-establish this principle occurred in 1989, when the Management Board was replaced by the NHS Management Executive (NHSME). Ministers are not members of the NHSME, which is now also physically separated, at its new headquarters in Leeds, from the politicians.

☐ *Planning, monitoring and review*

Throughout the 1980s the DHSS attempted to control health authorities more closely. In 1983, for example, manpower targets were introduced for each region. These targets represented a greater constraint than the previous system whereby the overall number of doctors and dentists was centrally controlled, leaving health authorities relatively free to determine the number and mix of staff.

The introduction of the annual review process during the early part of the decade, also promoted central intervention. According to Day and Klein (1985) the minutes of the annual reviews between ministers and regional chairman confirmed 'the picture of growing DHSS participation with service delivery at the periphery'. From 1986 the Management Board (and later the NHSME) began to conduct its own annual review, focusing particularly on managerial performance.

However, the review process may have been less effective than was commonly thought. Former health minister Ray Whitney (1988) has claimed that the reviews were not very effective, and were largely an exercise in 'cajolery rather than management'. Moreover, in some important specific areas of policy such as maternity services and preventive medicine, the evidence points to a clear failure on the part of the DHSS to promote an adequate response from health authorities in line with its stated priorities (House of Commons, 1986a, 1989d, 1990b). Other factors may also have inhibited centralisation. It has been argued that the reforms of the 1980s have seen a considerable delegation of responsibility downwards to the unit level, where medical power remains formidable. Finally, central government itself may well lack the ability to review local activities and promote change (NHSME, 1991b).

Nevertheless, ministers and civil servants have continued to intervene on detailed matters. The DHSS, and subsequently the Department of Health, was not content to give general direction to the service, but focused instead on specific targets. This was illustrated by the growing number of priorities identified by the department. Reflecting these national priorities, West Midlands Regional Health Authority identified fifty priorities in 1987; another, Oxford Regional Health Authority identified forty-six (Flanagan, 1989). As ministers themselves have subsequently admitted, such a large number of priorities in practice means in reality no priorities at all (Whitney, 1988).

Further changes to the planning system reflected the problems caused by the accumulation of specific priorities. Initially, the department's guidance consolidated earlier advice (DHSS, 1988a). This move was accompanied by procedural changes, aligning health authority annual programmes (short-term plans) more closely to budget allocations, in an attempt to harmonise planning and resourcing. Policy aims remained broadly the same as before, emphasising prevention, community care and so on. These were supplemented by specific service objectives, beginning with targets for surgical procedures such as hip replacements, cataracts, bone marrow transplants, and coronary artery bypass grafts.

Subsequently, the focus has shifted away from specific targets towards broader initiatives aimed at improving whole areas of service provision, such as maternity care, and overall standards of service, such as waiting lists. (DoH, 1989; NHSME, 1990, 1991a, 1992a). The Department of Health, through the NHSME, now focuses on a smaller number of priority areas as a basis for reviewing the performance of the regions, which in turn set the priorities of the districts. There has also been a greater emphasis on region-specific objectives and targets, to be agreed between the NHSME and each Regional Health Authority. On paper at least, this appears to be a more flexible and less centralised approach to the setting of priorities.

Other policy developments have also led to changes in the planning and review processes. The introduction of the internal market has led to the development of purchasing plans. These are drawn up by the District Health Authorities (DHAs) in light of regional and district priorities. The purchasing plan in turn provides a basis for the contracts between the purchasing authorities and the provider organisations. In addition, providers and purchasers are expected to co-operate with each other in the formulation of these plans.

The other major development that has impinged on the planning process is the government's national health strategy which has sought to place greater emphasis on health outcomes, that is, the impact of services on the health of the population. National targets for the reduction of illnesses such as heart disease for example act as a framework for the setting of local targets. Again, the DHAs, as purchasing authorities, are expected to address these considerations when drawing up purchasing plans.

☐ *Performance indicators*

Central intervention has also been enhanced in recent years by the availability of more information about the performance of health authorities. Performance indicators were introduced in September 1983. These indicators were grouped under the headings of clinical activity; finance; manpower; support services; and estate management. They were seen by some to be essentially a 'centre-run exercise focused on a narrow, finance dominated notion of performance' (Pollitt, 1985, p. 9).

The immediate impact of performance indicators was slight. Neither health authorities nor professionals took much notice of them. Planning and finance staff took them more seriously, however. Subsequently, the indicators became more refined and extensive, and new sets of performance indicators were introduced in 1985, 1986 and 1988. The later sets were influenced by the need to improve the use and collection of information in the NHS, in the light of the Körner reports (Windsor, 1986) and the national strategy for health services information (DHSS, 1986a). More recently, the development of performance indicators has been influenced by new initiatives such as resource management, medical audit, and the government's health strategy which is based on the need for information about health outcomes rather than on inputs or outputs.

Performance indicators are generally seen to be a centralist tool. Health authorities which perform less well can be identified and their managers held to account for performance. Performance indicators therefore dovetail neatly with the processes of accountability review and general management. However, continuing inaccuracies in the collection and processing of data generate a great deal of criticism (Skinner *et al.*, 1988). But even if the data improves there is no guarantee that the information will be properly used, or that performance will actually improve (Birch and Maynard, 1988).

Indeed, performance indicators may, in fact, be something of a double-edged weapon. Lowry (1988), for example, urges doctors to use indicators, in view of their potential to demonstrate the contribution of clinical activity. Rather than simply providing information to support the review process, performance indicators may become part of the process whereby doctors secure extra resources.

■ Conclusion

The Griffiths inquiry was at the centre of a reform movement aimed at altering the management process within the NHS. It is impossible to separate the impact of the specific recommendations of Griffiths from other changes, which have included the introduction of accountability reviews, performance indicators, the changes in health authority composition, resource management, medical audit, quality management initiatives and so on. Furthermore, the long-term implications of Griffiths are particularly difficult to predict. Many of the changes ushered in by

Griffiths will probably have even greater significance in future in the light of the government's White Paper *Working for Patients*, discussed more fully in Chapter 8.

The management reforms introduced by the Conservative government represented a departure from the earlier attempts at structural reform. The main aim was not merely organisational change, to produce a more coherent health service, but also cultural change, to make it more 'businesslike' and efficient. It has been widely recognised that such values will have to infiltrate the mind-set of clinicians before they can dominate the culture of the NHS. At present there is no hard evidence that such a cultural change has taken place, although a growing minority of doctors is supportive of the reforms.

Nor has the development of a professionalised management hierarchy as yet undermined the dominant interest in the NHS – the doctors. Some professional groups, such as nurses, have in some respects been weakened, at least initially. Yet the 'corporate rationalisers' (Alford, 1975) still have much to do to tame the medical 'professional monopoly' of the doctors. The reforms have not as yet produced a significant and unambiguous shift in the balance of power between doctors and managers.

Some argue that the foundation for such a shift may well, however, be in place (Harrison *et al.*, 1992). Given that local power has in the past been equated with medical power, this implies greater centralisation. Certainly, central government has more tools with which to monitor the NHS and promote action. But, ironically, many of the changes have promoted a greater delegation of responsibility to the unit level, where the medical profession remains fairly powerful. Moreover, as we have seen, doctors may be mastering the new managerialism by using performance indicators, resource management and medical audit to their own ends. If this becomes widespread, 'doctor-managers' could become a potent force.

The distinction between policy and management in the NHS still remains cloudy ten years after Griffiths reported. There is still no clear division between the responsibilities of the centre and those of the periphery. Time and again central government has interfered in detailed aspects of NHS management and has been unable or unwilling to confine itself to a strategic or co-ordinating role. The potential for detailed intervention is perhaps even greater now in view of the dominance of the business viewpoint (and by implication, government supporters) on the health authorities, although it remains to be seen how these members will react to interference from the central department and higher level authorities in the future. It is possible that they could 'go native' and bite the hand of patronage.

Finally, the politicians who head the service remain publicly responsible for NHS policy and funding, despite the increasing delegation of responsibility to NHS managers and health authorities. This trend, which began under previous governments, has no doubt been part of an attempt to avoid blame (Klein, 1983). But responsibility for the NHS is rather like throwing away a boomerang. When things go wrong ministers have great difficulty in distancing themselves from the problems of the service. As long as the NHS remains a national service, centrally-funded out of taxation, and as long as health care remains a political issue, responsibility for the service will continue to be focused at the centre. It is therefore not surprising that politicians have continued to intervene in matters identified by businessmen as the preserve of managers.

■ *Chapter 7* ■

Allocating Resources to Health Care

Resources can be allocated to health care by the state, by the market, or by a mixture of the two. Following the creation of the NHS, the public sector dominated health care to a greater extent in Britain than in most other comparable countries. The bulk of health care has since been financed out of general taxation. Within the NHS, as discussed in Chapter 4, resources were initially allocated on an historical basis; allocation was later based on estimates of need, in the form of RAWP.

Since the late 1970s, four major developments have had an impact on the operation of this public sector model of resource allocation. These are: the growth of the private sector; pressure to restrict public spending; the focus on greater efficiency and selectivity; and the introduction of internal markets into the NHS. The first three are discussed in this chapter, internal markets in Chapter 8.

■ Privatisation

The creation of the NHS reflected the established wisdom that the market was not an efficient allocator of resources (Honigsbaum, 1989, p. 45). Forty years on, the arguments against health care markets are still formidable, but, as we shall see later, political circumstances have increased the appeal of arguments in favour of market forces.

Traditional private markets, where health care is bought and sold as a commodity, fail on several counts (Normand, 1991). Markets like these are poor at allocating resources to those most in need of health care, but such a misallocation of resources is not confined to market-dominated systems of health care, such as that of the USA. As we saw in Chapter 3, the 'inverse care law' also applies to the NHS. The problems of misallocation are, however, exaggerated by market systems in a number of ways. First, in a private health care market, those who are ill are less likely to be able to afford the costs of treatment. This is partly because much illness is linked to socioeconomic status and poverty. It is also due to the commercial judgement of health insurers who fund private care. These organisations

146

have an incentive to protect their surpluses, usually by excluding subscribers who have a record of previous illness or who are likely to develop serious illness in the future.

Second, and following from this, the individual transactions in a private market cannot reflect the wider importance of health and health care for the whole community. Providers of health care will tend to locate where the population is generally prosperous, and poorer areas will be underprovided. Furthermore, if individuals cannot for financial reasons obtain the health care they need, this represents a social problem. The inability to obtain treatment could impose further costs on the community in the long run in the form of outbreaks of infectious disease, premature mortality and chronic illness. Taking a broader public health perspective, health care can be seen as a special good which should be allocated on the basis of need rather than on ability to pay.

Third, choice in a private market is limited by a number of factors. In particular, consumers (patients) lack information and expertise in health care matters: health care providers have a monopoly of knowledge and skills. This can lead to the exploitation of consumers and oversupply of services.

Fourth, health care systems dominated by the private sector tend to be fragmented, poorly planned and badly co-ordinated, with the result that the needs of the community are not adequately met. This again is not solely a feature of market systems, though it does tend to be exacerbated in systems where provision is determined by demand rather than need.

Finally, private health care markets are not very efficient. Bed occupancy rates are generally lower in private hospitals compared to the NHS and there is considerable overcapacity in the industry (Grant, 1985). Administrative costs also tend to be high in private health care systems. The share of administrative costs in UK private hospitals is around 18 per cent (Parker, 1988). Around a quarter of the cost of the US health care system is allocated to administration (Woolhandler and Himmelstein, 1991), while in the 'pre-reform' NHS, administrative costs accounted for just under 7 per cent of total spending (Office of Health Economics, 1984).

The experience of the USA is often held up by defenders of the NHS to be an example of the adverse effects of a health care system dominated by the private sector (Ginzberg, 1990). The USA spends almost a seventh of its national income on health care, about twice as much the UK. Health care costs in the USA are also rising dramatically, having doubled in the 1980s. Yet there is little evidence that the American system delivers higher standards of health care. Infant mortality is higher, and male life expectancy lower, in the USA when compared with the UK. There is also a good deal of evidence of unnecessary surgery and over-doctoring in the USA, as we saw in Chapter 3. Yet, paradoxically, around 37 million

Americans are uninsured (approximately 16 per cent of the population) and can only obtain basic care offered by the overstretched public hospitals.

☐ *Privatising the NHS?*

The conventional wisdom about the failure of private health care markets, bolstered by the American experience, has not prevented a move towards a greater role for the private sector. Yet Britain is not alone in seeking to alter the public/private mix in health care (Ham *et al.*, 1990; Newbrander and Parker, 1992). Nor is the growth in the private sector purely a consequence of a Conservative government: this sector began to expand before 1979, much to the annoyance of the then Labour government (Higgins, 1988, p. 77).

The Thatcher government gave private health care a significant boost by actively and enthusiastically pursuing policies which encouraged privatisation. These policies were rooted in the Thatcherite vision, discussed in Chapter 4. From this perspective the private sector was seen as being more efficient, better managed, and more responsive to the consumer. The public sector, on the other hand, was viewed as being insulated from competition and dominated by trade unions, and therefore inefficient, wasteful and unresponsive to the consumer.

However, the main obstacle for those who wished to see a greater role for the private sector was the popularity of the NHS. This remained high, even after the industrial strife of the 1970s. Certainly, the NHS had far greater support than the other nationalised industries, most of which were subsequently privatised.

Public opinion has represented a significant barrier to radical change in the public/private mix of health care. This was clearly illustrated in 1982, when the leaking of a report by the government's 'think tank', the Central Policy Review Staff (CPRS) suggested that the government might privatise parts of the NHS. The report argued that if the government were serious about their stated aim of reducing public spending, radical measures would have to be considered. It raised the idea of moving away from a tax-financed health service towards a private insurance system, and put the case for increased charges for health services, including charges for seeing a doctor.

The CPRS report, once in the public domain, caused the government considerable discomfort. According to Sir Norman Fowler, then Secretary of State for Health, the government had no intention of reforming the NHS in this way. His view was that the NHS should remain at the centre of the health care system. Fowler feared that, politically, the government would 'reap the whirlwind' if they were to be seen to be moving away from the NHS (Fowler, 1991).

Fowler also claims that the report had little support from the Cabinet. In the event, the hostile public response to the report forced ministers on to the defensive. This prompted the now famous statement by Margaret Thatcher at the Conservative Party Conference in October 1982, reassuring the public that the NHS was 'safe with us' and restating the principle that 'adequate health care should be provided to all, regardless of the ability to pay' (Thatcher, 1982).

The CPRS report was passed off by ministers as being politically impossible. However, it was revealed that Fowler's predecessor at the DHSS, Patrick Jenkin, had earlier established an internal inquiry of a similar nature. This inquiry, by a working party of civil servants drawn from the DHSS and the Treasury, assisted by two consultants from the private health sector, also cautioned against radical change in the funding of health care in the short-term. However, it did raise the possibility of a greater shift towards private funding in the long-term, with the development of voucher schemes to fund the care of the poor. But it was accepted that some services, such as public health functions and long-term care, would still have to be financed out of taxation.

While the Thatcher government was not prepared to pursue outright privatisation of the NHS, it was nevertheless actively undertaking a programme of what could be called 'creeping privatisation'. There were three main aspects to this. First, the attempt to introduce business-style decision-making, heralded by the Griffiths report, as discussed in Chapter 6; second, the introduction of compulsory competitive tendering for certain NHS ancillary services; and third, the expansion of private health care.

☐ Compulsory competitive tendering

Competitive tendering is when an organisation invites others to compete for the right to provide it with a particular service. In a public sector context, competitive tendering involves competition for areas of work currently performed within the public sector, between the existing workforce (known as the 'in-house' workforce) and private enterprise (Ascher, 1987). Each party sets out its 'bid' – a statement of what service it will provide and at what price. In theory, the bid that offers the best value for money will be invited to provide the service for a given period. At the end of this period a further competitive tender may be held, with other bidders perhaps taking part. Compulsory competitive tendering is where the public authorities in question are compelled to open up areas of work to this bidding process.

It should be made clear that competitive tendering, whether compulsory or not, does not necessarily lead to privatisation in a strict sense of the term. The service remains publicly financed even when the provider is a private firm. Second, as we shall see later, there is no guarantee that private firms will inevitably replace the in-house workforce. However, it would be wrong to assert that competitive tendering makes little difference. Irrespective of who wins, the process can produce changes in the delivery of services that can have potentially far-reaching consequences for patients and the workforce.

Before assessing the consequences of competitive tendering within the NHS, it is useful to sketch the political background to its introduction. The widespread industrial action in the NHS during the 1970s and the early 1980s demonstrated the ability of ancillary workers – cleaners, laundry workers and catering staff – to disrupt services. Compulsory competitive tendering was seen to be a powerful antidote to such action. Ministers believed that if more services were provided by private suppliers, the workforce would be smaller, fragmented, less militant and less likely to join a union. The competitive process would also be a major distraction for the in-house workforce, turning their attention away from the specific grievances that had prompted industrial action. Finally, the government was attracted to competitive tendering in view of its potential to reduce public spending. Ministers believed that the successful bids would be pitched at lower prices than the original budget for these services, so cost savings would be generated.

When the Conservative government entered office in 1979 the private provision of ancillary services was fairly limited, though not completely non-existent. Private firms provided around 2 per cent of NHS domestic cleaning services, 14 per cent of laundry services and less than 0.2 per cent of catering services. The introduction of compulsory competitive tendering in England and Wales in 1983 was intended to increase private sector involvement from this low base.

The main trade unions involved – COHSE and NUPE – opposed competitive tendering. There was also considerable opposition from some health authorities. Clinicians were also alarmed by some well publicised cases which indicated poor standards among some private contractors. For example, in 1985, Bromley DHA cancelled its contract with a private cleaning firm at Orpington Hospital following allegations of falling hygiene standards.

In the event, private firms secured only a small number of contracts in the first round of competitive tendering. Believing they were not competing on a level playing field, the private firms lobbied strongly for a change in the rules. Ministers then began to lean heavily on those health authorities that had awarded contracts to in-house bids. In some cases, ministers overruled the decisions made by district health authorities. Other changes were made to favour the private firms: ministers called for the removal of 'fair wages' clauses in service contracts (health authorities had earlier been prevented from binding contractors to the minimum terms and conditions of employment for NHS staff).

In light of these pressures, a greater proportion of contracts were awarded to the private sector. By December 1985, the private sector had secured 40 per cent of the contracts, the majority in cleaning services. But in the next round of tendering, the private sector share began to recede again – to around 30 per cent. Ministers responded by giving the Regional Health Authorities (RHAs) the responsibility of investigating complaints from private firms about the tendering process and powers to overturn the award of contracts by DHAs. RHAs began to use these powers. For example, in 1988, the North Western Regional Health Authority overruled a decision by North Manchester DHA to award a cleaning contract to an in-house bid (Moore, 1988). In spite of these added pressures, a majority of contracts so far have been won by in-house bids. By 1990 private contractors had secured only 23 per cent of the ancillary service contracts (McGregor, 1990).

☐ The costs and benefits of competitive tendering

The experiment of competitive tendering in the ancillary services has produced benefits. Government sources indicate savings of over £100m per annum from the tendering process (*Independent*, 15 June 1988, p. 6). Yet it is unclear to what extent these resources have been directed back into patient care. There has been a lower level of industrial action in the ancillary services, in recent years, and consequently less disruption of services. However, this is probably due more to the passivity of trade unions in general, the introduction of tighter rules regarding their conduct, and the economic climate of high unemployment than to the process of competitive tendering itself.

Against these benefits, there are some worrying problems. The majority of NHS contracts are concentrated in the hands of a small number of companies. In future these firms may raise the price of contracts in the absence of effective competition. Around two thirds of NHS cleaning contracts, for example, are held by only two firms. Three firms share 74 per cent of the market in laundering, while the share of the largest three players in the catering market is 81 per cent (McGregor, 1990).

There is also continuing concern that the financial savings from contracting have only been achieved at the expense of falling standards of provision. The Joint NHS Privatisation Research Unit – an organisation supported by the main unions involved in the health service – has recorded 103 failures (instances where standards are believed to have suffered as a result of the introduction of a private contractor) (Joint NHS Privatisation Unit, 1990; Newbiggin and Lister, 1988). This represents one failure for every four private contracts issued.

Predictably, the private contractors reject such allegations (Hall, J., 1990). The Department of Health, while admitting that almost 5 per cent of private firms have had their contracts terminated, are understandably keen to play down these findings. Even so, the problems associated with competitive tendering may not even be confined exclusively to the private sector. Pollock and Whitty (1990) examined a food poisoning incident at a psychiatric hospital in the south-east of England. They identified the inadequate level of staffing and poor supervision of catering staff as major factors in the outbreak. These shortcomings were attributed to a combination of factors: limited supply of labour, poor wages and conditions, and insufficient recognition of the problem of recruitment by managers.

This study suggests that competitive tendering, in view of its impact on terms and conditions of work and on staffing levels, is likely to have adverse implications for patient care, and that this applies just as much to in-house providers as private contractors. As Milne (1987, 1989) notes, competitive tendering often leads to pay cuts, worsening terms and conditions of work, and redundancies and resignations, even when a contract has been awarded to the in-house bidder. He does, however, note that a contract can be more efficiently monitored when it is awarded in-house and that adequate supervision may offset to some extent any decline in service standards.

Notwithstanding the potential benefits of competitive tendering, it is clear that serious problems can arise from a shortsighted pursuit of cost savings. This point has even greater significance now that health authorities are being encouraged to apply competitive tendering to clinical areas, including pharmacy, laboratories and renal dialysis as well as other non-clinical areas such as computing, portering and medical records. It is important that the lessons of competitive tendering in ancillary services are taken on board. In particular, it is vital that standards of service in these areas are protected, along with patient confidentiality and security, during the implementation of this new phase of competitive tendering.

☐ The growth of private health care

As we saw in Chapter 5, there are two ways of looking at the contribution of the private health care sector: the extent to which services are privately funded (by individuals, charities or insurance companies) and the extent to which they are provided by private-sector organisations (commercial providers, voluntary organisations and so on). No matter how one looks at private health care, its expansion over the past decade has been significant.

The Conservative government has been an enthusiastic supporter of private health care. As Rayner (1986, p. 440) has noted, 'the election of 1979 ended a period of outright hostility to private medicine'. Those wishing to see an expansion of the private sector had a powerful ally in Margaret Thatcher, who was both a supporter and a consumer of private medicine. There is no doubt that the Thatcher government wished to encourage a massive expansion in private medicine. Indeed, Gerard Vaughan, a junior health minister in the first Thatcher government, once voiced an expectation that 25 per cent of the population would have private health insurance by 1990. But, as noted earlier, the government was restrained by public opinion on this issue and had to tread carefully.

☐ Private funding

In 1979, the year the Conservatives were elected, approximately 4 per cent of the UK population were covered by private health insurance. Ten years later this had risen to 13 per cent. This trend was the result of a deliberate policy during the 1980s to expand private care (Higgins, 1988; Mohan, 1986). In the budget of 1981, employers were allowed to set health insurance premiums against corporation tax. Tax relief on health insurance as a fringe benefit was introduced in the same year for employees earning less than £8500 per annum. Tax relief on private health insurance was extended in 1989 to those over sixty years of age.

The fact that individuals are enrolled in private insurance schemes tells us little about the real extent of private-sector involvement in the funding and delivery of health care. After all, there is no guarantee that those having private insurance will make a claim on their policies in a given period. Nor is it certain that these individuals will opt for treatment in a private-sector facility when they become ill. To complicate matters further, the NHS itself has the largest share of private beds in the UK. Consultants have been allowed to practise private medicine within the NHS from the outset. Currently the NHS has over 3000 private beds, representing just under a quarter of the UK total.

Furthermore, many individuals pay directly for private health care, without the benefit of insurance schemes. In 1986, just over a fifth of private patients (excluding those having abortions) were self-financing (Nicholl *et al.*, 1989b). Patients also pay directly for low cost treatments. These include over-the-counter medicines (that is, bought without a prescription) and a wide range of appliances and therapies supplied by the private sector. Many also pay a contribution towards the costs of the NHS in the form of specific charges for services.

The increase in private payments during the 1980s has been considerable. Charges now contribute around 4 per cent of NHS income, twice the proportion of 1979. Increased charges for some services have significantly altered that balance of spending between the public and private sectors and for some represent 'back-door privatisation' (Birch, 1986).

In 1979 individual payments for NHS dental treatment represented 20 per cent of the total cost of the service, and this contribution had risen to almost 40 per cent by 1989. Prescription charges have risen by over 750 per cent since 1979, though a larger proportion of prescriptions (currently over 80 per cent) are exempt from the charge. The net effect has been a rise in patients' contribution towards NHS prescription costs, from 4 per cent in 1979 to around 8 per cent by the end of the 1980s. In addition, some medicines were removed from the NHS list of approved medicines in 1985 and must now be paid for in full, as with other over-the-counter medicines. In 1992 the government announced it would be extending this list further in an attempt to reduce drug costs. Furthermore, in 1989 charges were extended to eye tests and dental checks. These measures are discussed more fully in Chapter 9.

Another type of private funding is the contribution of charities and voluntary bodies. Such organisations have a long history of funding health services. Since the creation of the NHS, charitable funds have been mainly devoted to medical research and the provision of supplementary services for patients. Now there is real concern that private funds raised by charities are not merely providing optional extras for the NHS, but are, in fact, providing funds for core services. According to Fitzherbert and Giles (1990) appeals are increasingly being run to raise funds for hospital capital and running costs. These findings were supported by a further report which claimed that in the previous few years this trend developed further, with £370m annually being raised from charity, much of it for life-saving facilities (Fitzherbert, 1992).

The Conservative government has continually emphasised the importance of charitable contributions, and has encouraged donations through the tax system (for example, by giving tax concessions to charities and by introducing schemes such as payroll contributions). It has also encouraged independent fundraising by the NHS. The rules on hospital fundraising were simplified shortly after the Conservatives entered office. This was followed in 1988 by measures extending the powers of health authorities to develop commercial activities, such as the marketing of clinical services, video advertising in hospitals, and leasing space for shops, in an effort to generate income.

The extent of private funding of health care is shown in Table 7.1. From this it can be seen that private funding is higher in certain areas of care and treatment than in others. Private expenditure is relatively high in pharmaceuticals, ophthalmics and dentistry, abortion and long-term care of the elderly. It also represents a significant proportion of spending on elective surgery.

Table 7.1   *Public and private sectors in health care*

Care supplied by:		Care funded by			
		% public sector		% private sector	
		Public sector	Private sector	Public sector	Private sector
Elective surgery	1986	83	*	2	15
Long-term care elderly	1989	44	20	7	29
Acute psychiatric care	1989	93	*	*	7
Long-term mentally ill	1988	82	18	*	*
Long-term mental handicap	1988	82	18	*	*
Maternity	1987	99	*	*	*
Abortion	1988	41	6	*	53
General practice	1983	99	0	0	1
Pharmaceuticals	1988	61	0	5	35
Ophthalmics	1987	24	9	0	67
Dentistry	1987	62	0	27	10

Notes:

Figures have been rounded to avoid decimal amounts.

* indicates small percentage (less than 1 per cent).

Bases for comparison: surgery, abortions (cases); care of elderly, pharmaceuticals, dentistry, ophthalmics (cash); maternity (cases); acute psychiatric treatment, care of mentally ill and mentally handicapped (beds); general practice (consultations).

Source: Table compiled by Laing, 1989, p. 73.

☐ The relative contribution of the private sector: provision

Another way of looking at the contribution of the private sector is to look at the amount of money spent on private provision relative to the NHS. Laing (1990) has estimated that the private-sector share of UK hospital-based health care increased from 7.5 per cent in 1984 to 15 per cent in 1990. More specifically, there has been an increase of 48 per cent in the number of in-patients treated by private hospitals between 1981 and 1986 (Nicholl *et al.*, 1989a, 1989b). There has been an even larger increase (112 per cent) in private day-cases. In comparison, NHS in-patient numbers rose by 13 per cent and day-cases by 60 per cent over the same period.

Private-sector provision is extensive in the long-term care of the elderly, in pharmaceuticals, ophthalmics and abortion, which are also, as noted above, heavily financed by the private sector. Private provision, largely funded by the public sector, is also significant in other areas of long-term care (for example, mental illness and mental handicap). Commercial and voluntary residential homes now supply over half the places available in the UK compared with a third in 1979. During the 1980s the number of places available in local authority homes increased slightly and the number provided by charities fell, while those provided by the commercial sector more than quadrupled. The implications of this particular trend for the care of these client groups will be discussed more fully in Chapter 10.

A range of specific surgical interventions are also performed to an increasing extent in the private sector (not shown separately in Table 7.1). For example, 28 per cent of hip replacements and 16 per cent of varicose vein operations were performed in the private sector during the mid-1980s (Nicholl *et al.*, 1989b).

There are significant regional variations in the level of private health care provision. In some regions, namely the North West and South West Thames Health Authority regions, almost a third of patients underwent elective surgery (excluding abortions) in the private sector in 1986. In contrast, in the same year, only 6.3 per cent of patients did so in the Northern Region. This variation reflects the uneven distribution of private health care facilities in the UK. Around a third of districts are not served by a private hospital. Most private beds are concentrated in London and the South East. The North East Thames Region has forty-four private hospital beds per 100 000 population, while the Northern Region has only 5 per 100 000.

In addition to its efforts to encourage private funding, the Conservative government has actively promoted private provision of health care through a number of other technical changes. One such change was the modification of consultants' NHS contracts during the early 1980s which enabled them to perform more private work. Other changes had a rather more ambiguous impact on the private sector. The abolition of the Health Services Board in 1980 was such an example. This body was set up by the Labour government in the mid-1970s as part of a compromise on the heated issue of pay beds in the NHS. Its role was to consider the phasing out of NHS pay beds and to control the building or extension of private sector facilities.

The abolition of the Health Services Board was not necessarily to the long-term advantage of the private sector. The reason for this lay in the rather perverse impact of Labour's previous policy on pay beds and private medicine. The publicity relating to the phasing out of pay beds had led the private sector to expand its own facilities. The reversal of this policy raises the possibility that the private sector may face increased competition from the NHS. This prospect appeared likely as NHS hospitals began to view pay beds as a key part of their income-generation plans. The development of self-governing trusts (SGTs), which have greater freedom to determine the services they will provide, looks almost certain to exacerbate this situation.

☐ *Joint working arrangements*

Leadbeater (1990) has indicated the extent of co-operation between public and private sectors. By 1988, about half of the health authorities had used the private acute sector to care for NHS patients. A fifth had been involved in a joint purchasing or leasing arrangement for medical equipment. Another fifth had used private-sector screening services.

In addition health authorities have been directed to use private facilities as part of the drive to reduce waiting lists. In 1989 over 10 per cent of the funds provided by the government's waiting list initiative was spent on private hospital care.

Joint working arrangements are likely to increase with the advent of the internal market in the NHS, as the new purchasers of health care contract with private facilities. By the 1992–3 financial year the NHS was spending over £250m on health care provided by the private sector, a 25 per cent increase on the previous year. This figure excluded the purchase of care by GP fundholders, which was not known. The government encouraged further joint projects by raising the limit on private investment in the NHS. From 1993, new capital developments costing up to £10m can be financed by the private sector. It is also possible that the NHS will in future lease facilities from the private sector to a far greater extent. Even more controversially, it is possible that NHS services may in the future be run by private management.

☐ *The voluntary and informal sectors*

Voluntary and informal provision of services has grown over the past decade or so, again partly as a result of deliberate government policy. The voluntary sector as a whole receives over £2 billion per annum from central government. This figure has doubled in real terms in the past decade. Around £50 million is allocated to voluntary bodies in the field of health and personal social services. Most of this is funded by the Department of Health. The voluntary sector also receives funding from local authorities, the NHS and from the general public.

The voluntary sector has been supported by the government in other ways. In 1981 the DHSS explicitly told health authorities to collaborate more closely with the voluntary sector (DHSS, 1981c). Then, in 1986, the voluntary agencies were given a role in the joint planning of services alongside the NHS and local authorities. There have been other specific initiatives to encourage voluntary work. An example is the Opportunities for Volunteering scheme funded by the Department of Health. Under this scheme, operated by fifteen national voluntary bodies including MIND (The National Association for Mental Health) and Age Concern, unemployed people are encouraged to participate in voluntary work in the field of social care.

Most agree that the growth of the voluntary sector is, on balance, a favourable development. But there are dangers associated with an over-reliance on voluntary and informal provision. These dangers are discussed in Chapter 10 in the context of community care.

☐ *Implications of the expansion in private health care*

There has been a deliberate expansion of private health care since the late 1970s. What are the implications for the NHS and for health care in general? There is much disagreement about the impact of an enlarged private sector on the NHS. The view advanced by the Royal Commission on the NHS was that this impact, whether for good or ill, could largely be discounted because the private sector in the UK was small relative to the NHS. International comparisons reveal that the UK still has one of the smallest ratios of private to public health care expenditure. Even so, the growth of the private sector in recent years has been considerable and one can no longer ignore it.

One view, usually put forward by those on the political right, is that the growth of the private sector has had a significant and favourable impact on the NHS. According to this view, the private sector has acted rather like a safety valve for the overstretched NHS. One patient treated privately, it is argued, is one less on a waiting list. The co-operation of the private sector with the NHS waiting list initiatives is often presented as an extension of this symbiotic relationship. Another benefit claimed for the private sector is that it has provided a useful source of ideas for the NHS in its search for more efficient management systems. The private sector certainly has more experience in areas such as the costing and pricing of treatment, responding to the non-clinical needs of the consumer, and management information systems.

Yet there are reasons why the growth of the private sector may have an adverse impact on the NHS. Some believe that the private sector acts as a parasite, drawing resources out of the NHS (Widgery, 1988). There is some evidence to support this. In 1989, the National Audit Office (NAO, 1989a) found that the cost of treating NHS patients in the private sector was twice as high as the cost of treating them within the NHS. Such arrangements may be criticised as featherbedding the private sector, though it should be pointed out that the higher cost of treating NHS patients privately can be offset to some extent by the savings in overhead costs (such as the building of new facilities) which might have been incurred in treating additional patients within the NHS.

In the same report, the NAO expressed concern about the lack of monitoring of the private work done by NHS consultants. These sentiments were echoed in a report by the House of Commons Public Accounts Committee, the following year (House of Commons, 1990c). Indeed fears have been expressed that consultants have a vested interest in building up their waiting lists in order to produce a demand for private treatment, though this is difficult to prove. There have also been allegations that some consultants have not been fulfilling their contracts properly and that as a result NHS patients have been neglected. The government subsequently introduced detailed job plans for consultants and closer monitoring of their NHS commitments by health authorities.

A further area of concern is the impact of the private sector on nursing manpower within the NHS. Around a thousand nurses every year leave the NHS to work in the private sector and many more work for private hospitals on a part-time basis in addition to their NHS duties. Yet the private sector makes a negligible contribution to the training of nurses and their use is therefore effectively being subsidised by the NHS.

☐ *The future of the private sector*

It is possible that the growth of the private sector could have damaged the NHS in other ways. The fundamental principles of the NHS – a comprehensive service for all, free at point of delivery, regardless of ability to pay – may be undermined by a larger private sector (Iliffe, 1988). The breaching of these principles may have been assisted by other policies, such as public-spending restrictions and the introduction of internal markets, both of which have the potential to increase the role of the private sector. On the other hand, perhaps the private sector's ability to replace the NHS has been exaggerated. It may well be that the private sector is nearing the limits of its expansion. A study by the Institute of Health Services Management (IHSM, 1988) has argued that, even with radical changes to the NHS designed to create new opportunities for private enterprise, the private sector's share of total health spending would be unlikely to exceed 20 per cent of the total. Also, as Nicholl *et al.* (1989b) point out, the private sector is not geared up to perform complex, high-technology procedures on an appropriate scale. Its ability to diversify into these areas in order to compete with the NHS may, as a result, be limited.

Moreover, the private health sector has had its own crises of overcapacity and cut-throat competition in recent years (see Mohan, 1986; Higgins, 1988). Indeed, there are many divisions within the private sector, notably between the commercial (for profit) operators and the provident (non-profit) associations. The expansion of the commercial providers, many of them from overseas, has been well documented (Higgins, 1988). There have also been conflicts in recent years between the health insurers and the private hospitals over the pricing of operations and the reimbursement of fees. Economic recession has also hit the private sector hard, with many companies and employees cancelling health insurance plans in the light of business failures and redundancies.

Finally, as already noted, the recent NHS reforms may well have an ambiguous effect on the private sector. The market for private providers may expand, as the purchasers of health care buy care from this sector. But the creation of SGTs, on the other hand, has created a powerful set of competitors in the market for private and NHS patients against which the private sector will have to compete. The community care reforms, which are similarly based on a purchaser–provider model, may also provide both opportunities and pitfalls for the private sector. Under the new arrangements, local authorities will have to allocate a large portion of funding to the private sector. But at the same time the overall budget for residential care, where the private sector is at present strongest, is likely to be squeezed as the purchasing authorities seek to make their limited budgets go further.

■ Public expenditure on health care

The growth of the private sector is very much influenced by the state of the NHS and in particular by the resources at its disposal. The financial state of the NHS is in turn determined to a large extent by the general economic climate, and by the approach towards public expenditure taken by the government of the day. These factors set the framework within which the Treasury and the Health Departments bargain and negotiate over the size of the NHS budget.

The relatively poor performance of the British economy has often impinged upon the NHS. Webster (1988) has observed that the NHS had barely begun its life before it was overtaken by a crisis over expenditure. Periodic financial crises have generally produced two kinds of response: first, a search for supplementary or alternative sources of finance; second, an attempt to squeeze the existing NHS budget.

In 1951, the Labour government sought to offset the cost of the NHS by introducing patient charges for spectacles and dentures. Labour also paved the way for prescription charges, introduced by the incoming Conservative administration. The Conservative government explored the possibility of further charges, including the imposition of a 'boarding' charge for hospital patients. This option was returned to again and again by successive governments, including the Labour government of the 1970s. Because of anticipated problems involved in collecting the charge and its unpopularity with the public, this option was never taken up.

Governments have occasionally explored radical alternatives to the tax-funded system. As we have seen, the Thatcher government looked at the possibility of introducing an insurance-based system. This was not unprecedented. The Conservative government of Harold Macmillan examined the case for a national health insurance system during the 1950s. Plans to introduce such a scheme were abandoned in view of the likely public reaction, as the 1959 General Election approached. Alternative sources of finance were also considered (and rejected) by the Royal Commission on the NHS during the 1970s (Cmnd 7615, 1979).

Governments have also responded to the financial problems of the NHS by trying to squeeze its budget. This began under the first Labour government. Then in the early 1950s the Conservative government appointed the Guillebaud committee to review NHS spending. As already mentioned in Chapter 4, the government hoped that Guillebaud would provide arguments in favour of cutting back expenditure. However, the committee reported that the NHS provided good value for money, making it difficult to justify cut-backs.

The squeezing option was used more forcefully twenty years later, by a Labour government. During the mid-1970s, and in the face of a severe economic crisis, the Labour government was forced to cut back on public spending. Part of its strategy included the implementation of cash limits, which imposed a ceiling on budgets in the public sector. Cash limits applied to health authority spending, but not to the family practitioner services. The incoming Conservative government retained the system of cash limits, with some modifications, and sought to extend it to primary care, as we shall see in Chapter 9.

☐ The Thatcher government, public expenditure ☐ and NHS expenditure

The Thatcher government placed a great deal of emphasis on controlling public expenditure. This was central to its economic policy of reducing price inflation, and an important component of its aim of shifting the boundary between the public and private sectors. Initially at least, the government sought deep cuts in all spending programmes. It also brought in new mechanisms for regulating public spending, including the introduction of 'cash planning'. Under cash planning, budgets were now expressed in terms of money rather than volume of services provided. The main impact of this innovation was to squeeze budgets if inflation was higher than expected.

Although public expenditure after adjusting for inflation continued to grow during the 1980s, it fell as a proportion of national income from 43 per cent (1979) to 38 per cent (1990). This has since risen, partly as a result of falling national income during the recession years of 1990–3. This has in turn led to renewed pressures to reduce public expenditure.

It has been impossible to insulate the NHS from the constraining effect of tighter public expenditure policies. The health budget is simply too large to ignore. Yet despite the pressure on public spending the NHS share of expenditure has actually risen. The proportion of public spending devoted to the NHS, which had remained around the 10 per cent mark for most of the 1950s and 1960s actually rose from 11 per cent in 1981 to 14 per cent in 1990. This suggests that the NHS budget has fared well compared with other spending programmes. For example, the education and defence budgets remained at roughly the same proportion of public spending (11 per cent and 12 per cent respectively). Others declined – notably housing (from 3 per cent to 1.9 per cent of public spending) and transport (from 4 per cent to 3 per cent). Finally, the growth of NHS expenditure is illustrated by the substantial increase in its budget relative to average prices. Between 1980 and 1989 NHS spending rose by around 20 per cent in real terms – taking into account the change in average retail prices.

There are a number of reasons why the NHS budget has continued to grow in spite of the pressure on public spending. The constant interest of the media in health matters, and in particular the finance and funding of the NHS, has been a major factor. Any attempt to restrain spending has therefore taken place in the full glare of publicity, putting ministers on the defensive. As a result, the government has been forced to proclaim its commitment to greater rather than less NHS expenditure.

Meanwhile, the case for more spending has been bolstered by a vociferous lobby. This has included the main professional groups, such as the BMA and the Royal Colleges, and a wide range of patients' groups. Further weight has been added by Parliament, with widespread cross-party support for higher NHS spending, in both the Commons and the Lords.

☐ *Underfunding*

It is clear that the NHS has not suffered as badly as some public spending programmes. Yet a closer look at public expenditure on health care indicates that the growth rate is less dramatic than it first appears, for a number of reasons (Appleby, 1992). The first thing to note is that the growth in health spending in real terms is much smaller when one takes into account the rise in the cost of health services, which has in recent years risen faster than the average rate of inflation as measured by the retail price index (RPI). According to Appleby and Adams (1989) the inflation rate in health service costs, as measured by the Health Services Prices Index (HSPI) was higher than the RPI in seven out of ten years between 1980 and 1990. Between 1983/4 and 1989/90 the prices of hospital and community health services increased by 58.1 per cent compared with 44.4 per cent in general prices (Robinson, 1990). When deflated by the HSPI rather than the RPI, health spending shows a much less spectacular growth rate in the 1980s.

Robinson's calculations, which take into account these changes in the cost of services, show that overall spending on the NHS increased at an annual average rate of 1.8 per cent a year between 1979/80 and 1989/90. His figures also reveal a marked difference between funding increases in different parts of the service. The 'cash limited' hospital and community sector experienced a real growth of 0.9 per cent in 1980s, while the family practitioner services enjoyed a 3.1 per cent growth in resources during this same period.

The growth rate of 1.8 per cent is noticeably lower than the Department of Health's own assessment of what is required to maintain and improve the service in light of changing disease patterns, new forms of service delivery, demographic changes and developments in medical technology. The department has maintained that an average annual growth rate of around 2 per cent per annum is required to keep pace with these trends (House of Commons, 1986b, p. 26).

It is this 2 per cent figure which has provided the basis of the allegations about underfunding, and estimates of the amounts needed to rectify the situation. The House of Commons Social Services Committee stated in the late eighties that the cumulative shortfall meant that the NHS was underfunded by nearly £1.9 billion. The committee urged an injection of not less than 1 billion pounds over the following two years to help remedy the situation (House of Commons, 1988a). Estimates of this deficit have since grown even larger, with the National Association of Health Authorities placing the cumulative shortfall between 1980/1 and 1990/1 at £4.4 billion (NAHAT, 1990).

Those who argue for a higher level of funding for the NHS also find support for their case in international comparisons. Pritchard (1992) points out that, compared with mainland Europe, the NHS is 'unequivocally underfunded'. He points out that if the NHS were to match the German health budget its allocation would have to rise by a fifth. Figure 7.1 confirms that relative to most other comparable countries, the UK spends less on health care, both as a proportion of national income and in terms of expenditure per head of population.

Calls for extra funding to redress this shortfall have been rejected. More generous health settlements in the early 1990s were offset by costly new initiatives, not least the launch of the internal market. Increasing pressure on public spending in the early 1990s will restrict the health budget further. Wilding's argument (1992), that the restoration of economic deficits in welfare services becomes more difficult once a new baseline has been created, appears to have some foundation.

☐ *Rejection of the underfunding thesis*

There is a great deal of controversy about the adequacy of health spending, and the figures are open to a variety of interpretations. Critics of the underfunding thesis have played down the importance of international comparisons such as those shown in Figure 7.1. It is true that there are a number of problems associated with international comparisons of health expenditure: what may be categorised as health spending in one country may not be so regarded in another. The demands on the health services may vary between countries. Furthermore, the amount of money spent on health care may not necessarily be a good indicator of the quality and cost-effectiveness of health services.

Another point is that the level of UK public spending on health care (5.3 per cent of national income) is quite close to the average for all OECD countries (5.6 per cent). The main difference between the UK and most other comparable countries is in private spending on health care. Private health spending in the UK is still relatively small, despite its growth during the 1980s. For this reason, critics argue, it is more appropriate that the gap be closed by increasing private payments rather than by increasing public expenditure (Whitney, 1988).

The estimates of the year-on-year increases in expenditure required by the NHS have also been criticised. The 2 per cent 'target' increase in funding, based on rough estimates of the costs of new service developments, medical technology, population changes and so on, is very crude. This target takes no account of the extent to which the current budget is being spent effectively and efficiently (Haywood, 1990).

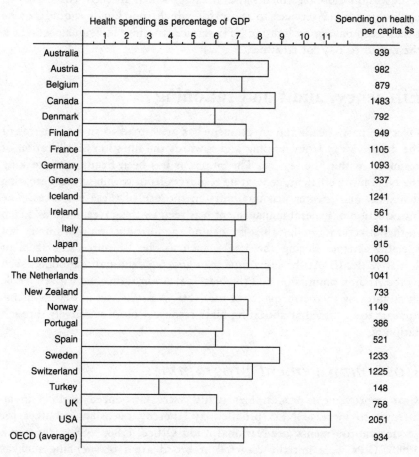

Source: OECD (1990).

Figure 7.1 *Cross-national comparisons of health expenditure (OECD countries), 1987*

Moreover, there is no guarantee that the existing level of resources, the baseline from which the target increases are calculated, is appropriate (House of Commons, 1988b, p. ix).

Underfunding exists where the existing level of funding is lower than that needed to provide an acceptable level of service. But what is an acceptable level of service? This is increasingly open to question. According to some, the gap between the demand for health care and the available resources is ever-increasing. As a result 'there is no longer any consensus about what constitutes the essential core of the NHS' (Thwaites, 1988).

Critics of the underfunding thesis point out that too much is expected of the NHS. The solution from this viewpoint is to improve the allocation of NHS resources through better financial management; by concentrating resources on those treatments and therapies which are most cost-effective; by limiting NHS services to those for which individuals should not be expected to pay; or by limiting NHS services to those individuals who lack the means to pay for treatment.

Efficiency, audit and rationing

Over the past decade the government has attempted to shift the terms of the debate away from funding and towards the question of allocation of resources within the service. The emphasis has been firmly upon making the NHS more efficient, generating resources from within to meet growing demands, and greater accountability in the use of these resources. The introduction of general management was seen by the government as a step in this direction. Similar aims lay behind the introduction of a number of specific schemes during the 1980s, such as the Resource Management Initiative (RMI). At the same time, new independent auditing bodies such as the Audit Commission and the National Audit Office were given a role in monitoring the performance of the NHS. A further set of developments appears to be aimed at allocating NHS resources more selectively through rationing.

Cost improvement programmes

Cost improvement programmes (CIPs) were introduced in 1984 in an attempt to increase NHS productivity, thereby releasing resources for service improvements (see National Audit Office, 1986, 1989b; Haywood, 1990). CIPs were initially targeted at broad areas of spending such as supplies and energy costs. On average, the level of cost improvements has been around 1.5 per cent of the previous year's budget. Recurrent cost improvements totalled over £1 billion in 1990/1 (NAHAT, 1990).

Although the intention was that the money released by CIPs would be used to fund patient services, there has been some concern that health authorities have not realised significant additional funding in this way. In particular, doubts have been cast on whether the reported cost improvements have actually been achieved in practice. There has been further criticism that CIPs have emphasised cost-cutting at the expense of efficiency and quality of service. By postponing expenditure in the short term, CIPs may raise costs in the longer term (National Audit Office, 1989b; IHSM/NAHA, 1989).

☐ *Efficiency scrutinies*

Efficiency scrutinies, introduced in the NHS in 1982 have been used to investigate areas of suspected inefficiency (Harrison, 1988a, p. 59). Such reviews are often called 'Rayner reviews' after the government adviser and businessman, Lord Rayner, who promoted their extensive use in central government. Rayner reviews begin with the appointment of a manager (or in some cases a small inquiry team) seconded from normal duties. The review then examines, within a given time limit, a particular area of health authority activity with a view to suggesting ways of achieving cost savings. In 1982 a Rayner review explored the costs of residential accommodation for NHS staff, pointing out that these facilities were not being used efficiently. This prompted the sale of such assets in some health authorities, amid much controversy. Rayner reviews have also been carried out into ambulance services, storage of supplies, catering and vacancy advertising.

Efficiency scrutinies have been placed on a more systematic basis with the creation of a value for money unit (VFMU) within the NHSME. The VFMU aims to promote local improvements in efficiency by indicating where savings can be made. In a recent report, the VFMU suggested that the boarding costs of patients in hospital wards could be almost halved by developing 'hotels' for post-operative care (DoH and OPCS, 1993b, p. 63).

☐ *The cost-effectiveness of care and treatment*

Other initiatives have focused upon promoting cost-effectiveness in clinical areas. In principle, resources can be released by reallocating them towards care and treatments which have been proved to be more cost-effective. As noted earlier, the Department of Health has encouraged and promoted medical audit. It has also backed a range of initiatives (for example, RMI, TQM and so on) aimed at monitoring the quality of care, assessing cost-effectiveness and measuring activity levels in relation to resources. The

Department has also recently established a national health technology assessment programme, which goes some way to addressing the concerns of those who have called for better evaluation of new technologies.

The extent to which these developments will actually lead to a more cost-effective service is at present uncertain. They certainly do represent a step in the right direction, provided they are not used as crude devices to curtail new service developments which might in the long run reduce costs.

☐ *Audit and monitoring*

As a national service, funded out of taxation, NHS expenditure is clearly a matter for Parliamentary scrutiny. The monitoring of NHS expenditure falls under the responsibility of two separate committees of the House of Commons: the Public Accounts Committee (PAC) and the Health Committee (formerly the Social Services Committee).

PAC is concerned with expenditure, accounting processes and procedures across the whole range of government spending. Its job is to ensure that public money has been properly spent and it has a watching brief against waste and inefficiency in government departments and agencies. PAC has often been critical of the Department of Health and its forebears. In 1990, for example, the committee was extremely critical of inefficiencies in the hospital building programme (House of Commons, 1990a).

The Health Committee is concerned with monitoring levels of expenditure within the broader context of government policy on health and therefore has more of a policy focus than does the PAC, although on occasion PAC has been highly critical of policies which have led to waste or inefficiency. For example, PAC has on a number of occasions criticised the Department of Health for not investing sufficient resources in preventive medicine (House of Commons, 1986a, 1989d).

Two other official bodies have played an increasing role in relation to monitoring efficiency in health policy and service provision in recent years. These are the National Audit Office (NAO) and the Audit Commission.

The NAO is a Parliamentary body which prepares the way for enquiries by the PAC (May, 1990). In addition, it has the power to make its own recommendations for improvements which it believes are necessary to improve value for money. It has published reports in recent years on issues such as the efficiency of operating theatres (NAO, 1991), the quality of clinical care (NAO, 1988b), and maternity services (NAO, 1990), among others.

The Audit Commission was originally confined to promoting value for money in local government. But even in this capacity it impinged on health issues in reports on community care, environmental health and housing. Since 1990, when the Audit Commission's brief was expanded to include the NHS, it has published a number of reports pointing out the scope for improvements in efficiency in areas such as primary care and day surgery (Audit Commission, 1990, 1992a and b). The Audit Commission also appoints the audit teams which examine health authority finances. In recent years these have begun to uncover evidence of waste, inefficiency and mismanagement in a number of health authorities (see Exhibit 7.1).

Exhibit 7.1   Financial mismanagement in the NHS

Two cases of financial mismanagement, which came to light in the early 1990s underlined both the importance of independent audit and the need for greater public accountability within the NHS.

1. Wessex Health Authority wasted at least £20m on its computer integration scheme during the 1980s. The contract to provide this service was initially awarded to a private company, but following lobbying of senior personnel within the health authority, the decision was reversed and the contract awarded to a rival bid which was fourth in the original list of possible contractors. Health authority members were not informed of this decision until months after the contract had been signed. It was also alleged that a former health minister and a senior member of the health authority, both of whom were connected to the companies which comprised the successful bid, had lobbied strongly in its favour.

   Interestingly, the district auditor's report which discovered this remained confidential until its existence was revealed by an investigation by the *Independent* newspaper and *Computer Weekly* magazine. The Department of Health clearly did not wish the contents to become public knowledge.

2. West Midlands Health Authority was accused of wasting money in connection with a contract, which ironically involved the hiring of efficiency advisers. Management consultants had been brought in from the private sector to advise on how to promote efficiency in supplies. In all £4m was spent on consultancy fees and other costs. This included annual expenses of £350 000 to cover the cost of high-quality accommodation, the hire of aircraft, and lavish entertainments.

   This was not the first time that this health authority had been accused of mismanagement. In 1990 the authority's decision to lend almost £1m to a computer software marketing company had been declared unlawful by the National Audit Office.

Sources: Independent, 15 April 1991, p. 2; 11 February 1993, p. 1.

One expects bodies such as PAC and the Health Committee to be critical of the government. After all, these committees are partly composed of MPs drawn from the opposition parties. However, the government does have some of its own supporters on these committees. In the case of the Health Committee, the government has tried to determine the composition of the committee and to influence its reports. The NAO and the Audit Commission are perhaps more independent in criticising the government and have done so on several occasions in the past. For example, both the NAO and the Audit Commission cast a cloud over the government's internal market reforms by pointing out shortcomings in financial and information management upon which the effective operation of the proposed internal market depended. (Audit Commission, 1991; NAO, 1989b).

Increased scrutiny of the NHS and health policy is undoubtedly a positive development. While encouraging audit, the government has to some extent been hoist by its own petard as auditors have uncovered evidence of waste and inefficiency, often related to the government's own reform programme (see Exhibit 7.1). It is perhaps not surprising to learn that the Department of Health, which has received much of the political fallout from these scandals, opposed independent audit when it was introduced in 1990 (Lawson, 1992).

☐ Rationing

More recently the focus has been upon reallocating NHS resources away from certain forms of care and treatment. There are two reasons for this. First, cost-effectiveness: there may be overall financial gains to be made by switching resources away from some treatments and towards others. A better service may result if ineffective treatments are discarded and the gains reinvested in those which are effective. A second reason for reallocating resources is that certain treatments, while effective, are not considered to be priorities. This is because the conditions which they cure or alleviate are not regarded as being life-threatening in a strict sense. These include cosmetic surgery, such as the removal of benign cysts, tattoos and so on, and infertility services. Painful conditions such as haemorrhoids, varicose veins and even arthritic joints are also considered by some to be of relatively low priority, although this is not to deny that such illnesses and conditions often seriously undermine the sufferers' quality of life.

Restricting or eliminating low-priority treatments on the NHS leads to rationing, in two ways. First, as services are restricted, waiting lists will tend to grow. This leads to a greater emphasis on how best to allocate treatment among those who need it. Rationing could take place on the basis of waiting times, or in relation to the severity of the case – as in the past. Or it could be based on an explicit assessment of the relative costs and benefits of treating each individual case as demonstrated in Chapter 3. Second, there is rationing by price. Patients could face the prospect of longer waiting lists, or, given the new directives on waiting times (discussed in Chapter 8) could end up being removed from waiting lists entirely. Alternatively, funding may be withdrawn for certain therapies with patients having little option but to pay privately. To some extent this is already happening in many areas of surgery, such as that for varicose veins and hip replacements. The restriction or elimination of treatment in so-called low-priority areas will exacerbate this situation. Of course, there will be many who simply cannot afford to pay and who will be forced to live with painful or emotionally stressful conditions.

The whole question of rationing has been stimulated by the advent of the internal market, which has forced the purchasing authorities to look more closely at priorities in the light of their limited budgets. The development of economic techniques such as the QALY and other evaluative tools has also generated interest, and controversy, about the possibility of rationing in the future. Rationing is explored further in the context of the internal market reforms in Chapter 8.

■ Conclusion

The expansion of the private sector and the increasing pressure on NHS resources has conjured up the nightmare scenario of the two-tier system. According to this scenario the NHS will in future cater only for certain client groups: the poor, the chronically ill, and accident and emergency cases, with the private sector providing a quick, efficient and consumer-sensitive acute service for the better-off. This is similar to the current situation in the USA, which combines high-cost, high-quality care for the better-off and inadequate services for the rest, but this scenario is unlikely to emerge in Britain, at least not in this crude form. The most likely outcome is a patchwork quilt of public and private services, with wide variations in the quality of service provided, between and within both sectors.

The private sector has grown considerably. In some parts of the country and in some areas of treatment it now rivals the NHS in terms of market share. The market is now a major allocative mechanism in health care, and with the advent of internal markets is set to become even more important in the future.

Further private sector growth will probably be insidious, taking the form of joint working with the NHS. This kind of development is likely to be further stimulated by the internal market and some of the other reforms mentioned above, although the private sector may have to fight the SGTs for market share. It is also possible through these changes that the NHS will be privatised from within, as the market ethos takes over. This may in the long run pave the way for the privatisation of SGTs.

The future of the private sector depends to an enormous extent on the level of NHS funding. Specific areas of care and treatment may be turned over to the private sector as public services are squeezed and rationed. As we have seen, the debate over public expenditure on the NHS is controversial. There is no agreement about the right level of funding. Meanwhile, the government has preferred, for obvious reasons, to focus on costs and efficiency rather than underfunding.

There is an element of truth in both arguments: the NHS is relatively underfunded and also could be more efficient. The provision of additional funds is not necessarily going to produce a more efficient service. But, on the other hand, underfunding can also be a source of inefficiency (Light, 1990b). For example, a short-term squeeze on funding may prevent the development of services – such as community-based care – which may in the long run prove to be more cost-effective.

It has been shown that the issues of privatisation, public expenditure and efficiency are closely interlinked. These interrelationships have been further complicated by the introduction of the internal market in health care, which combines public funding with a market allocation mechanism. It is to this remarkable new departure that we now turn.

■ *Chapter 8* ■

The Search for a Solution: Internal markets

In June 1987 the prospect of further upheaval in the British health care system appeared remote. The Conservative government, facing a General Election, proclaimed its devotion to the NHS, pointing out that health spending in the previous eight years had outstripped that of any previous governments, and that more patients were being treated than ever before. The party manifesto contained no radical plans for reform, though it did state that the NHS, while it was not a business, needed to be run in a more businesslike way (Conservative Party, 1987). Yet only a few months after the election, which returned the Conservatives to office once again, the NHS was again the subject of a controversial debate about its future. Within a year the government had set up a review of the NHS, with all options open for consideration.

■ The NHS: crisis and review

The government was forced into a corner by the growing catalogue of ward closures and postponed operations as health authorities sought to balance their budgets (Timmins, 1988). Two factors in particular were held to be responsible for the financial problems facing health authorities at this time. First, the deliberate decision by the government not to fund pay awards for NHS staff in full meant that health authorities had to meet higher wage bills, in part by cutting back on services (House of Commons, 1988a). Second, the effects of the RAWP system, which redistributed funds from areas which previously had been relatively well resourced. Health authorities in London were hit particularly hard by this.

The financial problems faced by the NHS during the winter of 1987/8 seemed to be the worst for many years. The media fuelled public concern by highlighting particularly emotive cases affected by the cut-backs. One such case was that of David Barber, whose heart operation at a Birmingham hospital was postponed five times, and who died following the delayed operation. Such cases were just the tip of the iceberg: one survey showed that over 3000 beds had been withdrawn in England due to shortages of cash or nursing staff (Timmins, 1988).

☐ *Political pressure*

The political pressure on the government intensified, and parliamentary activity began to focus sharply on the NHS (Duncan *et al.*, 1989). Between October 1987 and February 1988, fifty-two Early Day Motions were tabled in the House of Commons, drawing attention to closures and financial crises within health authorities. Ten adjournment debates focused upon problems in different parts of the country. There were also five full debates on the NHS, including two initiated by the Labour opposition. In addition, two of the House of Commons Select Committees, the Treasury and Civil Service Committee and the Social Services Committee, began inquiries into the state of the NHS.

Organisations representing the health professions and patients continued to voice their concern about the financial problems of the NHS. This came to a head in December 1987, when the presidents of three Royal Medical Colleges issued a statement claiming that the acute hospital services had almost reached breaking point. The entrance of the Royal Colleges into this controversial and highly public debate emphasised that the problems faced by the NHS were apparently of a different order from those it had faced before.

The combination of media coverage and pressure from the health care professions produced a response from the government in the form of an additional £100m for the NHS, most of which was aimed at averting ward closures. As it turned out, this was merely a stopgap. On 25 January 1988, Margaret Thatcher announced a review of the NHS during an interview on BBC TV's 'Panorama' programme. This was unexpected and surprised some members of her own Cabinet. However, according to former Chancellor of the Exchequer, Nigel Lawson (1992), the idea of a review of the hospital service had been put forward by the Treasury before the General Election. Ministers at the Department of Health also supported a review of the NHS. But, at this time, Thatcher did not. As the political pressure intensified later in the year, the Prime Minister apparently changed her mind, primarily, it seems, as a means of getting the issue off the political agenda.

☐ *The Prime Minister's review*

As Griggs (1991) has commented, the Prime Minister's review of the NHS was instructive of the government's policy-making style: speedy, secretive and loyal to Thatcher. The review team consisted of a small group of ministers drawn from the Treasury, the DHSS (later the Department of

Health), and the Scottish and Welsh Offices, plus Sir Roy Griffiths, the PM's adviser. It was supported by civil servants drawn from the departments concerned, plus a number of other political advisers. Thatcher chaired the committee and was able to exert a great deal of control over the direction of the review, particularly during its final stages (Paton, 1992).

Although the review was not an open exercise, individuals and organisations were invited to meet health ministers and to submit papers outlining their ideas for reform. The result was, to borrow Klein's phrase (1989b), 'an intense flurry of pamphleteering'. These proposals focused on two main areas: alternative systems of funding health care; and new mechanisms for allocating resources within the NHS.

□ *Funding*

There were many suggestions as to how to alter the funding system. Various schemes to increase private funding of health care were advanced by those to the right of the political spectrum (Green, D. G., 1988; Redwood, 1988). Former Cabinet Minister Leon Brittan (1988) proposed a state health insurance system that would encourage private funding, by giving those who contributed to a private scheme the opportunity to 'opt out' of the NHS. Other ideas put forward included granting tax relief on private health insurance contributions for the elderly (Brown *et al.*, 1988). This particular proposal was, in fact, later taken up by the government.

Other alternatives included a proposal for a specific health tax (Field, 1988, Owen, 1988). An earmarked tax for health, levied as a percentage of income, was appealing for a number of reasons. If fixed over a number of years, the revenue generated could provide a more solid basis for financial planning in the NHS. It was also believed that an earmarked tax would offer some protection for the NHS budget. A further argument in favour of this approach was that an explicit health tax would directly inform taxpayers about the cost of health services. On the other hand, it was naïve to think that earmarked taxes could be insulated from political decisions. The tax rate would reflect political expediency. Moreover, it was by no means certain that the tax would be set at a rate which would generate more funds for health care. Indeed, fewer funds might be available if the government had a commitment to low taxation or feared a hostile reaction from those who paid taxes. In any case, the proposal was unlikely to succeed given the long-standing opposition of the Treasury to all forms of earmarked tax.

In the event, the review rejected both insurance systems and earmarked taxes by accepting that the NHS would continue to be funded mainly out of general taxation. Indeed, a tax-funded system has a number of advantages (see House of Commons, 1988b). Most taxes raise funds on the basis of ability to pay, whereas health care is supposed to be allocated on the basis of need. This, in theory, benefits the healthy at the expense of the wealthy. The system not only distributes between rich and poor, but it also redistributes over the lifecycle. The majority of NHS spending (about 65 per cent) is on services for children and the elderly, while most taxes are raised from those of working age. Hence people contribute most to the service when they are earning (through direct taxes on income) and spending (through purchase taxes), and benefit most when their incomes and expenditure levels are relatively low. The system is equitable in that over the average individual's lifetime these contributions and benefits tend to level out.

The tax-funded health care system also represents a relatively cheap way of raising resources. Funds are raised as part of a general system of tax assessment and collection. Some of the proposed alternatives – particularly health insurance systems – would involve the creation of a new revenue collection system, and considerable additional cost and bureaucracy.

A further advantage of tax-funding is that it places an overall limit on health care spending. The competing bids of other public service programmes act as a powerful restraint on the health budget. Many would argue that this is a disadvantage, given the perceived need for more resources in health care. For a Conservative government, keen to restrain public spending on health care, this feature was a major plus and was the main reason why alternative sources of funding were rejected by the review.

☐ Internal markets

Having turned its back on alternative systems of funding, the review focused on the allocation of resources within the NHS. A number of schemes were put forward to introduce competition into the NHS. Competition and economic incentives were seen by a number of observers, largely on the political right, to be the spur for greater cost-efficiency and responsiveness to the consumer (Brown *et al.*, 1988; Butler and Pirie, 1988: Owen, 1988; Redwood, 1988; Whitney, 1988).

Such ideas were not brand new. The problem of perverse incentives within the NHS had been noted a few years earlier by an American academic, Alain Enthoven (1985). He believed that the NHS was caught in 'gridlock', a condition of general rigidity and inflexibility. Ministers were too closely involved with detailed service matters, while the health care professions resisted attempts to improve efficiency. Enthoven argued that better value for money could be achieved by improving economic incentives so that the most efficient providers were rewarded, claiming 'that there is nothing like a competitive market to motivate quality and economy of service'. He suggested the creation of an internal market in which health authorities would buy services from doctors and other health care providers on behalf of their resident populations as a possible remedy to the problems of the NHS.

☐ Health maintenance organisations

Enthoven's analysis drew heavily on the US experience, where greater competition had been introduced in the form of health maintenance organisations (HMOs). Individuals subscribe to an HMO, usually on an annual basis. If they become ill, the HMO provides care, either directly or by contracting with other providers. By the late 1980s around a fifth of the US population was enrolled in HMOs, and the scheme was heralded as a revolutionary development in achieving cost-effectiveness in health care.

Enthoven himself warned about the dangers of importing the HMO idea direct from the US, where more than half of health care is privately funded. Others, such as Petchey (1987) have argued that the HMO has a mixed record even in the US context. HMOs in particular tend to underprovide, particularly for the poor and chronically sick. Moreover, in recent years many HMOs have faced severe financial problems. Some have been taken over by other HMOs. The result has been a closure of facilities and a reduction in competition.

Nevertheless, many of the ideas submitted to the NHS review were based more or less on the HMO model. Goldsmith and Willetts' (1988) plan for a system of 'managed health care organisations' (MHCOs) is a fairly typical example. According to this scheme, MHCOs would take over the role of District Health Authorities and Family Practitioner Committees. They would be funded by tax revenues in order to purchase health care on behalf of their resident populations from hospitals, GPs and other health care providers. Subsequently, the private sector would be allowed to compete with the public-sector MHCOs for subscribers. Individuals would fund the difference between the premiums charged by MHCOs and the amount funded by taxation, generating additional health spending. The more radical HMO-type schemes did not ultimately receive the backing of the NHS review. There was, however, some support for fundholding schemes, which emphasised the gatekeeper role of the GP within the NHS (Bevan et al., 1988; Bosanquet, 1986; Culyer et al., 1988). Although details varied, these schemes were similar in principle: GP practices would receive a budget related closely to the number of patients on their lists; this budget would be used to pay directly for hospital and other health services; and GPs would compete for patients in order to generate revenue. Those practices which used their budgets most effectively would attract patients and expand; and those which were ineffective would contract and eventually go out of business.

The internal market was an idea whose time had come. It was later revealed that the government had earlier, in the mid-1980s in fact, toyed with the idea of an internal market. The NHS Management Board had explored this possibility in 1986, but rejected the idea as being impractical. It has also been alleged that the Conservatives considered putting a commitment to an internal market in their 1987 election manifesto (Owen, 1988). Since then, it appears that electoral victory and the financial and political problems of the NHS had caused the government to disregard caution.

■ *Working for Patients*

The government's health care review culminated in January 1989 with the publication of the White Paper *Working for Patients* (Cm 555, 1989). The White Paper covered a large number of issues, some of which continued earlier policy themes and initiatives. These included the extension of the Resource Management Initiative (RMI), the formal introduction of medical audit and changes in the composition of health authorities. *Working for Patients* also built on the government's reform of primary care, set out in an earlier White Paper, *Promoting Better Health* (Cm 249, 1987), which is discussed in detail in Chapter 9. Yet the core of *Working for Patients* did represent an important new departure: an internal market for health care, based on a system of contracting for services between purchasers and providers. The main proposals of the White Paper are shown in Exhibit 8.1.

☐ *Criticism of the White Paper: inefficient markets*

The central thrust of the White Paper – the internal market (see Figure 8.1) – suffered heavy criticism. As discussed in Chapter 7, there are strong arguments against the use of markets in health care. Although there are also potential benefits in employing market forces in this sector, these tend to be asserted rather than demonstrated (Hudson, 1992; Le Grand and Bartlett, 1993).

Exhibit 8.1 'Working for Patients'

The main areas of reform

(a) Changes at the centre

Within the Department of Health, the establishment of a new policy board responsible for strategic decisions and an NHS management executive, responsible for the running of the service.

(b) Health authorities

1. Regional Health Authorities to focus on monitoring performance, evaluating effectiveness and reviewing the state of their population's health, and to concentrate less on managing services directly.
2. District Health Authorities to delegate service delivery to hospitals wherever possible, and to set targets and monitor performance of providers.
3. Family Practitioner Committees to become more managerial in outlook and organisation (They were later renamed Family Health Service Authorities). FPCs to have extra responsibilities for monitoring GP budgets, prescribing and the quality of care provided by GPs. FPCs to be responsible to the Regional Health Authority rather than directly to the Department of Health.
4. The composition of Health Authorities to be altered. Health authorities to be smaller, comprising executive members (managers) and non-executive members appointed for their skills and experience. Health Authorities no longer required to include local authority representatives.

(c) The internal market

1. RHAs in future to receive funding for their resident populations, weighted by age and morbidity. Districts also to receive funding based on a 'weighted' resident population. Regions and districts to purchase services on behalf of their populations from providers in the public or private sector (see Figure 8.1 on p. 180)
2. Hospitals and community units allowed to apply for self-governing trust (SGT) status. Trusts remain within the NHS, but given much more freedom to buy and sell assets, to build up financial surpluses, to establish their own management structures, to employ staff, and to set pay and conditions. Trusts' income generated by selling services to the purchasers of health care (GPs, health authorities and the private sector).
3. GP practices with more than 11 000 patients (subsequently reduced to 9000 and later 7000) permitted to apply to manage their own budgets (fundholding). These GPs able to buy selected non-emergency services from providers (directly managed units, trusts, the private sector) on behalf of their patients. In addition, all GPs to have prescription budgets.
4. Purchasers and providers to operate on the basis of contracts specifying the price and level of the service provided (see Exhibit 8.2).

5. Capital charging. To encourage the efficient use of assets and to promote fair competition, NHS providers to be charged for their use of assets such as land, buildings and equipment worth over £1000.

(d) Hospital consultants and quality of service

1. Districts to agree 'job descriptions' with each consultant.
2. General managers to have a role in merit awards for consultants.
3. All hospital doctors would have to take part in medical audit.
4. Resource management to be introduced to all hospitals.
5. The Audit Commission, a body which investigates the efficiency of local government, to have its brief extended to the NHS.

(e) The private sector

1. People aged over 60 to be given tax relief on their private health insurance premiums.
2. Health authorities and GP budget holders encouraged to use private health facilities for their patients where this is cost effective. Further joint ventures between private and public sectors to be encouraged (see Chapter 7, p. 157).

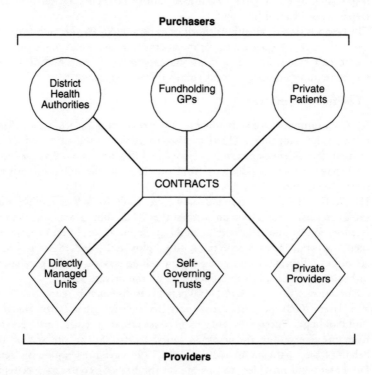

Purchasers

District Health Authorities

Fundholding GPs

Private Patients

CONTRACTS

Directly Managed Units

Self-Governing Trusts

Private Providers

Providers

Figure 8.1   *The internal market*

For Burke and Goddard (1990), drawing on Williamson's (1975) work on the comparative efficiency of markets and organisational hierarchies, there are strong reasons why health markets fail to deliver services efficiently. In Williamson's model, markets tend to be less effective than hierarchies in the following circumstances: where there are small numbers of specialist providers; where great uncertainty and technical complexity exist; where providers or purchasers can be tied into contracts for long periods; where there is imperfect knowledge about costs; and, where scope for 'opportunistic behaviour' exists. In these situations transaction costs are high and have to be offset against the possible benefits of a market. Burke and Goddard claim that an internal market in the NHS possesses these characteristics and is therefore likely to deliver services less efficiently than a hierarchical organisation (see also Bartlett, 1991).

These arguments were supported to some extent by the 'rubber windmill' exercise, a simulation of the internal market undertaken during 1990 (Office for Public Management, 1991). At the end of this exercise, the market became unworkable because the individual participants were pursuing their own self-interests without regard to an overall strategic or planning framework. The lesson of the 'rubber windmill' was that the market would descend into anarchy in the absence of regulation, clearly agreed health strategies, and explicit quality of service criteria.

☐ *Market power*

Others believe that an internal market will be affected by the same kinds of failure that plague private health care markets (see Appleby *et al.*, 1990; Robinson, 1990). In a private health care market there is an imbalance in the knowledge, information and power of consumers of health care (the patients) and those who provide health services. The internal market attempts to tackle this imbalance by creating purchasing authorities (such as GP fundholding practices and District Health Authorities) which have more clout than the average individual patient.

Even so, providers may still have the edge. This is because of the limited number of providers in any given locality. The deliberate policy of encouraging a smaller number of large district general hospitals has reduced the scope for competition in the supply side of the internal market. The private sector may, of course, provide additional competition, but the geographical spread of private facilities is uneven and this means that in some localities, particularly in the North, competition is very limited.

For many, market forces do not guarantee that the interests of patients are upheld. Indeed, there are strong reasons for believing that a market system could undermine the interests of patients. One of the main principles of the internal market is that money follows the patient. In theory the most efficient providers of health care will attract the greatest amount of revenue because they give the best value for money in the eyes of the purchaser and an acceptable service from the point of view of the patient. But in practice the internal market seems to reverse this. Patients instead follow the contracts negotiated between purchasers and providers. If a purchasing authority does not have a contract with a particular provider, its patients can have great difficulty in obtaining treatment from that provider, even if it is cost-effective and appropriate. This appears to be a major restriction on the choice of both patients and non-fundholding GPs. It also raises the possibility of inconvenience for the patient, particularly where the chosen hospital is some distance away.

Stories of patients being transported long distances for treatment as a result of the internal market have perhaps been exaggerated. Yet they are not entirely without foundation. The White Paper contained no guarantees that patients' interests would be protected when contracts were drawn up. The role of community health councils (CHCs) – the patients' watchdogs in the NHS – was not clarified. Indeed, in the restructuring of health authorities which followed the White Paper, many CHC representatives were prevented from attending meetings and many others were kept in the dark about health authority contracting decisions. Nor are the new 'business-like' health authorities likely to be in a better position to judge matters from the perspective of the patient. Indeed, the removal of local authority representatives from the health authority boards distances them further from the people they serve. The impact of the market upon patients is further explored later in this chapter.

☐ Quality and access to services

The reforms also raise questions about the impact on the quality of services. There has been concern that the purchasing authorities would place their contracts on the basis of price alone, in the absence of regulation from some central authority (Scrivens and Henneh, 1989). Yet price is not inevitably a good indicator of quality. In the absence of information about quality, purchasing authorities have no alternative but to purchase care on the basis of price information. This has given rise to fears that high-quality, high-cost producers will lose out in the market-place and that low-cost, low quality providers will emerge victorious.

A further problem associated with health care markets is that of access. Markets do not allocate resources equitably, on the basis of need. Some argue that market forces heighten the impact of the inverse care law: where good medical care is allocated to those least in need (Tudor-Hart, 1971).

Even in a publicly-funded health care system, allocation by market forces could create perverse incentives. Patients with extreme (and costly) medical needs could be regarded as 'bad for the budget' and may even be denied access to care. This practice is a feature of market-style health systems (Weiner and Ferriss, 1990).

Some American commentators have been at pains to point out the dangers of market forces as allocators of health care. Donald Light (1990a) has claimed that the British government imported American ideas without considering the problems associated with markets. He goes on to observe that there are important differences between the UK and the USA which could lead to unforeseen problems. For example, a shortage of suppliers in the UK compared with the USA makes it more likely that a 'seller's' market would emerge in the UK.

Ironically, at the same time as the UK was considering the introduction of market forces into the NHS, the United States was debating the future of its own system. Many observers believe that the increased competition during the 1980s failed to solve the problem of rising health care costs in the USA (Wood, 1990). Meanwhile, the opportunity of access to health care deteriorated as the uninsured population rose. Pressure for reform subsequently led the US government to consider a reorganisation of health care.

☐ *Incentives*

Some commentators strongly believe that both the achievements and the fundamental principles of the NHS have been seriously threatened by the introduction of an internal market. McLachlan (1990), for example, is not alone in his assertion that the NHS has in the past provided a relatively cheap yet effective service (see also Owen, 1988; Paton, 1992). This achievement, it should be noted, has been based largely on the efforts of health care professionals, in the absence of financial incentives.

For McLachlan, the reforms introduced by *Working for Patients* damage the existing incentive structure within health care. He has argued that the reforms fail to recognise that those who work in the NHS do not in general respond to crude financial incentives. Such incentives cut across and undermine traditional values which motivate health professionals, such as dedication, trust, a sense of vocation and self-improvement.

This may appear to be a rather rosy view of professionalism, particularly from the point of view of the political right and anti-professionals such as Illich, discussed in Chapter 3 (see p. 69). But nevertheless McLachlan raises a crucial point. People working in the NHS have been motivated by other factors over and above financial incentives, and it is important that these are recognised. Above all, one should not dispense with values which maintain and improve a caring, high-quality health service, by simply imposing new incentives which, if not properly thought out, may work against the grain, producing an inferior service.

☐ *Planning*

There has also been a great deal of concern about the impact of the internal market on the planning of health services (McLachlan, 1990; House of Commons, 1989b). Certainly, a market approach, with its numerous buyers and sellers of services and its absence of formal command structures, does appear to confound planning. Moreover, many other countries are moving away from the kind of fragmented structure created by *Working for Patients* in an attempt to improve planning (Paton, 1992, p. 72).

However, some believe that the division between purchasing authorities and providers may actually improve planning (Ham and Mitchell, 1990; Ham and Matthews, 1991). Freed from the responsibilities of managing service delivery, purchasers may be in a better position to evaluate the health needs of the population and to plan and commission services accordingly. It is also possible that a more appropriate mix of health care may result from, for example, altering the balance between budgets for prevention, care and treatment.

Planning is not necessarily incompatible with the market. What the government envisaged was a type of business planning for the NHS, with the main actors in the market, the purchasers and providers, rather like firms in the business sector, developing their own plans in the light of market conditions. Yet it has become clear that these plans must be reconciled within an overall health strategy. The government has subsequently tried to encourage a form of co-operative planning through changes to the planning process, as we discussed in Chapter 6. Furthermore, the publication of yet another White Paper in 1992, on the subject of health strategy, reflected a recognition that the market could not operate in the absence of health objectives and targets. This initiative is discussed further in Chapter 11.

■ Implementing internal markets

The timetable for the implementation of *Working for Patients* was short. The government intended that the main elements of the programme would be in place within two years. There was a strong feeling, particularly among the health care professions, that the reforms should at least be piloted and tested before continuing any further towards a market system. Indeed, one of the main exponents of the internal market, Alain Enthoven, was himself concerned at both the pace at which the government intended to proceed and the lack of evaluation of the reforms. He was also critical of the government's specific proposals, in particular GP fundholding and tax relief on private insurance for the elderly (May, 1989). Nevertheless, the government continued to resist an extension of the proposed timetable. It was also hostile to independent evaluation of the reforms. However, there was some backtracking on these commitments at the implementation stage, as we shall see in a moment.

Most of the government's plans required legislation. The main vehicle for this was the NHS and Community Care Act which became law in June 1990. Despite the controversy surrounding the reforms and the hostility of the main organisations representing health professions and workers, the government steered its legislation through Parliament fairly smoothly. It was helped by its large majority in the House of Commons and by the skilful use of parliamentary rules that severely curtailed debate: 252 new clauses and amendments to the legislation went undebated while 100 government amendments were carried in one vote. A few minor concessions were made along the way. For example, under pressure from the professions, the government agreed to establish a statutory Clinical Standards Advisory Group to evaluate the impact of the reforms upon standards of care in the NHS.

☐ The steady state

Despite the smooth passage of the legislation, opposition remained. At this stage the government appeared ready to consider the problems of implementing the reforms. At the same time ministers started to play down the 'market' element in the reforms, speaking of 'managed competition' rather than internal markets. As the government began to distance itself from the market language of the White Paper, it also became clear that the pace of the reforms was slowing, and that important developments were being undertaken at the implementation stage (Butler, 1992).

There was some backtracking on the funding of health authorities. Their budgets were to be based on the size of the resident population, adjusted to take account of health care needs, a system known as 'weighted capitation'. Weighted capitation was to have been introduced within two years. But the government feared this would lead to a dramatic fall in the demand for some services, in particular those provided by the larger London hospitals. Therefore it was agreed that health authorities in London would be granted extra resources as a cushion in the short term. At the same time, an inquiry was established into the future of health services in the capital. This represented an attempt to plan the rationalisation of London hospitals rather than to allow the market to prompt the closures directly. These developments effectively slowed down the movement to weighted capitation and this will not be fully implemented until 1998 in some regions. By 1993 one in six health authority budgets were still at least 6 per cent higher or lower than the weighted capitation targets set by the Department of Health. One in ten were at least 9 per cent over or under target (NAHAT, 1993).

□ Health care in London: the Tomlinson report

The problems of London's health care system are well known. First, there is an imbalance between the existing pattern of health services and the health needs of the population. London is relatively well provided for in terms of acute hospital care, having around 25 per cent more acute beds than the average for England. The size and importance of the acute sector in London reflects the historical importance of the capital as a centre for medical education, research and specialisation. On the other hand, London has relatively poor primary and community health care facilities. In particular, there are a large number of GPs working on their own. Such GPs are often housed in unsuitable premises and have fewer support staff when compared with the national average. There is also a shortage of nursing and residential accommodation for the elderly in the capital.

Second, the London population has complex health needs. There is great social deprivation in the capital, which generates a wide range of health problems. In particular, there is a large homeless and rootless population. There is also a large ethnic population, which has diverse needs. To add to this, London has a great influx of visitors on a daily basis, tourists and commuters, who may require health care in the event of accidents and emergencies.

Third, there is a great variation in the quality of care within as well as between the hospital, primary and community care sectors. In addition, health services in the capital are regarded as high in cost, and in many respects inefficient. Londoners have longer hospital stays on average than patients outside the capital (around 10 per cent longer on average), though this is to some extent a consequence of poor community and primary care provision. London hospitals are also relatively expensive to run, and have higher-than-average staffing costs.

Finally, London's health care system is plagued by poor planning and weak co-ordination. Specialist services are often duplicated, while other services are patchy and fragmented, and there is poor co-ordination between the various sectors of health care. The situation is exacerbated by the division of responsibility for health and social care in London among a large number of Regional and District Health Authorities, Family Health Service Authorities and local councils.

The problems of health care in London are not new and have been well documented (Benzeval, Judge and New, 1991). Yet little was done to resolve the situation until it became exacerbated by two factors. First, in the late 1970s, there was the introduction of RAWP, which moved resources away from the London health authorities that had historically received relatively generous budget allocations. This shortfall prompted health authorities in London to cut back on acute services during the 1980s.

The second factor was the internal market, which meant that in future London hospitals would have to compete with each other, as well as with other hospitals outside the capital. The internal market makes the London hospitals vulnerable in two respects. First, the duplication of services in London suggests that the market will be fairly competitive there, driving prices (and revenues) down for all providers. Second, London hospitals are disadvantaged by the relatively high cost of providing services in the capital. Purchasing authorities have begun to transfer at least some of their resources to lower cost providers, some of which are located outside London.

The net effect of this has been market-led rationalisation, with London hospitals contemplating closure in the face of falling demand, but with no guarantee that primary and community care services would expand accordingly. The government responded to this politically sensitive situation by embarking on a planned rationalisation programme for the capital's health services. In 1991 Sir Bernard Tomlinson was appointed to report on how this could best be achieved.

The thrust of Tomlinson's report, published the following year, was that primary care should be expanded at the expense of the acute sector (Tomlinson, 1992). The report suggested that as many as 2500 hospital beds needed to be cut. This was broadly supported, though many worried about acute facilities being closed before primary care facilities had been properly developed. More controversial were the specific proposals for closing acute units. Tomlinson argued that at least ten hospitals – including the prestigious St Bartholomew's (Bart's) teaching hospital – should close, and that others should merge.

The government undertook a period of consultation following the Tomlinson report. This exercise was marked by intense lobbying by hospitals, trade unions, professionals and patients most affected by the rationalisation plan. It was widely expected that the government would dilute the Tomlinson recommendations in the light of this campaign. However, the government's response, published in February 1993 (DoH, 1993), upheld the inquiry's broad conclusions, while adopting a cautious and low-profile rationalisation programme in an attempt to defuse the political campaign to save the hospitals. Some of the threatened units (such as St Bartholomew's) were given a stark choice of whether to merge, shrink or close. Implementation of the rationalisation plans was delegated to a special implementation group, while rationalisation of specialist services was subjected to a further review of services in the capital. This process took place within a fairly tight timetable, a matter of months. The government sugared the pill with an extra £170m for primary care initiatives aimed at reducing the pressure on the acute sector in the short term.

The situation in London is often depicted as being a special case. Certainly, the problems of the capital are more severe than those faced by other cities in the UK, but these problems are not unique (Maxwell, 1993). All major cities face, to some extent, health problems related to social deprivation, the particular health needs of ethnic minorities, imbalances between primary and hospital care and so on. Moreover, the acute sector outside London faces similar consequences with respect to the internal market. If, as seems likely in the future, purchasers begin to switch contracts to lower-cost providers and lower-cost services (such as day-surgery), and from hospital to community-based provision, the Tomlinson axe will be applied more widely throughout the hospital sector in the UK.

☐ Contracts

Another sign of the slackening pace of the reforms lay in the guidance given to the health authorities. In effect, this advice proposed a 'steady state', with new contracts reflecting the current pattern of services (DoH, 1990a). Health authorities were also encouraged to use block contracts in preference to other types of contract (see Exhibit 8.2). These would create a much more predictable situation. Health authorities were also told that the new contracts would have to mirror the current referral patterns of local GPs unless there were compelling reasons not to do so (DoH, 1990b).

It also became clear that the freedom of the self-governing trusts (SGTs) would be limited (DoH, 1990c; Hughes and Dingwall, 1990, p. 1770). Ministers have the power to set the financial objectives of trusts, to set

---

Exhibit 8.2   Contracts for health care

There are three main types of contract:

1. **Block contracts**. The provider receives a fixed payment for services given. The numbers and types of cases treated under the contract are not specifically designated.
2. **Cost and volume contracts**. Providers receive a fixed sum for a basic level of treatment, and receive extra payments for treating patients beyond this level.
3. **Cost per case contracts**. Providers receive an agreed price for each case treated.

It should be noted that NHS contracts are not enforceable through the courts (Hughes, 1990). Disputes over contracts are referred to Regional Health Authorities, or ultimately to the Department of Health.

---

limits on their borrowing, and to control their financial surpluses. They also appoint some of the members of the trust management board. Ministers can, if they wish, dissolve a trust. The government also made it clear that trusts would have to provide services designated as being essential by the relevant health authority.

The introduction of the NHS trusts was staggered. Only fifty-seven units in England were granted trust status in the so-called 'first wave' beginning in April 1991. These were joined by another ninety-nine in the following year, and a further 137 in 1993. Together these formed a formidable bloc of providers, consuming over two-thirds of the total NHS budget. It is anticipated that the vast majority of providers will in future take the form of SGTs.

The GP fundholding scheme was implemented at a slower pace. Only 306 GP practices, covering 6 per cent of the population, adopted fundholding in the first year. Following the second wave of GP fundholders, which became operational in April 1992, around 3000 GPs had fundholding status, covering about 14 per cent of the population. By 1993 a quarter of the population were covered by fundholders and this is expected to rise to around 50 per cent by 1995.

The reforms were introduced at a slower pace than the government had originally envisaged. The rhetoric of the market was being played down. It is also clear that the internal market was more centralised and more closely regulated by the Department of Health and the regional health authorities than many of its more enthusiastic supporters believed should be the case. The reasons for this are discussed below.

☐ *The political context*

Changes at the top provide a possible explanation of why the government applied the brakes to reform. In early November 1990, Kenneth Clarke, who had steered through the legislative changes, was succeeded as Secretary of State for Health by William Waldegrave, who displayed a much more conciliatory approach than had his predecessor. The replacement of Margaret Thatcher as Prime Minister by John Major a few weeks later brought a similar change in style at Number 10 Downing Street, with Major presenting himself more convincingly as a supporter of the NHS, and of public services generally.

Although it is possible that the implementation of the NHS reforms was affected by these changes in political office, it is doubtful that they were crucial. Department of Health guidance slowing down the reforms, mentioned earlier, was issued before Margaret Thatcher's resignation.

Perhaps more important than changes in personality at the top were the electoral consequences of reform. Conservative MPs, many of whom had faced a great deal of pressure from constituents on the subject of the NHS, were well aware that the reforms were highly unpopular. Opinion polls consistently showed that between a half and three-quarters of the public were opposed to the reforms. Worse still for the government, the NHS remained high on the political agenda during 1990 and 1991 as a general election approached. Attributing a number of by-election defeats directly to the NHS reforms, Conservative MPs urged Ministers to avoid anything that might provoke public hostility and cause electoral defeat.

Health Ministers responded by issuing a booklet, at an estimated cost of over £2m, aimed at alleviating public concern (DoH, 1990d). The booklet explained the reforms, carefully avoiding commercial or business language. It was heavily criticised as a propaganda exercise and a waste of resources.

The public remained opposed to the reforms, according to most opinion polls. Meanwhile, the organisations representing NHS professionals and workers kept the issue very much in the public eye and accentuated the electoral problems for the government. The heat of the anti-reform campaigns did cool slightly following the changes at the Department of Health and in Number 10. The main professional associations enjoyed a more constructive dialogue with the government, although they continued to oppose both the principle and the detail of the reforms.

Practical as well as political difficulties acted as a constraint on the reforms. NHS managers, many of whom supported the changes, told the government that its timetable of reform was hopelessly unrealistic. In their view, the infrastructure of the internal market, the staff, computers, procedures and above all the financial management systems necessary for an internal market to operate, could not be in place in time. This view was shared by the Social Services Committee (House of Commons, 1989b), the Audit Commission (1991), and the NAO (1989b). Eventually this message was accepted by the government, which was already well aware of the political problems of moving ahead too quickly.

☐ The impact of the internal market

Despite the 'steady-state' approach, the introduction of the internal market in April 1991 was accompanied by dramatic headlines. First, a number of Trust hospitals – notably Guy's and Lewisham Trust in London and Bradford Royal Infirmary, announced between them almost 1000 redundancies. This led to predictions that the trust hospitals would be at the forefront of staff cuts, and generated widespread fears about service levels.

The focus on hospital trusts continued, with concern that many of the newly-created trusts were not financially viable. The Health Committee expressed concern about the future extension of trust status on this and other grounds. Its report, published in the run-up to the general election was toned down following pressure from Conservative members of the committee (House of Commons, 1991). Subsequent reports from the committee (House of Commons, 1992) have identified three major problem areas associated with the creation of trusts. First, the potential loss of strategic planning implied by the fragmentation of the service into trusts. Second, problems associated with the dismantling of national pay and conditions. Also, in this category, issues such as job security and the imposition of so-called 'gagging' contracts which prevented staff from speaking out on trust policies. Third, the lack of public consultation and accountability within the new regime.

The government responded to this criticism in three main ways. First, by allocating reserve funds to regional health authorities, which could be used to support trusts in a financial emergency. Second, by publishing crude activity statistics which suggested that the new trusts were outperforming the directly managed units (DMUs) (NHSME, 1992b). Total activity in NHS trusts reportedly rose by 8.2 per cent compared with an increase of 6.9 per cent in DMUs. Third, the NHS Management Executive issued a document which encouraged purchasers to be more sensitive to local needs. This will be discussed later (see p. 196).

☐ Fundholding

The impact of GP fundholding has been mixed. Although fundholders' budgets so far represent a small proportion of health authority financial allocations, around 2 per cent in 1992/3, providers have been fairly sensitive to their needs (NAHAT, 1993). At the margin, these revenues are very important in enabling providers to balance their books. As a result, GP fundholders found that they could negotiate favourable contracts, and that their patients benefited from a quicker and more flexible service for non-emergency care. Meanwhile, there was evidence that patients of non-budget-holding GPs were waiting longer for operations, irrespective of their needs (see, for example, *Independent*, 3 May 1991, p. 2). The Department of Health convened talks with the Joint Consultants' Committee in an attempt to reassure the public that patients would be admitted on the basis of clinical needs and a code of practice was subsequently implemented. But as the internal market developed, allegations that fundholders' patients received priority treatment returned.

An independent report on the experience of the first wave of GP fundholders could throw no light on this problem (Glennerster, Owens and Matsaganis, 1992). Nor did it find any evidence that fundholding GPs were discriminating against 'expensive' high-risk patients, as some had suggested might happen. The report accepted that the benefits of fundholding, such as shorter waiting times and a more responsive service for patients, were largely confined to the fundholding practices. But it went on to argue that in the longer term all practices (including those GPs who remained non-fundholders) could benefit from the efficiency stimulated by fundholding.

However, Glennerster and his colleagues did not give fundholding an entirely clean bill of health in their report. Flaws were identified in the allocation of resources to GPs, which reflected historical costs rather than the efficiency of practices or their patient's needs (see Day and Klein, 1991). A number of problems were also identified in relation to the contracting process, with some providers remaining hostile to the demands of GP fundholders.

The Audit Commission (1993a, 1993b), in a review of purchasing authorities, also recognised the benefits of fundholding. However, it also identified a number of crucial problems. The Audit Commission believed that an extension of the scheme in its present form could be problematic, for a number of reasons. First, GP fundholders were not integrated within a strategic framework. They could therefore frustrate national and local policy objectives by pursuing their own narrow self-interests. This echoed earlier criticisms from health authority managers, who believed that fundholding was a threat to the coherent planning of services (NAHAT, 1992).

Second, the Audit Commission was concerned about the lack of accountability of fundholders. Forty practices had made surpluses of over £100 000, while a number of others had mismanaged their resources. One practice, in Sheffield, had its fundholding status removed after over-spending by £100 000. Such cases reflected the difficulties experienced by some GPs in managing the fundholding process.

The Audit Commission called for closer co-operation between GP fundholders and other purchasers. One way forward is joint purchasing, discussed on p. 195 below, where district health authorities and FHSAs pool their resources and share knowledge in an effort to commission appropriate patterns of services for their populations. Another idea is 'practice-sensitive purchasing', where local GPs are closely involved in decisions about the commissioning of services for their patients. (Starey *et al.*, 1993; Ham, 1992; Morley, 1993). These schemes attempt to retain the benefits of fundholding, such as flexibility and responsiveness, within a broader framework of planning and accountability.

☐ The wider impact

Further evidence sheds light on the wider impact of the internal market. The NHS Management Executive published a review six months after the creation of the internal market, covering the period April to September 1991. This report, not surprisingly, proclaimed the reform to be a success. It documented a 3.7 per cent increase in patients treated, a fall (by 8000) in the number of patients waiting over two years for treatment, and record levels of childhood immunisation (NHSME, 1991c).

Critics have pointed out that these improvements could not be attributed to the reforms, for a number of reasons. First, some of these statistics, particularly the increase in patients treated, were part of long-term trends. Second, the internal market had been held in a 'steady state' for the first year and hence market forces had not been fully unleashed. It was far too early to judge whether it was a success or a failure. Third, in the run-up to the general election the government had spent money on the NHS, both to ease the implementation of the reforms and to reduce waiting lists. Extra funding rather than increased efficiency was the most probable cause of the trends identified by the government during the first year of the internal market (Radical Statistics Health Group, 1992).

During the second year, however, the brakes which had been applied to the internal market were relaxed. Cost and volume contracts began to replace some of the block contracts, based on past levels of treatment (NAHAT, 1993; Harrison and Wistow, 1992), and a further generation of fundholders entered the market. Although at the time of writing a comprehensive, independent evaluation of the second year has yet to emerge, there were indications at this stage that the market was beginning to operate as intended. Patient activity increased during 1992/3, and providers often exceeded their contract specifications in terms of numbers of patients treated (NAHAT, 1993).

However, towards the end of the 1992/3 financial year, hospitals began to run out of money. As contracts were fulfilled, treatment for non-urgent conditions was cut back. A survey by the 'Today' programme, broadcast on Radio 4 on 1 February 1993, found that 60 per cent of acute-hospital trusts were in this position. Operations were cancelled and waiting lists began to rise once again. The restrictions on treatment towards the end of the financial year did not seem to apply to the patients of GP fundholders, however. Indeed, in a number of hospitals, managers told surgeons to give preference to these patients in an attempt to generate extra revenue. This appeared to contravene the code of practice on admissions, mentioned earlier, and fuelled once again allegations of a two-tier system.

Rather than bridging the gap between needs and resources in health care the internal market began to expose the lack of resources relative to need. Indeed, over two-thirds of health service managers believed that the internal market alone could not solve the fundamental problems of underfunding (NAHAT, 1992). Given the limit on resources, purchasing authorities have had no alternative but to use their budgets as a device to ration care. It is to this development that we shall now turn.

☐ Rationing

It was pointed out in Chapter 3 that rationing is not a new concept within the NHS: what is new is the shift towards *explicit* rationing. As the internal market emerged it was likely that rationing would become increasingly explicit, as purchasers explored ways of maximising the use of their limited budgets. In 1991, for example, North West Thames RHA announced plans to restrict treatment for minor conditions such as benign cysts, wisdom-tooth removal and varicose veins. Other health authorities began to reduce (and in some cases, to end) so-called low priority treatments, such as cosmetic surgery and fertilisation programmes. Even so, there was little evidence at this stage that consistent criteria for rationing were being applied (Harrison and Wistow, 1992). Techniques such as QALYs were explored, but with caution. Moreover, for obvious political reasons the Department of Health was not prepared to give a clear lead in stating which procedures should or should not be available on the NHS.

A further aspect of rationing within the internal market concerns patients whose treatment is not covered by existing contracts. These are known as extra contractual referrals (ECRs). In theory, purchasers retain a reserve to pay for such cases, but in practice the pressure on these funds is enormous, raising the possibility that some patients will simply not obtain NHS treatment in that particular financial year. According to NAHAT (1993), most health authorities have increased their ECR budgets to meet the demand. Even so, between April and September 1992 over 7000 ECR cases (a fifth of the applications for non-emergency treatment) had been refused. The majority of these (70 per cent) did, in fact, obtain NHS treatment, often at the providers' expense. The fate of the remainder was largely unknown, although at least 200 ECR cases were known to have been refused treatment because the purchasing authority lacked funds. Subsequent guidance from the Department of Health ruled this to be an unacceptable reason for refusing ECR cases. A major worry about ECRs is that treatment appears to depend on a mixture of luck and the lobbying power of GPs and consultants. This is not dissimilar to the pre-market situation, where a patient's access to treatment often depended on who their doctor was, where they lived, and the type of treatment they required. Some have called for clear agreements or 'protocols', to ensure that ECR funds are distributed more rationally (Salter, 1992).

☐ *Other implications*

The internal market gave rise to other developments which should be mentioned. The implementation of the reforms required a considerable investment in management systems and personnel. Not surprisingly, the number of NHS managers rose, from 4610 (1989) to 12 340 (1991). Over the same period, the number of administrative and clerical staff went up by 9 per cent, while the numbers of nursing and midwifery staff fell, by 1.5 per cent.

The infrastructure required by the market was not cheap: over £257m was spent on implementing the reforms (House of Commons, 1991, p. xii). The cost was a cause for concern, even among managers (NAHAT, 1992). Once the market was operating, further structural changes also took place and mergers between DHAs became commonplace (Ham and Heginbotham, 1991). Before the reforms began in 1989, there were 190 DHAs. It is anticipated that by the late 1990s, there could be less than a hundred. Ironically, these authorities will be similar in size and number to the much-maligned Area Health Authorities (AHAs) abolished by the Conservatives in 1982. The main reason given for such mergers is that larger purchasers are in a stronger position relative to providers. Merging may also counteract the leverage of GP fundholders in the internal market.

A further development has been the emergence of joint purchasing arrangements between DHAs and the Family Health Service Authorities (FHSAs) which are responsible for family practitioner services. The government for a long time has resisted mergers between FHSAs and DHAs. However, it encouraged the development of formalised joint purchasing arrangements, or 'health commissions' as they are also known. There were forty such arrangements in England by the middle of 1993. Supporters of joint purchasing argue that they will produce more effective planning and better integration of primary and hospital care services (Audit Commission, 1993a).

Virginia Bottomley, who succeeded William Waldegrave as Secretary of State for Health after the 1992 election, was responsible for implementing the structural changes that followed the introduction of the internal market. In 1993 she announced a number of changes to the NHS market structure. New legislation was proposed to enable FHSAs and DHAs to merge. While the RHAs, which had been criticised by the NHS trusts for 'over-regulating' the market, are to be slimmed down and eventually abolished. Most of their functions will in future be undertaken by eight regional directorates based on the NHSME regional outposts (see p. 107).

☐ What about the patient?

There is a feeling that the internal market has neglected patients' desires and interests and the public has been opposed to the reforms. There has been little consultation with patients on specific plans to confer fundholding or trust status. Neither patients nor their representative bodies – the CHCs – have a right to participate directly in the contracting process. Even those on the radical right have commented about the weakness of patients and the lack of consumer responsiveness in the new NHS (Green *et al.*, 1990).

Health authorities are now encouraged to pay attention to 'local voices' and to become 'champions of the people' (NHSME, 1992a). But this operates very much on the basis of the 'supermarket model' of consumerism, mentioned in Chapter 3. The emphasis is upon monitoring local opinion through various forms of market research rather than upon public consultation and participation.

During the 1980s there were some positive moves to improve the rights of patients. For example, since 1987 patients have been able to obtain access to medical records held on computer. This right was extended to manual records compiled from November 1991. However, access to medical records can still be refused if the doctor feels that it may cause serious harm to the patient or a third party.

The introduction of the Patients' Charter in 1992 was also heralded as an attempt to redress the balance in the patients' favour (DoH, 1991). This initiative was part of a wider strategy – the Citizens' Charter – geared to making the public sector more responsive to the consumer. The Patients' Charter sets out a number of national rights and service standards that patients can expect. Since 1992, local health authorities have been expected to produce their own local charters, geared to their specific circumstances.

Seven out of the ten rights set out in the national Charter previously existed. These included the right to be registered with a GP, and the right to treatment on the basis of need, regardless of ability to pay. Three new rights were created. First, that no patient should be on a waiting list for treatment for more than two years. Second, that detailed information should be available about local health services (including waiting times and quality standards). Third, that patients should have a full and prompt investigation of complaints.

No one disagrees with these rights in principle. Yet there are doubts that they will be realised in practice. The rights set out in the Charter are not legal rights. Patients who feel that they have been denied their rights can ultimately take the matter up with the Chief Executive of the NHS. It should be noted that many of the existing rights – the right to a GP, for example, – are not upheld in practice. Many homeless people, for example, find it difficult to register with a GP because they have no fixed address.

There is also cynicism about the service standards that are contained in the Charter. Some of these have been seen as being purely cosmetic exercises – for example, the naming of nurses responsible for each patient. Others are regarded as a major step forward if properly implemented. Waiting times at out-patient clinics – a regular source of irritation – are limited by the Charter to within thirty minutes of a specific appointment time. But there are worries even about such apparently reasonable targets. It is believed that the outcome for patients may well be undesirable if the focus of concern moves away from the comfort and care of the patient towards the achievement of crude, mechanistic targets such as waiting times.

Indeed, there are important lessons to be learned from the experience of implementing the 'right' to a maximum two-year waiting time for treatment. The Department of Health decreed that this limit be in place by March 1992. By this time according to official figures, no patients were waiting beyond twenty-four months (DoH and OPCS, 1993b). The reduction in two-year waits from 50 000 in March 1991 to zero a year later was accompanied by an equally dramatic fall in the number of patients waiting between one and two years. However, the total number of patients waiting for treatment remained fairly constant, at over 900 000. This was because those waiting under a year during this period (the largest category on the waiting list) had actually increased, by approximately 5 per cent. In the year since the general election in April 1992 overall waiting lists have risen, for reasons outlined earlier. In March 1993 the number of patients on waiting lists stood at 992 324, an increase of over 8 per cent since the election.

Opposition parties have alleged that these figures underestimate the true size of waiting lists and that the figures are manipulated for political reasons. In some hospitals it appears that minor conditions, which cost less to treat, are being dealt with ahead of more serious cases. There is also evidence of patients awaiting minor surgery being removed from waiting lists. In some places, hospitals have begun closing waiting lists for non-urgent cases (*Independent*, 6 November 1991, p. 4).

The waiting lists saga demonstrates how crude targets can in certain circumstances operate against certain patients. More generally, the Patients' Charter, though in principle a step in the right direction, is unlikely to benefit all patients. The most articulate and vociferous are likely to be the main beneficiaries.

Despite more than a decade of reform, the patient appears to have little power and to be a fairly low priority (Harrison *et al.*, 1992). This is illustrated by the rising tide of complaints within the NHS, which reached record levels in the early 1990s. The Health Service Commissioner, who investigates maladministration in the NHS, received 1176 complaints in 1991/2, an increase of almost 20 per cent on the previous year. Over half these complaints were upheld. The General Medical Council also experienced a similar rise, receiving 1301 complaints against doctors in 1991/2. In addition, Family Health Service Authorities, District Health Authorities and hospitals are receiving between them over 50 000 written complaints each year.

The number of complaints is to some extent a reflection both of the willingness of individuals to complain and of the effectiveness of complaints procedures, as well as standards of service. It is widely accepted that a systematic reform of complaints procedures is long overdue, the main criticisms being that there are too many separate complaints systems, that the processing of complaints is slow, that procedures are intimidating to patients, and that there is little scope for redress or compensation within these various systems. During the 1980s improvements were made to complaints procedures. In 1988 the DHSS specified clearer procedures for health authorities to follow when dealing with complaints and the government subsequently outlined plans to make it easier to complain about family practitioner services, as will be seen in Chapter 10. In addition, the Patients' Charter, as noted earlier, set out the right to have any complaint fully and promptly investigated.

Even so, these attempts at reform were not systematic. They failed to address the fragmented nature of complaints procedures and the relative weakness of patients when faced with bureaucracy and professional power. Patients' groups and consumer bodies have continued to lobby for further change, in particular the establishment of an independent inspectorate to monitor and investigate complaints (National Consumer Council, 1992; Association of Community Health Councils, 1992).

There are a number of other ways in which patients could exert influence over health care (see Exhibit 3.4 on p. 56). Better consumer appraisal is essential, but this is only one component of a more responsive, better-quality health service (Steele, 1992). There has to be more participation in health care by patients and by their representatives to give voice to patients' desires, interests and needs. Many go further and argue that only through empowerment, by giving patients a real say in decisions affecting them, will the balance ever be redressed between patients and providers of health care (Shearer, 1991; Winn, 1990).

■ Conclusion

One of the most common sentiments expressed following the establish-ment of the NHS review in 1988 was that the strengths of the NHS should not be overlooked in seeking a short-term remedy to some of its problems (House of Commons, 1988b). Despite the radical zeal with which the Prime Ministers' review began its work, this message seems to have been taken on board. What eventually emerged was a much more centralised, more regulated and politically-controlled system than the free-marketeers could stomach. Insurance schemes were spurned, and taxation remained the cornerstone of NHS funding.

Even so, the internal market reforms, while impure from a radical right perspective, nevertheless have fairly wide-ranging implications for health care. The system is very much a leap in the dark. The 'steady state' which accompanied the introduction of the market is being replaced by a more dynamic situation where eventual outcomes defy accurate prediction. As Butler (1992) observes, it is simply too early to draw a line across the balance sheet and to say unequivocally whether the reforms are good or bad. The potential benefits – in terms of responsiveness to patients, flexibility and greater efficiency – are certainly worth striving for. In places, these desirable objectives are actually being achieved. But the reforms also involve considerable risks, some of which are clearly evident. The extension of trust status and GP fundholding produces fragmentation and difficulties in the planning of services. The market tends to exaggerate the problem of unequal access to care. Furthermore, the costs of operating the internal market are substantial and ongoing, and may not necessarily be outweighed by the benefits of improved efficiency.

Perhaps the most serious risk of all is that the internal market may have a dynamic of its own. If things do begin to go wrong the process may be irreversible. The victory of the Conservative Party at the 1992 General Election has assured that the reforms are here to stay for the foreseeable future. Opposition parties and professional groups realise that they have little alternative but to work with the new system. Problems that arise will be dealt with by regulating rather than replacing the market. But should the political will to replace the internal market emerge in the future, the clock cannot simply be turned back. The internal market has injected commercial values into socialised health care. The development of this new culture of care, and the entrenchment of market arrangements, underpinned by the vested interests of the 'winners' in the market-place, will make it extremely difficult, if not impossible, for any future government that wishes to get the genie back into the bottle.

■ *Chapter 9* ■

Care in the Community: Primary Health Care

Health care systems throughout the world are developing and extending care based in the community. Community care is seen as being a more appropriate response to growing and increasingly complex health care needs. It is also viewed as a better way of using scarce resources, resulting in a more cost-effective, though not necessarily a less costly, service.

Community care as a concept is open to a variety of interpretations (Higgins, 1989), yet most would agree that the community care ideal is based on a number of fundamental principles: a greater emphasis on care and support in the home; a greater reliance on caring professions practising outside large institutions, and the mobilisation of the community itself, both individual and by collective effort, to care for those in need.

In the past, health policy has been overwhelmingly concerned with hospital services (Stowe, 1989). The relative importance of the hospital sector has been underlined by the large proportion of health care resources devoted to it (see Figures 5.5 and 5.6 on pp. 116–17). Meanwhile community-based care has had a much lower status, lower priority, and a less than adequate budget.

Arguments for a shift in resources from the hospital sector towards community-based services for groups such as the elderly and the mentally ill, have been around for years. The need for a network of good community health services for everyone, not just the vulnerable, has also long been recognised. From the late 1970s such arguments began to carry greater weight within the government as the search began for ways of reducing the pressure on public finances. Community-based care raised the prospect of reducing the cost of hospital care in a variety of ways, creating a powerful incentive to press ahead with such a policy. There were two main aspects to this policy. First, the reform of primary health care – which is the subject of this chapter. Second, the development of social care in the community, explored in Chapter 10.

■ The nature and significance of primary care

Primary care covers all the services provided by the family practitioner services (FPS) – general practitioners (GPs), dentists, pharmacists and opticians. It also includes the care provided by community nurses and midwives, health visitors, and other professions allied to medicine which operate in the community, such as chiropodists and speech therapists. Primary care is provided in a range of non-hospital settings including doctors' surgeries, clinics, special institutions for the handicapped and disabled, and in patients' own homes (Hicks, 1976). It incorporates a range of services which include health maintenance, prevention of illness, diagnosis and treatment, rehabilitation, pastoral care and certification of illness (Pritchard, 1978).

Around 90 per cent of illness is managed outside hospital, and the workload of the primary care services has increased in recent years. The number of GP consultations rose by over a fifth between 1979 and 1992, while the number of prescriptions issued rose by 27 per cent (DoH and OPCS, 1993b). District nurses treated 10 per cent more people in 1988 than ten years earlier. Over the same period the number of people seen by health visitors increased by around 14 per cent.

There are a number of reasons why the primary care workload has increased. First of all, the decline in the number of available beds in the NHS (see Figure 9.1) has placed a premium on the use of the existing capacity. Hospitals now discharge patients much earlier than was previously the case. In 1978 the average length of stay for acute patients was 9.8 days. By 1989 this had fallen to 7.1 days (DoH and OPCS, 1993b). As patients are discharged more quickly there is an increasing need for aftercare and rehabilitation services provided in the community. The increase in day-surgery has similar implications. Between 1978 and 1991, the number of day-cases has more than doubled, to well over a million each year. The proportion of day-cases has risen, from under 10 per cent of acute cases in the 1970s to around 20 per cent today, and will rise further. The development of new minimally invasive therapies (MIT) of the kind discussed in Chapter 3 makes the expansion of day surgery inevitable (Audit Commission, 1990, 1992b).

Other trends have placed the primary care services under greater pressure. The promotion of community care among the elderly and other vulnerable groups, such as the mentally ill, has increased the demand for primary care. The increasing emphasis upon the prevention of illness has further added to the workload.

■ Reforming primary care

Primary care has been regarded as a relatively neglected area, with considerable scope for improvement (Marks, 1988; Cmnd 7615, 1979;

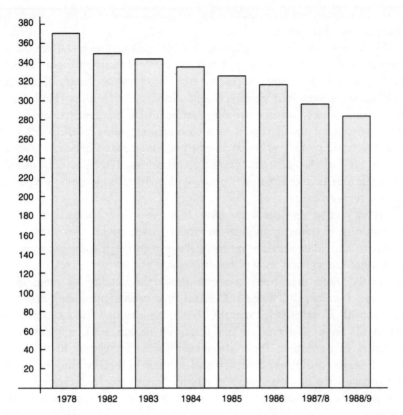

Source: Department of Health.

Figure 9.1 *Hospital beds (000s): average number available daily (all specialities), England*

Taylor, 1988). Criticism has fallen into three main categories: professional rivalries; poor management and co-ordination; and problems relating to the quality of services.

Primary care involves a wide range of professionals, who often have different views and ideas about what is best. Attempts to improve co-operation and co-ordination between these professionals led to the development of the primary health care team (PHCT) (Ministry of Health, 1963). This involves the attachment of nurses, health visitors, midwives and in some cases, social workers, to GP practices. While the PHCT was a step forward, it became obvious that such arrangements sometimes failed (DHSS, 1981b). GPs tended to dominate, much to the annoyance of the other professions, thus undermining co-operation. PHCTs were rarely based on explicit agreements about each participant's role. This often led to a lack of co-ordination and a failure to recognise mutual responsibilities.

There has also been a general lack of management responsibility in primary care. In England and Wales the NHS authorities most concerned with primary care were formerly the Family Practitioner Committees (FPCs), since renamed Family Health Service Authorities (FHSAs). The FPCs' task was to administer the contracts of GPs, dentists, pharmacists and opticians. They did not have a clear management role. To complicate matters further, other primary care professions such as district nurses were employed by the District Health Authorities (DHAs). Collaboration between DHAs and FPCs was poor, with neither body being prepared to accept responsibility.

Primary care services have also been poorly co-ordinated with the community services provided by local government. Attempts to co-ordinate and plan services more effectively through joint planning have had a limited impact, as will be shown later.

Finally, there has been concern about the quality of primary care services. The Royal College of General Practitioners, in giving evidence to the Royal Commission on the NHS, mentioned unacceptably low standards in a minority of practices. There has been a great deal of criticism in particular about the quality of primary care in inner cities, where needs were often complex and services limited (Cmnd 7615, 1979). To some extent this was also a resourcing problem; the increased demand for primary care services was not matched by an appropriate rise in funding.

☐ Primary care and the Conservative government

Primary care issues emerged from time to time during the 1960s and 1970s, but in the 1980s they reached the top of the agenda. The conservative government took a close interest in developments in this field, believing that primary care had the potential to reduce the demands on the hospital service by providing alternative forms of care and support. As this care was often seen as being low-cost, this raised the opportunity of reducing the financial burden of the NHS. Attention was also focused on the 'gatekeeper' role of the primary care services, and in particular the GPs. This role also had an impact on costs, by regulating access to other forms of care, such as hospital services and medicines.

Ministers also realised that a great deal primary care expenditure – namely the spending on family practitioner services – was difficult to control. During the 1980s, this category of spending grew by more than 3 per cent in real terms. This reflected the clinical decisions of the practitioners concerned, as such expenditure was not subject to the cash limits imposed on health authorities since the 1970s. Above all, the government feared that attempts to restrain spending in the hospital sector would be offset by increased spending in the primary care sector. Indeed, in 1982 the DHSS appointed a team of management consultants to inquire into the feasibility of imposing cash limits upon the family practitioner services. As will be discussed below, some categories of spending were later subjected to cash limits.

The government was also critical of the quality of management in primary care. The problems of co-ordination and the lack of management responsibility in this sector have already been mentioned, but during the 1980s ministers focused particularly upon the failure of FPCs to undertake strategic and financial management. They were also concerned about the lack of financial and managerial accountability in this sector, and were frustrated by both the independence of the family practitioners and the inability of FPCs to influence their performance.

Other considerations drew the government towards primary care. Charging for primary care appeared, on the whole, to be less contentious than levying charges upon hospital services. Ministers believed that the imposition of charges encouraged individuals to take more responsibility for their own health and also contributed to the cost of NHS. It was also believed that charges would discourage unnecessary and excessive use of NHS services. Finally, primary care was seen as being an area where private care could be encouraged, and where greater competition and wider consumer choice could be introduced.

■ Promoting Better Health

The Conservative government's approach to primary care reform was initially rather piecemeal. In 1984 the opticians' monopoly over the supply of spectacles was abolished. The government subsequently removed the entitlement to NHS spectacles, replacing this with a voucher system. A year later, the pharmacists' contract was renegotiated, in an attempt to reduce costs. At the same time, the government sought to reduce the cost of NHS medicines by introducing a limited list. This restricted the freedom of GPs to prescribe medicines in certain categories, including decongestants and cough remedies. In a further attempt to make savings on the drugs budget the government sought to drive down the price of prescription medicines in negotiations with the pharmaceutical industry. It also maintained a policy of raising prescription charges substantially year by year.

A limited reorganisation of primary care was also undertaken during the mid-1980s. The FPCs were freed from health authority control and became directly accountable to the DHSS (and in Wales, to the Welsh office). In addition, they were given new responsibilities to plan and develop primary care services. The FPCs were required to collaborate with DHAs and local authorities and to this end were granted membership of joint planning bodies in 1985.

Later in the decade, the government's policies for the future of primary care were outlined in the White Paper, *Promoting Better Health* (Cmd 249, 1987). Its main proposals are shown in Exhibit 9.1.

The White Paper was preceded by two official documents, which had produced a great deal of debate about the future of primary care. These were the government's Green Paper, *Primary Health Care: An Agenda for Discussion* (Cmnd 9771, 1986) and the report of a review into community nursing, *Neighbourhood Nursing: A Focus For Care* (DHSS, 1986b). We shall now briefly examine the reforms proposed in these documents.

☐ *The Green Paper*

Three highly controversial proposals were contained in the Green Paper. First, a commitment to introduce a good practice allowance (GPA) for GPs satisfying certain criteria. These criteria included the availability of GPs to patients, the extent to which they offered screening and preventive services, and their attendance on postgraduate education courses. In the event, the government did not introduce the GPA, though it did introduce financial incentives for specific activities such as screening, immunisation, health promotion, postgraduate education and so on. The tightening up of eligibility for the GP basic practice allowance (BPA) was also very much in line with the principles of the GPA.

A second measure – the creation of health care shops – also created controversy. The government suggested the possibility of allowing other bodies to provide integrated primary care services. This was seen as an attempt to introduce private enterprise into the provision of primary care.

Indeed, it was envisaged that in the longer term primary care professionals would be employed by 'businesses' providing a comprehensive range of services in return for a single capitation fee. This approach, which surfaced later in the wider debate about the internal market, was based on health maintenance organisations.

Exhibit 9.1 'Promoting Better Health'

Consumer choice

- The procedure for changing doctors to be altered (permission from current doctor no longer necessary).
- The procedure for making complaints against family practitioners simplified (oral complaints allowed, complaints period extended to thirteen weeks).
- More information on practices to be made available (opening hours, services offered by practices and so on).

Health promotion/illness prevention

- Targets (with financial incentives) for GPs to encourage immunisation, vaccination and screening.
- Fees for GPs performing health checks on new patients.
- Amendments to GPs' terms of service to clarify their role in relation to health promotion and prevention of ill-health.

Remuneration of doctors

- GPs to receive a higher proportion of their income from capitation fees (that is, the fee received for each NHS patient).
- Tighten the qualifying criteria for the GPs Basic Practice Allowance by raising the minimum number of patients on the GPs lists (from 1000) and the minimum number of hours spent on direct services to patients (from 20 hours) and making payment dependent on the doctors carrying out prevention and health promotion work.
- Financial incentives for GPs carrying out minor surgery, comprehensive care for the elderly, and child health surveillance.
- Financial incentives for GPs working in deprived areas.
- A new postgraduate allowance for GPs to encourage regular training and education throughout their careers.

Dentists

- Renegotiation of dentists' contracts to place greater emphasis on prevention.
- Initiatives to increase funds for water fluoridation and to promote dental awareness among the young, particularly in deprived areas.

Primary health care teams

- Removal of restrictions on types and number of staff employed by GPs. Part of the costs of employing health care staff reclaimable. Additional resources to be allocated for this purpose.

Family Practitioner Committees (now Family Health Service Authorities)

- FPCs encouraged to collaborate with other NHS agencies.
- FPCs to have increased responsibilities for improving practice premises, allocating resources for practice staff.
- FPCs, in conjunction with DHAs, to agree appropriate targets for disease prevention.
- FPCs to monitor performance of family practitioner services.
- FPCs (along with DHAs) to ensure cost-effective use of hospital facilities.
- FPCs to develop systems to encourage more effective and economic prescribing by GPs.
- FPCs to undertake evaluation of public attitudes in order to ensure that such views are taken into account.
- FPCs to identify underprovision of dental services and to have the power to inspect dental surgeries.

Charges/Finance

- Charges to be imposed for optical and dental checks.
- Dental charges to relate more directly to treatment received.
- The amount of money available for directly reimbursed GP expenses provided by FPCs to be cash-limited (including the employment of ancillary staff, improvement grants for premises, and loans for new premises).
- General Practice Finance Corporation (which provided loans for GP practices) to be privatised.

Other items

- Encouraging the use of information technology in primary care.
- Encouraging women to enter and remain in general practice.
- Distribution of GPs to be determined locally.
- Retirement age (70) specified for GPs and dentists.

The idea of health care shops was not taken up in the White Paper, but the government did try to encourage more private-sector funding of GP surgery premises, by privatising the General Practice Finance Corporation, which provided government loans for GPs. The implication of this was that in future more private capital would be used for surgery developments.

A third area of controversy was the proposal that the prescription charges for medicines should be more closely related to their cost. This was not pursued by the White Paper. Instead, the government sought to raise extra revenue from the optical and dental services by imposing a charge on eye tests and dental check-ups, a move which proved as controversial as the original proposal.

Despite these changes the main principles underlying the Green Paper remained largely intact. *Promoting Better Health* demonstrated that the government was still keen to introduce into primary care a greater emphasis on economic incentives, clearer accountability, a new style of management, and increased private expenditure.

☐ The Cumberlege report

The report of the Community Nursing Review, known (after its chairperson's name) as the Cumberlege report (DHSS, 1986b), had a less direct impact on policy. This report explored the problems of primary care from a different perspective. Most of its attention was directed to two main problems: the fragmentation of primary care, and the failure to maximise the contribution of the nurses in the community.

The Cumberlege report recommended a reorganisation of community nursing on the basis of small local areas called 'neighbourhoods' containing up to 25 000 people. Each neighbourhood nursing service (NNS) would integrate the work done by nurses and would plan and organise services on the basis of local needs.

The report sought to establish a more equal relationship between nurses and GPs. It argued for explicit agreements between the NNS and GP practices, establishing the objectives for each primary health care team and clarifying the various roles of the team members. It also urged the ending of subsidies for GPs to enable them to employ their own nurses. The report also called for nurses to be given greater responsibilities, including the power to prescribe drugs.

The Cumberlege report redefined primary care in terms of community nursing, and was, given the power of the medical profession, politically unrealistic (Allsop, 1986). Its recommendations represented a sharp challenge to the GP-centred system of primary care. The government was not prepared to challenge medical power in this way and did not back the central recommendations of the Cumberlege report. It passed the buck to health authorities, asking them to review their services at a local level in the light of the review. Some DHAs did respond positively by reorganising their community nursing service in line with the Cumberlege recommendations. By 1988 around a third of DHAs had developed models of primary care based on the neighbourhood nursing service (Martin, 1992).

The government also explored the possibility of expanding nurses' powers. Community nurses were granted limited statutory powers of prescription in 1992, although the implementation of this measure has been delayed for financial reasons. In other respects, however, the recommendations of the Cumberlege report were not heeded. The GP was still seen as the 'leader' of the primary care team. This was bolstered by the government's encouragement of GPs to employ their own nursing and other staff directly.

■ Criticism of the primary care reforms

The transformation of primary care from a backwater to the forefront of health policy-making in the 1980s may be seen as a positive development. Despite the consensus on the importance of primary care, there has been specific and continuing criticism of the government's reforms. These can be summarised under six headings: the narrow definition of primary care adopted; the negative impact of charges; the inability of FPCs, and their successors, the FHSAs, to manage primary care; resourcing problems; the continued fragmentation in primary care; and finally the problems surrounding the introduction of new contracts for primary care professions.

□ *Narrow definition of primary care*

For many observers the government's definition of primary care has been too narrow (Marks, 1988). The government has defined primary care as the activities of particular professionals: GPs, community nurses and so on. Such an approach contrasts sharply with that adopted by the World Health Organisation (WHO, 1978) which incorporates activities that contribute to health, but which are not necessarily undertaken by trained health care professionals.

The WHO concept of primary care is based on an explicit aim to shift the balance significantly towards primary care and away from hospital and institutional care. The WHO suggests a number of practical developments to this end. These include the promotion of self-help; the integration of medical care with other social services; environmental improvements; the promotion of good health rather than simply good health services, serving the needs of the underprivileged and under-served groups in the community; and, finally, allowing the wider community to participate in the planning and delivery of health services (Ashton and Seymour, 1988).

In light of this broader concept of primary care, Britain has a mixed record. The government has encouraged health promotion and self-help, but it has been less concerned about the health of the underprivileged, as we shall see in Chapter 11. In addition, the notion of consumer choice has been given given far more weight than has community participation.

There has also been a failure to recognise that other professionals and agencies outside the health sector might have a role to play in primary care. Essentially, the government's primary care reforms have concentrated on the NHS, and in particular on the family practitioner services, as the principal means for improving primary care. Moreover, these reforms have been implemented apparently without regard to other important policy developments, such as the internal market, the Griffiths review of community care in the late 1980s, and the national health strategy.

☐ *Charges*

The government's decision to impose charges on optical and dental checks was heavily criticised. Indeed, many of the government's own supporters were critical of charges when they were debated in Parliament. During the passage of the legislation in 1988, twenty-two Conservative MPs voted against the government, though this rebellion was insufficient to prevent the measure becoming law.

The government, in its defence, argued that priority groups were exempt from the new charges. It also conceded exemptions as the legislation passed through Parliament. (As a result children, students up to the age of 19, and those receiving social security income support can obtain exemption from both charges; expectant and recent mothers and 16- and 17-year-olds, are exempt from the dental charge; and those already suffering from severely impaired eyesight, or who have a family history of diseases related to blindness, such as glaucoma and diabetes, are exempt from the eye test charge.)

Ministers claimed that the charges were modest – £3 for a dental examination and around £10 for the eye test, and reflected the principle that individuals should take responsibility for their own health. They argued that the imposition of charges for optical and dental checks did not represent a radical departure from the existing policy of charging for prescriptions and appliances.

Both dentists and opticians claimed that the charges would discourage individuals from having such tests. They pointed out that this could undermine the government's own emphasis on preventing illness. If people were discouraged, serious illnesses such as oral cancer and glaucoma might go undetected. Delayed treatment would be both more costly and less effective than intervention made possible by early detection of these illnesses.

Following the imposition of these charges, the number of eye tests fell significantly (by 30 per cent). This may partly have been due to patients bringing forward their tests to avoid the charge, yet, two years after the charge was imposed, the number of eye tests was still well below the 1989 level. The number of people having dental examinations also fell over the same period. Two years after the introduction of the charge, dental checks were just under 10 per cent down on the 1988/9 baseline. The number of courses of adult dental treatment also declined significantly over this period. However, in the following year this figure surged above the original baseline, indicating that the impact of the (smaller) dental charge may be much weaker in the longer term.

The imposition of charges for primary care raised fears about the privatisation of services in this sector. Increased charges for appliances, medicines and dental treatment, coupled with the introduction of charges for eye and dental checks, were seen to be the thin end of the wedge which would lead eventually to payment for medical and nursing services. Critics believed that this breached a fundamental principle of the NHS – the availability of treatment irrespective of ability to pay.

☐ *Family practitioner committees: fit to manage?*

In 1985, as noted earlier, the government gave FPCs a more independent and pro-active role. There were worries that an extension of this role, as envisaged in *Promoting Better Health*, would be difficult to achieve. The National Audit office (NAO, 1988a) found that FPCs had experienced difficulties in producing adequate plans for service development. The NAO was critical of the level of resources available to FPCs in view of their additional responsibilities, and believed the level of management training for FPC personnel was inadequate.

The NAO criticised the arrangements used by the DHSS to monitor and review FPC performance. It found that the DHSS had not given clear guidance to FPCs on policy objectives. On a more optimistic note, its investigation did reveal good progress in computerisation which, it was believed, would be useful in regard to health screening programmes.

An earlier investigation into FPCs by Allsop and May (1986) also identified shortcomings. FPCs were shown to have inadequate levels of staffing, training and a general lack of resources to perform their new role. Allsop and May also found that FPCs had few sanctions which they could use to influence practitioners. They had responsibility without power. In spite of these difficulties there was evidence that some FPCs were making a real effort to work with practitioners to raise standards and improve services. The National Audit Office, in its inquiry, also found examples of good practice, attributing these achievements to the drive and enthusiasm of these particular FPCs.

In the aftermath of *Promoting Better Health*, the FPCs were given new financial powers (see Exhibit 9.1 on p. 207). They now exercise more discretion over the allocation of funds for GP staff and the development of premises. This creates some potential for greater practice accountability, though at present only 10 per cent of FPC (now FHSA) funds are allocated on a discretionary basis. The extent to which practices can be held accountable in this way depends on the degree to which they need these resources (Huntington, 1993).

Further changes were aimed at strengthening the management role of FPCs. Griffiths-style general managers were introduced in 1989 and shortly afterwards the composition of the FPCs was altered in an attempt to improve their managerial function. The new bodies, subsequently renamed Family Health Service Authorities (FHSAs), were slimmer and contained fewer representatives drawn from the professions.

Working for Patients (Cm 555, 1989) reiterated the importance of FHSAs in relation to the monitoring of family practitioner contracts, quality of service, and GP drug budgets, yet at the same time their independent role was undermined by this White Paper. FHSAs once again were brought under the wing of health authorities, now being accountable to the RHAs. The internal market also appeared to threaten the FHSAs' position. They did not have the purchasing power of the DHAs, and have entered into joint arrangements in an attempt to share service provision, as will be discussed below. Furthermore, the development of GP fundholding in the early stages largely bypassed FHSA management. Regional health authorities have played the main role in establishing the GP fundholding scheme, and are also responsible for allocating fundholders' budgets, although in more and more cases these tasks are being delegated to FHSAs.

☐ Fragmentation

The reforms introduced by *Promoting Better Health* have failed to tackle one of the major problems of primary care, namely the fragmentation of responsibilities among different agencies and professions. The division between FHSAs and DHAs has been identified by many observers as being a major obstacle in the co-ordination of primary care services. Despite the introduction of new arrangements for collaboration in 1985, obstacles remained (National Audit Office, 1988a). In particular collaboration has been made difficult by the fact that most FHSAs do not share a common boundary with a single health authority.

There has been a good deal of support for merging FHSAs (and their predecessors, the FPCs) with DHAs. The House of Commons Select Committee on Social Services (House of Commons, 1986) argued that there was no logical reason for keeping them separate. Echoing an earlier recommendation by the Royal Commission in 1979, the committee called on the government to review the relationship between the two agencies and to consider the likely benefits of amalgamation. Such a move was also supported by the Cumberlege inquiry (DHSS, 1986b).

Many DHAs and FHSAs have since joined forces, some producing joint plans for purchasing services, as was already noted in Chapter 8. The Department of Health, which has in the past opposed amalgamation, has now decided to allow these authorities to merge.

The improved co-ordination of primary care which could result from these new arrangements may not overcome the professional rivalries that have exacerbated the fragmentation of services in this sector. Poor levels of collaboration between GPs and community nurses were still apparent by the late 1980s (Bond, Cartlidge and Gregson, 1987). The government's apparent solution to these problems was to support a GP-centred approach.

Promoting Better Health was almost exclusively focused on the GP service, and some of its proposals clearly encouraged a GP-led service. For example, GPs were given incentives to increase the employment of nursing staff in their practices. The number of practice nurses in England and Wales subsequently doubled, from 5000 to 10 000, between 1988 and 1990. There has been some criticism of this trend, largely on the grounds that the distribution of these new posts has occurred in a haphazard fashion, without regard to need (Audit Commission, 1993b). This criticism echoes the view of the Cumberlege report, which, it will be recalled, argued for the phasing out of subsidies for GP-employed nurses, and in favour of explicit agreements between the primary care professions.

The movement towards a GP-led primary care system looks set to continue with the development of GP fundholding. Since April 1993 fundholders have received budgets to purchase community health services for their patients. Fundholders cannot at this stage employ health visitors and district nurses but such a move cannot be ruled out for the future. It may be unnecessary, however, if GPs can secure the type and range of services they require through the purchasing process.

☐ Resources

The government's original review of primary care appeared to be directed at restraining expenditure. Yet when the reforms were unveiled in 1987, it was announced that expenditure on family practitioner services would be increased. Moreover, between 1979 and 1991, the share of the NHS current expenditure allocated to primary care increased, and currently about a third of NHS expenditure (excluding capital spending) is spent on primary care.

There have been doubts about the adequacy of primary care funding in view of increasing demand for services (discussed earlier). In addition, as with the NHS budget in general, the rising cost of services has eaten into the primary care budget (Audit Commission, 1992a). The real increase in resources for primary care, relative to the volume of services required, is therefore much lower than the government's expenditure statistics suggest. Moreover, the shift in resources from hospital to primary care may also have been exaggerated: the hospital sector takes the lion's share of capital resources, and when these funds are taken into account, the movement of resources between the two sectors is fairly marginal.

As noted earlier, the government's interest in primary care was raised initially by the fact that the budget for the family practitioner services was 'open-ended'. *Promoting Better Health* represented an attack on this principle by cash-limiting the funding of GP practice staff, improvements to premises, and the building of premises.

There were further developments in this direction with the introduction of the indicative prescribing scheme in 1991. The aim of this scheme was to place 'downward pressure on expenditure on drugs' (Cm 555, 1989; DoH 1990e). FHSAs now monitor prescription budgets set for each GP practice. These budgets are not strictly speaking cash-limited; they may be exceeded, but GPs who persistently exceed their budgets have to explain why, and can face financial penalties. GP fundholders, on the other hand, receive a budget for drugs as part of their overall allocation. They are permitted to increase spending on drugs by reducing expenditure in other areas, if they wish to do so.

☐ Contracts

The most acrimonious criticism of the government's plans for primary care surrounded the details of the new GP contract. The government's plan was to create financial incentives to encourage doctors to perform certain tasks such as screening, immunisation, health checks, minor surgery, health promotion, and child health surveillance. Under the terms of the new contract, which came into force in 1990, GPs receive a larger proportion of their income from capitation fees (the money they receive for each NHS patient). This proportion was raised from 46 per cent to 60 per cent of the GPs' average income. The capitation fee is higher for elderly patients. GPs practising in rural areas or in areas of deprivation also receive a larger payment.

The GPs have been highly critical of the new contract. They support the movement towards prevention, health promotion, and improvements in the quality of care, but have expressed concern about the way in which the contract seeks to achieve these aims.

First and foremost, GPs claim that the introduction of incentives undermines their clinical judgement on a day-to-day basis. They hold reservations about the impact of increased competition for patients, implied by the changes in both capitation fees and in the procedure for changing doctors. GPs feel this places more emphasis on window-dressing than on the quality of services delivered. It has been argued that few patients will act as consumers in the new general practice 'market' (Leavey *et al.*, 1989). There are fears also that increased competition might encourage 'doctor shoppers' – people who switch doctors on a whim. A further possibility is that the practices which attract more patients could end up with longer lists, leading to a fall in the standard of service. Meanwhile, the less successful GPs might eventually 'go out of business'; the net result being fewer practices and longer lists.

Second, GPs have been concerned about the extra workload brought on by the new contract. GPs now have to be available for longer periods; they are expected to provide health checks for the over-75s annually and health checks for other adults every three years. They must produce more information about their practices for both the public and the FHSA. Some GPs have also complained that the introduction of financial incentives for carrying out night visits, child health surveillance, minor surgery, health promotion and screening forces them, by economic necessity, to work long hours.

Third, some of the incentives built into the new contract appear to have perverse implications for patient care. Payment for health checks, for example, may lead GPs to spend too much time on the 'worried well'. This promotes a kind of inverse care law, where the healthy receive more attention than the sick. Indeed, one study has found that the likelihood of a patient accepting an invitation to attend for a health check is inversely related to the risk of that patient having a heart disease (Waller *et al.*, 1990).

Fourth, it has been argued that some of the targets set out in the revised contract are rather crude. In the original plan, a GP who immunised 90 per cent of the children on his or her list would receive £2000, but would get nothing if the proportion immunised fell below this threshold. The government subsequently introduced a second, lower, target (70 per cent), yielding a smaller monetary reward (£700). This still means that a GP immunising 68 per cent of the children on his or her list would receive the same – that is, nothing – as one who did not immunise any patients. This creates a discentive, which may lead GPs who are unable to reach the target to reduce their efforts to immunise. The same arguments apply to cervical cancer screening, where GPs receive monetary rewards for hitting targets of 80 per cent or 50 per cent of their female patients.

There have also been fears that patients might be excluded from practice lists if they jeopardised the achievement of the targets set for immunisation and cervical cancer screening. Shortly after the new contract came into operation, two council housing estates in Carlisle were excluded from a practice list, allegedly for this reason, though following considerable media attention this decision was reversed. There is no clear evidence as yet on the extent to which the new contract is leading to exclusion. However, there are worries that moves in this direction could be hastened by fundholding, which, according to some, creates an incentive to exclude high-risk patients.

A further criticism of the proposed targets is that they take little account of the environment in which GPs are working. Targets for immunisation and cervical screening are much harder to attain in inner-cities, for example. The government did introduce a new weighting for doctors practising in deprived areas, but this did not remove the fears of inner-city GPs, who felt that these payments did not fully compensate them for the disincentives faced by such practices. Similarly, there have been complaints from doctors in rural areas, who also face more difficulties in attempting to provide services (such as health promotion clinics, for example) which attract financial rewards under the new contract.

The new contract was the subject of considerable friction between the Department of Health and the BMA. Some concessions were made (as in the case of the revised immunisation and cervical screening targets, mentioned above). Yet this did not prevent GPs rejecting the new contract by 3 to 1 when the issue was put to a ballot. Eventually the government imposed the contract, which further strained relations between the medical profession and the government. Subsequently, however, the government has adopted a more conciliatory tone and made a number of adjustments to the contract, including some concessions for rural practices.

Other primary care professions also negotiated changes to their contracts in the aftermath of *Promoting Better Health*. In contrast to the acrimony surrounding the GPs' contract, these changes were made in a more relaxed atmosphere, though in the case of the dentists, the implementation of the new contract has subsequently produced much controversy. The 1990 contract moved dentists a small way towards a capitation-based system, but in 1991/2 there was a disagreement between the profession and the Department of Health over the level of payments under the new scheme. The result was that many dentists began to deregister NHS patients and others refused to admit new NHS patients. This caused a great deal of public concern, and to defuse the crisis the Department of Health initiated a review of dental remuneration.

■ The future of primary health care

It is widely accepted that good primary health care provides the key to a better health service. Expansion of this sector is a more appropriate, and in the longer term may also be a more cost-effective, development. Although the benefits of primary care are well known, it is only recently that it has come to the forefront of policy-making and been the subject of wider debate and reform. While this is a positive move, opportunities to improve primary care have been missed. The government has taken a narrow view of primary care: it has preferred consumer choice above consumer participation, and has failed so far to integrate its reforms in this sector with other key developments in health policy, such as community care, the internal market, and public health.

Little has been done to resolve the problems of inter-agency collaboration. A similar story is revealed in relation to community care for specific client groups to be discussed in Chapter 10. The changes did not address the question of professional rivalries either. The government did not seek to establish a consensus, but merely infuriated every professional group. Nurses were offended by the rejection of Cumber-lege, and GPs offended by the imposition, and dentists by the implementation, of new contracts.

The government did provide more resources for primary care, but relative to the demand for these services, and given the appetite of the acute sector for capital resources, there was little change in the balance of resources consumed by the two sectors. The introduction of the internal market may well have a greater impact. Primary care is likely to expand as budget holders seek out more cost-effective forms of care. The market does seem to have produced new pressures for change, as the case of London's health care, discussed in Chapter 8, clearly shows. However, this does not remove the need for proper planning. The shift from hospital to primary care needs to be resourced adequately, planned strategically and managed effectively.

■ *Chapter 10* ■

Care in the Community: Social Care for Client Groups

The heaviest users of health services include the elderly, mentally ill and handicapped people, physically disabled people, and children. Together, the elderly and children account for 60 per cent of the expenditure on hospital and community health services (HCHS). A tenth of HCHS expenditure is allocated to services for the mentally ill and a further 5 per cent to services for those with learning difficulties. In addition, these client groups require a wide range of social care and support, including income maintenance, appropriate accommodation, and practical help and advice.

It has long been recognised that these client groups require special attention. Yet there are many equally well-known problems involved in developing an adequate network of services for them. Individuals within these groups often have multiple health and social problems, and their needs are complex. Many are vulnerable and dependent. To add to these difficulties, the existing pattern of services has often been poorly matched with their needs. The NHS, as we have already noted, has traditionally been geared to the provision of acute services while in many cases social services, social security and housing provision have failed to provide an appropriate pattern of services for the groups mentioned above. The services provided for these groups have often been of poor quality, particularly those for the elderly, mentally ill people and the mentally handicapped – the so-called 'Cinderella services'.

Since the 1960s, however, successive governments have declared the development of these services to be a priority. Three main aims have underpinned government policy. First, to shift resources from the acute sector towards the care of these groups. Second, to improve the co-ordination of health services, social services and, more recently, private provision. Third, to develop caring services for these groups in the community rather than in hospital.

■ Community care policies

Government policy on community care is often traced back to a speech in 1961 by the then Health Minister, Enoch Powell, in which he announced the running down of the large mental hospitals. Official thinking had been moving in this direction for some years previously. In 1954, for example, a government report had favoured community care for the elderly (Ministry of Health, 1954). The Guillebaud Committee, which inquired into the cost of the NHS, had also earlier made out a case for community care on both humanitarian and economic grounds (Cmd 9663, 1956).

□ *Arguments for community care*

Throughout the 1960s, a broad consensus developed, and care in the community was seen as being a more appropriate and more effective form of care. The poor standards of care for many long-term patients became increasingly evident. This was confirmed by a series of cases which came to light during the late 1960s involving the maltreatment of patients in long-stay hospitals (Robb, 1967; Martin, 1984). These cases were seen as being typical of the standard of institutional care, and reinforced the notion that community care was a more humane policy.

Supporters of community care argued that it avoided the dependency which patients often experience in institutions. By integrating these individuals within the community, it was believed they could achieve their full potential with a degree of independence. At the same time, it was thought that the location of patients in the community would make it more difficult for society to ignore them and their needs, since they would no longer be hidden away from public view in institutions.

Finally, community care was supported on economic grounds; institutional care is certainly expensive. According to the Audit Commission (1986), for example, elderly people could be cared for in their own homes at less than half of the cost of a bed in a hospital geriatric ward. It is this economic argument which has been the main driving force behind the development of community care policies in the 1980s. Yet, as we shall see later, the cost argument is not as clear-cut as it seems at first glance.

□ *Community care in the 1960s and 1970s*

Despite the growing support for community care during the 1960s it remained largely a paper policy. The policy was reiterated in the early

1970s with the publication of White Papers on services for the mentally handicapped (Cmnd 4683, 1971) and the mentally ill (Cmnd 6233, 1975b). It had been accepted by this time that for community care to become a reality the main agencies involved (the NHS and the local authorities) would have to collaborate far more effectively. To this end a system of joint planning was introduced in 1974, involving the creation of Joint Consultative Committees (JCCs) which consisted of health authority members and local authority councillors. These were later supplemented by Joint Health Care Planning Teams consisting of officers drawn from both authorities. In a further development, financial incentives were introduced in 1976 in an attempt to promote collaborative projects. Joint finance became available, enabling health authorities to make annual grants to local authorities and voluntary organisations wishing to establish community-based schemes, such as the establishment of day-centres, for example.

The government also planned to shift resources towards community services used by the elderly, the mentally ill, the mentally handicapped, the physically handicapped, and children. These priorities were set out in a policy document (DHSS, 1976a). However, in the following year these expansionary commitments were toned down, largely as a result of public expenditure constraints and protests from the acute sector (DHSS, 1977).

The squeeze on public spending by both the Labour government of the late 1970s and its Conservative successor strongly inhibited the development of community care services. Health authority budgets were used to maintain the existing pattern of services rather than to expand community-based services. Expenditure on personal social services in fact increased in real terms by 20 per cent in the period 1975/6 to 1980/1 (Webb and Wistow, 1983) though it appears that funds were not allocated in response to changing needs, priorities or policies relating to care in the community, and did not ensure a constant level of service output. Indeed, the impact of expenditure constraints tended to squeeze out the most cost-effective forms of community care. This was due to the reduction of expenditure on relatively easy targets, such as home help services, which provided crucial support to many of those being cared for in the community.

The Thatcher Government and community care

The Thatcher government was keen to promote community care, for a number of reasons. Community care was viewed as a means of saving public money in health and social care. Such a policy created opportunities to shift the burden of responsibility for care from the state to the individual. It also had the potential to stimulate private provision of care.

☐ *Encouraging community care*

The government set out its proposals for transferring patients out of hospital into the community in a number of policy documents during the early 1980s (DHSS, 1981c,d; Cmnd 8173, 1981). Out of this emerged specific programmes such as the Care in the Community Initiative. Under this particular scheme the NHS could allocate limited funds to local authorities, and also voluntary organisations, in order to fund services for long-term patients who were released into the community. At the same time the government relaxed some of the rules on the joint finance scheme, in an attempt to stimulate its use.

The take-up of joint finance had been disappointing. Local authorities feared the longer-term financial burden implied in the acceptance of such grants, which only supported projects for a limited period (Green, 1986; Webb and Wistow, 1983). The problems surrounding joint finance persisted throughout the 1980s. It was later discovered that most of the funds had been used by the NHS for its own schemes, rather than to promote an expansion of local authority social services (Wistow *et al.*, 1990; NAO, 1987).

☐ *The voluntary and commercial sectors*

The Thatcher government sought to promote the private provision of community care in a number of ways. Voluntary organisations involved in community care received increased funding from central government. The importance of their role was also reiterated in policy documents, and health authorities were urged to co-operate with them (DHSS, 1981c). In 1985, voluntary organisations were included in the joint planning process, along with the NHS and local authorities. At the same time a statutory duty was placed on health authorities to consult the voluntary sector.

Informal care by families, friends and neighbours was also encouraged. The government stressed that the care of the elderly and of other vulnerable groups was a community responsibility and that 'care in the community must increasingly mean care by the community' (Cmnd 8173, 1981, p. 3). For many, this meant a heavy individual responsibility. There are over six million informal carers in Great Britain regularly looking after sick, disabled or elderly persons. A quarter of them spend at least twenty hours a week caring for someone. Most carers, around 58 per cent, are women: a quarter of women in the 45–64 age group are carers (Green, H., 1988).

A further strand of government policy has been to promote commercial residential care for the elderly, the chronically ill, and people with physical handicaps. Figure 10.1 illustrates the extent of this growth. Commercial provision of residential care now represents just under half the total. On top of this, the commercial sector in 1989 operated an additional 88 600 nursing home places. In the same year there were 10 400 places in voluntary nursing homes and 80 000 NHS beds available for geriatric patients and the elderly mentally ill. When these are added to the residential care figures, the total public-sector supply of long-term institutional care represents 43 per cent of the total places available. The voluntary sector has a 10 per cent share, while the commercial sector holds the largest single share, at 46 per cent.

The expansion in commercial care for the elderly was given an important boost by changes in social security regulations in 1980. These changes allowed the elderly to claim social security to cover the costs of residential care. As a result, the amount of social security expenditure rose

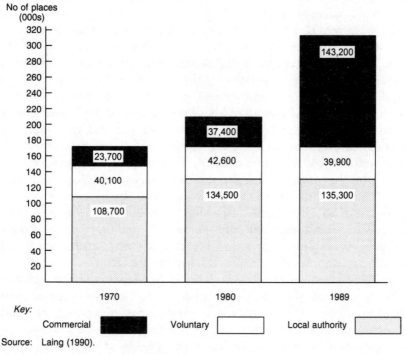

Figure 10.1   *Places in residential homes, by sector*

dramatically, from less than £20m in 1980 to around £700m by the end of the decade. At the same time, the proportion of elderly residents paying directly for care in private homes fell. By the end of the 1980s only 40 per cent were self-financing (Laing, 1990).

■ Community care: a growing problem

Despite the government's encouragement of community care, serious problems became increasingly evident as the 1980s progressed. The main concerns fell into four categories: the adequacy of community care standards; the role of the voluntary sector; problems associated with planning; and problems of funding.

□ *Adequacy of community care standards*

In 1984 the government responded to worries about standards in private residential care homes for the elderly by passing new legislation. Under the Registered Homes Act 1984, local authorities were given powers to register and inspect residential care homes. The monitoring of standards in nursing homes, however, is a health authority responsibility. This division of responsibility has since been criticised on a number of occasions (DHSS, 1988b; National Institute for Social Work, 1988). So far the government has resisted calls for the regulation of the two sectors to be integrated.

Small homes with less than four residents were excluded from the 1984 Act. Yet there was much concern about standards in these homes (Social Services Inspectorate, 1988). Furthermore, the Act did not apply to residential care in the public sector, despite evidence of poor standards here as well (Day, 1985). More recently, the government has responded to demands for the independent registration and inspection of local authority homes (National Institute for Social Work, 1988). Local authorities now have to establish arms-length inspection units to examine standards in both private and local authority homes. In addition, recent policy developments explored later in this chapter may encourage local authorities to dispose of their own residential care facilities.

The lack of adequate community facilities for mentally ill and mentally handicapped people was also clearly evident. Most observers agreed with the conclusion of the Social Services Committee that 'the pace of removal of hospital facilities for mental illness has far outrun the provision of services in the community to replace them' (House of Commons, 1985, p. xviii). According to Groves (1990), nearly 100 000 long-stay patients have been discharged into the community over the past thirty-five years, while only 4000 places have been created in local authority hostels. As these discharges have not been monitored, no one knows what has happened to this 'invisible cohort', although there are strong reasons for believing that many of these people are homeless and destitute, or in prison (Weller, 1989; Coid, 1984).

A third area of concern about standards centred on informal carers and their burden: carers often cope unaided. Support services are poorly developed and there is a lack of respite care available to carers. Of those who care for someone for twenty hours a week or more, only one in twenty find it relatively easy to arrange for alternative care of two days' duration. Around a fifth find it difficult or very difficult to arrange such cover, while 44 per cent find it impossible to make such arrangements (Adams, 1991).

The burden of caring, often without outside help, has implications for the health of carers. Approximately a tenth of men and a quarter of women who care for the elderly suffer from fatigue. Around a third of female carers (against only 8 per cent of male carers) face a loss of social opportunities. It has been estimated that around 10 per cent of carers have serious health problems of their own (Green, H., 1988; Adams, 1991). This is quite possibly due to the burden of caring itself. A survey of the Carers' National Association membership revealed that two-thirds had become ill after caring for sick, elderly or disabled friends or relatives (*Guardian*, 22 May 1992, p. 4). The same survey found that half had financial problems, which added to the level of stress. This seems to confirm the view of the Royal College of Nursing that 'the quality of life for the carer can be more impaired than the person for whom they are caring' (Royal College of Nursing, 1990).

☐ *The role of the voluntary sector*

Voluntary organisations have a key role to play in improving and complementing public-sector care and in promoting health. Yet the growing emphasis on voluntary welfare provision has raised the possibility of replacing NHS and local authority community services. This is seen by some observers to be a kind of back-door privatisation, and by others as a crude way of saving public money (see Johnson, 1989; Deakin, 1991).

The voluntary sector is not equipped to take over large areas of service delivery; it cannot provide a comprehensive or a universal service. Voluntary organisations are not directly accountable to the public or to Parliament. Furthermore, by allowing voluntary organisations to substitute for public services, they inevitably enter into a closer relationship with the government. There is a real danger that this will in turn undermine their most attractive features: their independence, flexibility and adaptability.

Indeed, voluntary bodies are anxious about allegations of privatisation (Taylor, 1988). Few, if any, seem to relish the prospect of displacing public sector provision. Most voluntary organisations prefer to talk of a partnership with the public sector rather than of replacing it.

There is a good deal of scope for improving the partnership between the public and the voluntary sector in health care, and a number of obstacles have been identified. Fears about the substitution of statutory services by the voluntary sector, mentioned above, can create an unhelpful atmosphere of mutual suspicion. There has also been a general lack of understanding about roles and working practices, which has on occasion made it difficult to establish an effective partnership between the statutory and voluntary sectors. Effective working relationships between the two sectors have also been undermined by the sheer diversity of the voluntary sector. The NHS often finds it difficult to relate to such a large number and wide range of groups.

NAHA and NCVO (1987) have made a number of recommendations in an attempt to surmount these barriers. These include the adoption by health authorities of an explicit policy on the voluntary sector; the appointment of voluntary sector liaison officers within the NHS; better consultation processes involving the voluntary sector; and more information-sharing between the two sectors. The same report urged voluntary organisations to operate through 'umbrella bodies' to overcome the problems which health authorities faced in dealing with large numbers of groups, to develop a better understanding of NHS structures, and to identify and develop contacts with key health authority personnel.

☐ The failure of joint planning

As we have seen, governments have tried to encourage collaboration on community care between the health authorities and local authorities through joint planning. During the 1980s the Family Practitioner, Committees (and their successors the Family Health Service Authorities, FHSAs) and the voluntary sector were brought into this process. Yet studies of joint planning have continued to expose serious shortcomings in the system. It is clear that the creation of formal planning systems was not sufficient to guarantee effective collaboration.

Collaboration has often failed because of the contrasting organisational cultures and structures of the NHS and local authorities. As a result, certain needs have often been defined in different ways. For example, the majority of health authorities have tended to regard the elderly mentally ill as part of the psychiatric service, while local authorities preferred to view them as part of their services for the elderly (Health Advisory Service, 1987). Related to these different perspectives are the professional rivalries which exist between NHS and local government staff, which have also provided considerable obstacles to effective planning and co-ordination in the past (Green, 1986).

There are further problems with the planning process (National Audit Office, 1987). These include problems caused by the different planning timescales of the two authorities and differences in accountability and management structures. In many areas, difficulties arise because local authorities and health authorities no longer have coterminous boundaries, although some observers are less convinced that the establishment of common organisational structures and boundaries would necessarily improve the situation (Challis *et al.*, 1988).

The poor quality of joint planning is still evident (Audit Commission, 1992a). Discussion at Joint Consultative Committees (JCCs) tends to be dominated by marginal issues and specific projects rather than strategic issues. Important areas of concern between the local authorities and the NHS, including policies for people with disabilities, for example, are not covered sufficiently, and in some cases not discussed at all.

The weaknesses of joint planning leads to poor co-ordination of services. A study of elderly people has shown that social services and health authorities liaise regularly in only 7 per cent of cases where individuals are receiving care from both agencies (Davies *et al.*, 1990). Similar problems of co-ordination at grassroots level have been shown to exist for other client groups such as the mentally ill, mentally handicapped people, the physically disabled and children at risk (Audit Commission, 1989; Beardshaw, 1988; Health Advisory Service, 1987; House of Commons, 1985; Brent Borough Council, 1984). The result for the user of these services is a piecemeal, fragmented and incoherent service.

Most enquiries into co-ordination and collaboration have stressed the need to clarify responsibilities in relation to community care. The Social Services Committee called in 1985 for social care for mentally handicapped people to be financed and administered by local authorities. The Audit Commission (1986) argued that local authorities should be responsible for the mentally and physically handicapped, with the NHS retaining responsibility for the mentally ill, while the needs of the elderly would remain a joint NHS/local authority responsibility.

At this stage such plans did not appeal to the government. Instead, the shortcomings identified in the collaborative arrangements were tackled by strengthening rather than replacing the existing system. Plans were drawn up to involve senior health authority members and local authority councillors to a far greater extent. Attempts were also made to clarify the responsibilities for joint planning and the implementation of collaborative strategies and programmes. Before long, however, the government was forced to consider the question of responsibilities, as will be discussed later.

☐ *Funding*

A fair amount of controversy has surrounded the level of funding allocated to community care, and the way in which these funds are spent. As we have seen, one of the main arguments advanced in favour of community care is that it raises the prospect of saving money by replacing 'high cost' institutional care with 'low cost' community services. This argument has been strongly contested. In 1981 a study by the DHSS found that for some people community care was neither cheaper nor more effective than institutional provision, and that in some cases low-cost care in the community was inadequate (DHSS, 1981a). The Working Group on Joint Planning (DHSS, 1985) also thought that it was unsafe to assume that community care was a cheaper option. The Social Services Committee (House of Commons, 1985) directly questioned the principle of cost neutrality – that the shift towards community care could be achieved without adding to public expenditure. It went on to argue that a community care policy based on a cost neutral assumption was not merely naïve, but positively inhumane. It became increasingly obvious that if community care was to be provided adequately, the cost of care would have to rise, at least in the short-term, as new services became established and old institutions were gradually run down.

At the same time there was wide agreement that a great deal of the present budget for long-term care was being spent inefficiently. According to the Audit Commission (1986), two-thirds of the government budget for the care of the elderly, the mentally ill, and people with mental and physical handicaps was spent on residential care. The Audit Commission believed that many of these individuals could be cared for in their own homes at lower cost. There was, however, some uncertainty about the extent to which individuals could be moved into the community. Bradshaw and Gibbs (1988) found that only 7 per cent of a sample of elderly people had been inappropriately admitted to residential care. However, the same study also discovered that a further 10 per cent of residents would not have required admission to residential care if there had been adequate support services in the community.

Despite uncertainty about levels of institutionalisation, the conclusion that the present system of funding discouraged the development of community care was inescapable. The Audit Commission (1986) estimated that around £500m was spent on care funded through the social security system, much of this financing institutional care for the elderly in private residential homes. The major growth area, as noted earlier, was the commercial sector. For many this was an unwelcome trend. Yet it was not so much the amounts of money involved that raised eyebrows, but the fact that the trend apparently lacked purpose and direction.

Within government circles there was a great deal of concern about the sharp rise in the cost of residential care. Under pressure from the Treasury, health ministers established an internal inquiry into funding. This was followed by an inquiry by Sir Roy Griffiths, the Prime Minister's adviser on health care, and architect of the new management arrangements in the NHS which were discussed in Chapter 6. The Griffiths' review of community care made a number of recommendations, some of which caused the government considerable discomfort and embarrassment, which will be discussed in due course.

■ Griffiths' community care reforms

□ *The report*

The Griffiths report set out three guiding principles on which to base community care policy (DHSS, 1988b). First, that the right services should be provided early enough, to the people who need them most. Second, that these people should have more choice and a greater say about how they are helped. Third, that people should be cared for wherever possible in their own homes, or in as near a domestic environment as possible so that hospital, residential, or nursing home care could be reserved for those whose needs cannot be met in any other way.

Griffiths sought to achieve these ends first of all by allocating clear responsibilities for services. At the top, the report recommended, a minister responsible for community care. At the local level, local authority social service departments were viewed as being the best organisations to take a lead role in identifying needs, setting priorities, and developing plans for community care. At the individual level, Griffiths proposed case managers to co-ordinate the assessment of needs and arrange appropriate packages of care.

In an attempt to encourage community care, Griffiths proposed that the perverse incentive in favour of residential care should be removed, by reducing social security payments for those in residential homes to a basic level. The balance (the care element) would then be paid by local authorities on behalf of those individuals who, on the basis of assessment, actually needed residential care. For those who did not require residential care, the care element could be used to purchase an alternative package of services in the community. These services would be provided by the local authorities themselves, the NHS, and the private sector.

Exhibit 10.1   The Griffiths review of community care

Terms of Reference

- 'to review the way in which public funds are used to support community care policy and to advise . . . on the options for action that would improve the use of these funds as a contribution to more effective community care'.

Main Recommendations

- A clearer role for central government, including the creation of a Minister in the DHSS publicly identified as being responsible for community care.
- Social services departments identified as the lead agencies in community care. Their tasks: to identify needs, devise packages of care, and co-ordinate services. They should develop local plans for community care in consultation with health authorities, housing authorities, voluntary bodies and private providers of care.
- Where appropriate, specific care managers should be assigned to each case, to assess individuals' needs and to arrange packages of care.
- Social services departments should be given an enabling role. They should ensure that services are provided, within budgets, by private or public sectors according to where they can be provided most economically and efficiently.
- Social services departments' plans for community care should be reviewed and approved against national objectives, and alongside the plans of health authorities.
- A specific grant to local authorities for community care should be made available from central government, covering a significant proportion of the costs of an approved programme. This funding should be 'ring-fenced' in order to prevent it from being spent on other services.
- The perverse incentives which have led to the expansion of residential care should be removed. Social security payments should be limited to a basic level only, the balance paid by local authorities on the basis of individual care assessments.
- Collaboration at local level on training matters is necessary in order to prevent insularity of professions and promote mutual understanding of each profession's role.
- A need for a new multi-purpose auxiliary force of carers to be given limited training and to give practical help in the field of community care.

Griffiths envisaged that central government would provide a substantial chunk of the resources needed to arrange care packages. These resources would be subject to central government approval of local authority community care plans. The local plans would in turn be drawn up in consultation with the other authorities and agencies involved in the provision of community care services, such as health authorities and the private sector.

☐ *The reaction to the Griffiths report*

The reaction to Griffiths' proposals was mixed. Understandably, local authority social service departments were largely in favour. The review after all, had given them a key responsibility in an area of service expansion. According to one survey, 91 per cent of social services directors were in favour of the Griffiths review's recommendations, as were 69 per cent of local authority Social Services Committees (Hunter *et al.*, 1988). In contrast, the health authorities were less happy. Only 46 per cent of health services managers and 28 per cent of health authorities expressed positive sentiments regarding the changes.

There were a number of reasons for this. Health authorities feared the impact of a substantial loss of resources (around 20 per cent of their budgets) following the designation of local authorities as the lead agencies in community care. Some had genuine doubts about the competence and will of local authorities to implement Griffiths' proposals.

The private residential care sector was also worried about the implications of Griffiths. Many within the industry believed that it would lead local authorities to withdraw funding from residents in private homes, thus leading to closures. Many client group organisations also feared that a sudden withdrawal of funding from the residential sector would propel vulnerable people into the community before proper support services had been developed.

Others within local government also had reservations, believing that increased central control would be the result of the proposed planning and review process and the system of specific grants for community care. There were particular worries that a hidden agenda of privatisation was behind the recommendations that local authorities should seek an enabling role. Local authorities were also rather cynical about the government's willingness to provide an adequate level of resources. The Griffiths report, while denying that the review was a cost-cutting exercise, said nothing about the overall level of resources required to implement the changes, which lay outside its terms of reference.

These doubts were offset to some extent by relief that at last the government was taking a serious interest in community care. Moreover, there was broad support for many of the ideas put forward by Griffiths, such as a minister for community care, the ring-fencing of central funds for community care, the strategic role of the local authority, and the arrangement of care packages for individuals. Indeed, the last two of these recommendations were also backed by an official enquiry into residential care. The Wagner report, which had been commissioned by the DHSS and reported around the same time, thereby added further weight to Griffiths' recommendations (National Institute for Social Work, 1988).

☐ *Implementation*

There was, however, considerable opposition to the Griffiths report from within the government itself. Since taking office in 1979, the Thatcher government had harboured a suspicion of local government and in particular its spending ambitions. The Prime Minister and some of her senior colleagues were therefore unhappy at the recommendation to grant local authorities a key role in the new regime. This recommendation also horrified right-wing pressure groups close to the government. Both the Adam Smith Institute (1989) and the Institute for Economic Affairs (1989) subsequently came up with alternative plans to reform community care without expanding the local authority role.

The delay caused by internal battles within the government over the Griffiths report was considerable. The *Economist*, observed that the government had held on to the original Griffiths report for sixteen months: longer than it took the author to research and write it (*Economist*, 20 April 1991, p. 27). Eventually the government published its response in the form of a White Paper, *Caring for People* (Cm 849, 1989).

According to Kenneth Clarke, the then Secretary of State for Health, the White Paper was 'eighty per cent Griffiths'. The White Paper upheld Griffiths' central idea that the lead responsibility for community care should be given to local authorities and it backed the widely supported principle of case management. But there were a number of concessions made to those who had expressed concern about some of the review's recommendations.

First, Griffiths left open the question of how to deal with those already in residential care. The government seized on this deliberate omission, and attempted to placate the private residential sector, as well as some of the elderly and other client groups, by protecting those already in residential care from the changes. These become known as 'preserved rights' residents. Second, the government did not back the idea of a minister responsible for all aspects of community care at a national level. Indeed, such a move was rendered virtually impossible by the division of the DHSS in 1988. The government offered consolation by identifying community care as a specific responsibility of a junior minister at the Department of Health. But this responsibility excluded the social security aspects of community care, which now came under the new Department of Social Security.

Third, the government refused to accept the proposal to grant specific 'ring-fenced' community care funds for all client groups. Only services for the mentally ill would receive such grants, and these were to be channelled through to local government from health authorities. The decision not to 'ring-fence' all community care funds evoked strong opposition from local authorities. Three years later the government backed down on this question, when it announced that during the first few years of the policy, local authorities would not be able to use central government funds earmarked for community care for other purposes.

The White Paper also stressed privatisation far more heavily than Griffiths had done. The Griffiths report clearly wished to encourage private provision, in circumstances where this was more economic and efficient than direct provision by the public sector, but the report did not openly advocate the widespread replacement of statutory services by the private sector. The government stated that maximum use should be made of the private (that is, commercial and voluntary) sector, and sought to enforce this through a planning and review system. At the same time it was decided that council-run homes would not receive the residential allowance – a housing cost element for each resident. This placed them at a disadvantage compared with commercial and voluntary homes, and provided an incentive for councils to privatise their homes, or place their residents in the private sector.

The importance of the private sector was further underlined during the implementation of the reforms. The Department of Health required local authorities to allocate 85 per cent of any new money they received from central government towards services provided by the private sector. This '85 per cent rule' was designed to protect the private residential sector to some extent from the loss of 'new business' and to promote the gradual expansion of private community-based services.

In the words of the then Labour spokesman on local government, David Blunkett, the local authorities had been handed a 'poisoned chalice' by the government. They were to be given the responsibility for community care, but would not be given adequate resources to do the job. Moreover, the role which had been given to local authorities – effectively that of purchasers in a community care market – gave further scope for privatisation of service provision, not just in residential care but also increasingly in domiciliary and other home support services, such as home helps. This generated much concern within local government, and discussions with the government over the detailed implementation of the White Paper became increasingly acrimonious.

Many of the problems of implementation were highlighted by the House of Commons Social Services Committee in a series of reports in the 1989/90 session of Parliament (House of Commons, 1990d–h; see also the government response – Cm 1343, 1990). The Committee believed that the government was unrealistic in expecting the new structure for community care to be in place within such a short space of time.

Despite these reservations, the government pressed ahead with legislation in the form of the NHS and Community Care Act of 1990 (the same legislation that enacted the internal market reforms announced in *Working for Patients*, which was discussed in Chapter 8). But towards the end of 1990, health ministers announced that they would be delaying the implementation of most of the community care provisions until April 1993. The main reason was not the failure to secure agreement with the local authorities on the details of implementation; it was the wider issue of local government finance which derailed the government's plans. The government had miscalculated the levels of the community charge, the local tax which replaced domestic rates. The result was higher-than-expected bills, which would have been even higher had the community care reforms been implemented. It was estimated that if the reforms had gone ahead, around £15 would have been added to each community charge bill in 1991/2. Given the proximity to a general election, political expediency dictated that the reforms should be shelved.

☐ After the election

Following the Conservative victory at the 1992 General Election the government became worried once again about the introduction of the community care reforms. Yet again, this was related to local government finance. Ministers were worried that the new council tax would be as unpopular as its predecessor, the community charge, if higher bills resulted from the community care reforms.

In December 1992 the Department of Health announced a transfer of funds from the social security budget to the local authorities in the form of a special transitional grant (STG). In the initial three-year period the local authorities will receive over £1.5 billion in 'ring-fenced' STG from April 1993 to help them cope with their new responsibilities. The concern about the adequacy of these funds remained (House of Commons, 1993). The transfer of funds, moreover, was to depend on local authorities reaching agreement with health authorities on two main issues: strategies for placing people in nursing homes; and the integration of arrangements for discharging people from hospital with the new care assessment procedures. In order to be eligible for funding, local authorities had to secure agreement by December 1992. All of them, in fact, met this deadline.

Earlier, in April 1992, all but one local authority had published their community care plans. These and future plans will be monitored by the Social Services Inspectorate within the Department of Health. It now appears that the planning and review process is not as centrally controlled as originally envisaged. The government, for the moment, seems happy to allow health and local authorities to find their own working arrangements for implementing the reforms. There is no requirement that joint plans be produced, although some local authorities and health authorities have developed such plans. While some welcome the flexibility that such an approach may bring, others feel that a more rigorous framework of planning and collaboration is required at the local level if the aims of the community care policy are to be realised (House of Commons, 1990f).

The government intended that the first year of the community care reforms would take the form of a 'steady state', rather like that which followed the introduction of the NHS internal market. The '85 per cent rule' and 'preserved rights' for existing residents, discussed earlier, represented a clear attempt to prevent radical changes taking place immediately. The transitional arrangements set out in the STG also discouraged a shift in provision, by funding local authorities partly on the existing pattern of social security spending. In addition, the Department of Health urged local authorities to be cautious about developing innovative community care schemes in the first year.

It seems likely that the impact of the reforms will be spread over subsequent years. There have been some immediately apparent consequences, however, which deserve a mention. Services for those with alcohol and drug problems appear to have been hit quite badly by the changes. In a number of cases those requiring help have experienced delays due to the new assessment procedures, and in at least one case such delay has led to a fatality.

Drug and alcohol services, and other care services which cater for a rootless or homeless population, have faced other difficulties in the light of the changes. Such services are often seen by local authorities as being of low priority, and some agencies have had their budgets drastically reduced since April 1993. In addition, the new system of funding which allocates resources on the basis of the users' place of residence is obviously inappropriate for services catering for the homeless and rootless, who have no permanent base and who often seek help far away from their original residence.

There was also a great deal of concern in the months following the introduction of the reforms about the whole question of caring for mentally ill offenders in the community. This was heightened by the publicity given to several serious offences, including murder, committed by mentally ill people who had been recently discharged from institutions. These events could not be attributed directly to the community care reforms, although services for the 'homeless and rootless' mentally ill have been threatened by the new funding arrangements in similar ways to the alcohol and drug agencies. These cases, however, did raise broader issues about whether community care was appropriate for individuals who remained a danger to themselves and to others and about the adequacy of supervision arrangements for mentally ill people discharged into the community.

■ Conclusion

Delay has constantly dogged the implementation of community care. Community care strategies in Britain have moved at different speeds, reflecting the diversity of policy in different areas (Hunter and Wistow, 1987 a and b). It is generally recognised that progress has been slower in Scotland (particularly with respect to the mentally handicapped) and faster in Wales, when compared with England.

One reason why community care has been subject to such delays lies in Griffiths' comment that it is a 'poor relation; everybody's distant relative but nobody's baby' (DHSS, 1988b, p. iv). A similar point could have been made about primary care, which, as shown in Chapter 9, has also suffered from neglect in the past.

Community care, like primary care, has moved up the political agenda in the 1980s. Both have completed a move from the backstage to the forefront of policy development, yet the increased attention given to these issues may have been, from the point of view of some commentators, for the wrong reasons. As Langan (1990) has commented in a review of community care policies, 'the central concern of the government is not to improve the quality of community care, but to reorganise community care in the interests of reducing overall social services expenditure'. Others, particularly those in the labour and trade union movement, point out that it is easier to privatise primary and community services than mainstream hospital services.

Recent policies have certainly reflected the desire of the government to privatise community provision, yet it is by no means clear what will happen in the longer term. The community care reforms may produce an expansion of publicly-funded care by highlighting the gap between resources and services, leading to pressure for greater public funding (Levick, 1992). Moreover, the assessment of needs, which forms an important part of these reforms, may give individuals a right to care which they previously did not possess. If this is upheld it will be incumbent on the authorities to arrange adequate levels of provision, a development the government certainly did not intend.

The future is highly uncertain. The introduction of competitive market forces into both primary care and community care is, as in the acute sector, a leap in the dark. A number of observers – including the Health Committee – have expressed their doubts as to whether increased competition in health and social care will actually improve service quality, efficiency and consumer choice (House of Commons, 1990 e, f, g; 1993). Indeed, it is entirely possible that the market reforms in both these sectors of care could produce more rather than less bureaucracy, and less rather than more choice for service users.

■ *Chapter 11* ■

The Health of the Nation

For most of this century, health policy has been concerned mainly with the provision of health care rather than with the promotion and maintenance of good health. Public health medicine, with its emphasis on tackling health problems through prevention and early detection of illness at the community level, has played second fiddle to the mainstream biomedical approach, which focuses more narrowly on the manifestation, diagnosis and treatment of disease in individuals.

The public health approach has not always been subordinate. In Victorian times there was a very clear emphasis on public health. Reforms introduced by the Victorians provided a legislative and administrative framework, in the form of the Public Health Acts of 1848, 1872 and 1875, which acted as a firm basis for improvements in the nation's health. Moreover, in recent years the public health approach has undergone something of a revival. It is now realised that many of the challenges facing the health system, outlined in Chapter 1, require a much more broader approach than simply expanding health services. Public health is now firmly back on the political agenda.

This chapter is divided into three main parts. First, there is a discussion of the decline of the public health approach in the present century and its recent revival. This is followed by an account of the Thatcher government's response to the need for a public health strategy during the 1980s. Finally, the British government's current health strategy is examined, along with its future prospects.

■ The fall and rise of public health

□ *The decline of public health*

During the early years of the twentieth century, the emphasis began to shift from public health towards the provision of health care and, in particular, hospital services. This reflected the growing role of the state in promoting, financing and providing health care services, which culminated in the creation of the NHS after the Second World War (Brand, 1965).

In the post-war period, the reorganisation of responsibilities within central government sharpened the focus on health services. By the 1950s, the main department responsible for health policy, the Ministry of Health, had lost many of its wider public health responsibilities, including housing and water, to other departments. As a result, health policy at a national level became increasingly concerned with the development of services. In Klein's (1980) words, 'Britain had a health service but no policy for health.'

As the century progressed, health policy at a local level also focused increasingly on service provision. In consequence, the Medical Officers of Health (MoH), created by the Victorians to act as guardians of the public health at a local level, also became more service-orientated. Moreover, the status of the MoH deteriorated as local authorities were dispossessed of health functions in the post-war period. The removal of municipal hospital services from local authorities following the creation of the NHS began a period of separation between the community and hospital services to the detriment of the former. Reorganisation in 1974 further reduced the health service functions of the local authorities by transferring all but environmental health and personal social services to the NHS.

The 1974 reorganisation also abolished the post of MoH, replacing it with the community physician employed by the health authorities. Community physicians were mainly concerned with service planning and had a place on the newly-created consensus management teams. Though it was intended that the status of the new community physicians would be higher than that of their predecessors, the MoHs, this move did not halt the long-term decline of the public health doctor (Lewis, 1987). The final straw came with the Griffiths management reforms, which restricted the role of the community physician and led in some authorities to the abolition of their posts. Public health medicine had plummeted to an all-time low.

☐ *The need for a public health strategy*

In retrospect, the movement away from a broad public health philosophy was a mistake. In the early 1970s there was a growing recognition that the burden of illness in modern societies required something more than a narrow medical response. Since then, the need for a public health strategy has become even more evident.

In Chapter 1, it was pointed out that the bulk of the illness burden in the developed world is in the form of chronic diseases, and that the UK is no exception. However, many of these chronic diseases may be reduced to some extent by taking preventive action at the community level. These diseases include heart and circulatory diseases, cancers and respiratory diseases. But the value of preventive action is not confined to chronic disease alone. Many acute health problems, some of which cause premature death and permanent disability, are also preventable; these include deaths and injuries caused by accidents and violence, and infectious diseases.

We shall shortly explore the broad types of action which can be undertaken to prevent illness and death, but before we do this it is important to examine the most significant causes of mortality and morbidity operating at the social level. These causes can be divided into three categories: lifestyle, environment, and deprivation.

□ *Lifestyle*

The way in which people live their lives has an important bearing on their health. Smoking, poor diet, alcohol abuse and 'unsafe' sexual habits have been identified as being among the most important lifestyle factors affecting health.

- Smoking-related diseases kill approximately 100 000 people each year (Royal College of Physicians, 1983b). In addition to its role in heart disease, smoking is a causal factor in respiratory illnesses such as emphysema, bronchitis, and cancers of the throat and lung; lung cancer alone kills 40 000 people a year in the UK. In addition, smoking during pregnancy can damage the foetus. Recent evidence on the impact of passive smoking suggests that non-smokers may also be at risk (Independent Scientific Committee on Smoking and Health, 1988). Smoking-related diseases are relatively difficult to cure – lung cancer survival rates are quite low – and therefore the most cost-effective strategy to deal with the health problems associated with smoking is prevention: to persuade people to give up the habit.
- Diet is also an important lifestyle factor affecting health, (BMA, 1986a; WHO, 1988). Diet is associated with around 35 per cent of all cancers (Doll and Peto, 1981), including bowel cancer, the second largest cause of death from cancer in the UK (Royal College of Physicians, 1981). It is believed that bowel cancer may be prevented by increasing the consumption of fibre in the diet.

  Diet is also implicated in heart disease (British Cardiac Society, 1987). High blood cholesterol has for some time been recognised as a major risk factor for heart disease. Blood cholesterol can be reduced by increasing dietary fibre, by reducing total fat consumption (particularly saturated fat, which is derived mainly from animals) and by drugs. However, this situation has been complicated in recent years by evidence linking low cholesterol levels to other causes of morbidity and mortality, including cancer. Attempts to lower cholesterol levels across the board may well reduce heart disease but could exacerbate other health problems (Dunnigan, 1993). High blood pressure, another major risk factor for heart disease and for stroke, may also in some cases be related to diet – the excess consumption of salt can raise blood pressure in some individuals. Obesity is also held to be a risk factor in heart disease, stroke and cancers (Garrow, 1991), though the extent of its contribution, and indeed the causes of obesity, are often disputed, as was shown in Chapter 2.

- Alcohol is implicated in a wide range of health and social problems including accidents, violent assaults, mental illness, and a range of physical disorders and illnesses (Baggott, 1990; Faculty of Public Health Medicine, 1991a). One estimate – from the Royal College of General Practitioners (1986) – puts the annual number of deaths from alcohol abuse at 40 000. The cost of alcohol abuse to society has been estimated at almost £2000 million per annum (McDonnell and Maynard, 1985). There appears to be a general relationship between the level of alcohol consumption in a society and the level of alcohol-related problems. The doubling of the amount of alcohol consumed per adult in the UK over the past thirty years has been matched by a growth in alcohol problems over the same period.

- Sexually transmitted diseases (STDs), as noted in Chapter 1, have risen dramatically in the post-war period. The recent emergence of AIDS has made the prevention of STDs a crucial issue (Hancock and Carim, 1987). As yet, no one is sure of the exact proportion infected with HIV who will go on to develop AIDS; most recent estimates suggest around a third (Adler, 1987). As there is no cure at present for those infected, this leaves prevention as the only feasible way of tackling the disease.

☐ *Environment*

- Accidents are a major cause of illness and death. As we saw in Chapter 1, much of this toll involves young people and is road-traffic related. Around 5000 deaths every year result from road accidents, with a further 5000 caused by accidents in the home, and 500 deaths from accidents at work. Most accidents are preventable by altering the environment within which people live and work, and by educating individuals about risk.

- Pollution and contamination, are regarded as being major health problems (Hall, R. H., 1990; WHO, 1986). Air and water pollution can have a significant detrimental effect on the health of the population, particularly in the case of children and the elderly. However, the ways in which environmental pollution damages health are complex. It is not always possible to identify a simple causal process. For example the link between lead in car exhaust fumes and mental health problems in children (Wilson, 1983), or the relationship between pollution and asthma, are based on circumstantial evidence. Yet in such cases preventive action may be judged necessary because the potential consequences of inaction are so serious.

A further form of pollution is contamination in the agricultural and food industries (Cannon, 1987; Millstone, 1986). Pesticides, food additives and modern food production techniques have been associated with a wide range of health problems. In addition, the growth in food poisoning in recent years has also been attributed to such technologies (House of Commons, 1989c).

☐ *Deprivation and material conditions*

- As was shown in Chapter 1, there are wide variations between the social classes in terms of their relative mortality and morbidity. This suggests that social deprivation and differences in material conditions are responsible for at least some of the burden of illness. What in fact lies behind social variations in health, morbidity and mortality is the subject of controversial debate. It is widely accepted that specific social conditions such as poor housing (Lowry, 1991) and unemployment (Smith, R., 1987) are associated with with ill-health. Limited educational opportunities have an impact on social deprivation and may therefore contribute in varying degrees to ill-health within the population (BMA, 1987). Low incomes are also a probable factor, as indeed is income inequality. As noted in Chapter 1, research into the health of civil servants at different grades has revealed that employment grade and salary are strongly related to health status (Marmot *et al.*, 1991). Cross-national research has also revealed a link between income and health inequalities (Wilkinson, 1992). Later in this chapter there will be a closer examination of the impact of deprivation on health in the light of the wider social and economic policies pursued by the Conservative government during the 1980s.

Although it is useful to categorise possible causes of ill-health under these three headings, in practice the distinctions blur. Health problems rooted in deprivation, for example, are linked to unhealthy lifestyles.

Smoking is now a predominantly working-class habit (OPCS, 1992), while only the better-off may be able to afford a wholesome diet. Similarly, environmental factors are related to lifestyles. The use of the motor car, a major cause of both pollution and accidents is clearly related to the individualistic and materialistic lifestyle of modern industrialised countries. There are also many important forms of illness, notably mental illnesses such as anxiety and depression, which cannot be attributed wholly or directly to specific lifestyles, environments or material conditions, but which nevertheless may be preventable by concerted action in all three of these spheres.

☐ *Public health strategies*

Governments in industrial countries have recognised the need to tackle the social and environmental roots of ill-health. Policy-makers' attention may have been attracted to the academic debate over the role of social factors in ill-health and the relative effectiveness of medical and social intervention. But more significant, perhaps, is a belief that preventing the onset of illness could reduce health service costs. The potential for savings is illustrated by the case of heart disease, which costs the NHS £500 million every year, and the government a further £250 million in sick pay (National Audit Office, 1989c), although it has been pointed out that other costs are incurred by a healthier population in the longer term (Normand, 1991); as people live longer, the cost of services for the elderly is likely to rise.

There is still considerable room for disagreement on the precise relationship between social and environmental factors and ill-health, and how these problems should be tackled. Many governments have in recent years devised strategies which seek to prevent health problems and to identify conditions at an earlier stage, where treatment is more likely to be effective. Essentially, these strategies have three main elements (Smith and Jacobson, 1988).

First, *education* – to inform and persuade individuals to adopt healthy lifestyles and reject or moderate habits which may harm health – such as smoking and heavy drinking, for example. Education may also be aimed at groups and private institutions in an attempt to encourage voluntary collective action to prevent ill-health. Examples include the promotion of alcohol awareness and smoking bans in the workplace.

Second, *clinical prevention*. This includes services to monitor health and detect illness at an early stage. For example, the provision of screening facilities to detect the early signs of breast and cervical cancer. Also included in this category are other preventive clinical interventions such as immunisation against diseases such as mumps, measles, whooping cough and rubella (German measles).

A third part of any public health strategy is *intervention at the social and environmental level*. This involves government and other public authorities in adopting policies to tackle the causes of ill-health. The state has considerable legislative and financial powers to encourage health. It can, for example, ban or restrict activities which are harmful to health, or impose penal taxation upon such activities. It also has the capacity to co-ordinate national and local policies in order to ensure that health objectives are not compromised. The state also has the strength and legitimacy to restrict and regulate powerful vested interests whose activities may undermine public health, such as the alcohol, tobacco and food industries. Third, the state can arbitrate between individuals' rights and liberties. Some individuals in a liberal society may choose to indulge in health-damaging behaviour even when fully informed. These rights, however, impinge on others. The current issue of smoking restrictions in public places is a good example of how the state has to balance the conflicting rights and interests of its citizens.

☐ *Public health revival*

Policy-makers in many countries began to explore public health strategies during the mid-1970s. This was a period of severe economic crisis, which led to a squeeze on publicly-funded health services, and a search for more cost-effective health strategies. In the UK the Labour government published a consultative document, *Prevention and Health: Everybody's Business*, in 1976, which identified the following items as being key areas for future action: inequalities in health status; heart disease; road accidents; smoking-related diseases; alcoholism and mental illness; drugs; diet; and venereal disease. The tone of this document was not prescriptive; it aimed to promote discussion rather than to outline a programme of action.

It was expected that the government's subsequent White Paper (Cmnd 7047, 1977) would set out such a programme. In the event, this was a rather cautious document which failed to articulate a coherent public health strategy. Central government instead took a passive rather than a strategic role in the development of public health activities. Expenditure on health education was increased but interventionist measures were avoided. The government was also reluctant to provide extra resources to encourage prevention, refusing, for example, to divert resources from high technology medicine.

The Thatcher government and public health

☐ *Public health policies*

The Thatcher government gave added impetus to prevention. It initially put its faith in high-profile health education. The government spent around £2 million on drug abuse campaigns in the early 1980s. This was later exceeded by expensive campaigns on heart disease and AIDS. Spending on mass media health education campaigns rose from £1.6 million to £11.4 million per annum between 1979 and 1988 (Whitehead, 1989). In 1993, the government planned to spend over £20 million on such campaigns.

In addition, high level ministerial committees were established to discuss specific prevention issues such as AIDS, and drug and alcohol abuse. These committees in turn developed a number of policy initiatives. In the case of alcohol abuse, for example, the ministerial committee produced a list of policy initiatives, most of which were subsequently implemented. These included a tightening of the rules governing alcohol advertising, further restrictions on drinking and driving, and the encouragement of local inter-agency collaboration on alcohol problems (Lord President of the Council, 1991).

The Thatcher government actively supported clinical prevention by encouraging screening programmes for breast and cervical cancer. This included a national breast cancer screening programme costing around £100 million. 70 per cent of all women between the ages of 50 and 64, the age group invited for breast cancer screening, now attend. In addition, around £30 million per annum is spent on cervical cancer screening for women. Between 1976 and 1989, the proportion of women screened rose from 13 per cent to 21 per cent. The establishment of a nation-wide computerised call–recall system for cervical screening has helped raise this proportion further to over 70 per cent in 1991.

The shake-up of the primary care services, in the form of the White Paper, *Promoting Better Health*, also emphasised clinical prevention. This initiative, discussed in Chapter 9, led to the introduction of financial incentives for GPs for achieving target rates for child immunisation and cervical cancer screening. GPs were also encouraged to monitor the health of patients and to undertake health promotion clinics.

Despite the Thatcher government's apparent encouragement of preventive medicine, critics attacked its policies on a number of grounds (Public Health Alliance, 1988; Smith and Jacobson, 1988). The main criticisms were as follows.

☐ Education and clinical prevention

While the government's enthusiasm for health education and clinical prevention was applauded, there were some reservations. The emphasis on high-profile health education campaigns was criticised, and there was particular criticism of the government's drug abuse campaign, which some believed might be unhelpful as it reinforced the 'heroin addict' stereotype. At the same time the government expressed its hostility to low-profile community education campaigns, which form a useful part of a prevention strategy.

There was also criticism of the government's policy on screening services. While recognising that breast and cervical cancer represent major threats to women's health, some commentators have argued that the potential benefits of such screening programmes are low, in terms of numbers of lives saved relative to the resources invested (Barclay, 1989; McCullough, 1989; McCormick, 1989). Screening often fails to detect problems. One in five women screened will not have their cancers detected; on the other hand, in 95 per cent of cases where problems are found, the abnormality will be non-cancerous. This creates unnecessary anguish for women, and in some cases, unnecessary treatment as well.

The emphasis on GP-based health promotion was also criticised as being too narrow in its focus. Subsequent evaluation of health promotion in general practice revealed that the benefits had been modest relative to the cost, estimated at over £200 million (*Daily Telegraph*, 19 July 1993, p. 7).

A further line of criticism levelled at the policy on prevention was that, despite the rhetoric, little was being done to redress the imbalance between prevention and treatment services. A report on coronary heart disease by the Public Accounts Committee of the House of Commons (House of Commons, 1989d) revealed that only £10 million was being spent on prevention of this disease, compared with £500 million being spent on treatment services.

☐ Individual responsibility

The government accepted that many health problems were associated with social habits such as drinking, smoking and poor diet, but it took a rather narrow view of how such lifestyles had developed, attributing them largely to ignorance. There were fears that this emphasis was tantamount to 'victim blaming'. One minister in particular, Edwina Currie, was heavily criticised for her reported comments regarding diet (Currie, 1990).

An alternative view, noted earlier, is that lifestyles, environment and social conditions interact in a complex manner. Policies which simply try to change lifestyles through informing and educating the population may well be ineffective in the absence of a wider commitment to ensure that social conditions and the environment are conducive to the development of responsible and healthy lifestyles (Smith and Jacobson, 1988; Public Health Alliance, 1988).

For example, in order to prevent smoking-related diseases it may be necessary to regulate more effectively the marketing activities of the tobacco industry. Norway, for example, has operated a comprehensive Tobacco Act involving a total ban for nearly two decades on the advertising and promotion of tobacco products. Britain has avoided taking such a step in the face of considerable pressure, as will be seen later.

Intervention to protect public health proved less compatible with the Conservative government's philosophy. Its attachment to free markets bolstered a resistance to intervention in commercial aspects of ill-health. Previous governments were also reluctant to tackle those industries whose products and practices are connected with public health problems, namely the alcohol, tobacco and food industries. It is easy to understand why. Profits from alcohol and tobacco companies total over £2 billion per annum. These products also raise around 9 per cent of tax revenue. The food industry, on the other hand, accounts for approximately 10 per cent of manufacturing output and employment (Millstone, 1986). These industries are wealthy; they have considerable political leverage and can persuade governments not to intervene in their commercial affairs (Taylor, 1984). They also make considerable contributions to Conservative Party funds and this may in part explain the added reluctance of a Conservative government to adopt policies hostile to their interests.

☐ Social and economic policy

There has been a great deal of criticism of the impact of the Thatcher government's social and economic policies upon public health. Economic policies such as deregulation have been blamed for inadequate health and safety standards. The rapid increase in food poisoning has been blamed partly on weak regulation of the food industry.

Another main feature of government policy in the 1980s – privatisation – may have had an impact on health. Most of the utility companies increased prices following privatisation. They also appear more ready to disconnect services to those who fail to pay their bills. Perhaps the privatisation of the water authorities has attracted the most concern, however, given the importance of water availability, price and quality in the maintenance of public health.

The general aim of government policy in the 1980s was to improve economic incentives. This actually led to a greater degree of inequality. In income distribution the top fifth received 42 per cent of disposable income in 1986 compared with 38 per cent in 1976. The bottom fifth received 6 per cent of income compared with over 7 per cent ten years earlier. Subsequent taxation and social security changes in the late 1980s widened this gap even further. By 1989, 12 million people (22 per cent of households) were living on below half the average income, compared with 5 million people (9 per cent of households) a decade earlier (Department of Social Security, 1992).

The government has denied that material inequalities are a direct cause of ill-health. While accepting the existence of health inequalities, the official line has been that the variation between the health of different social classes can be explained in other ways, and indeed, there *are* alternative explanations which can be used to explain health inequalities (Carr-Hill, 1987).

It has been argued, for example, that the method of measuring class – by occupation – artificially exaggerates inequalities in health (Illsley, 1986). Misrecording of occupations may also contribute to the distortion of these figures. It is worth noting that the mortality rates are calculated on the basis of the occupation of the deceased taken from the death certificate. Previous occupations, which might have placed people in a higher social category, are not therefore taken into account.

Accurate measurement of health inequalities over a period of time is difficult, and reclassification of occupations has added to these difficulties. The changing size of the social classes themselves (between 1931 and 1981 social class V shrank by 55 per cent while social class I grew by 217 per cent) also means that over time one is not comparing like with like. The widening gap between the social classes may therefore be a reflection of the growth in the upper/middle classes and the shrinkage of the working class. Recent studies however, suggest that even when the changing size of classes is taken into account, health inequalities remain significant (Pamuk, 1985; Goldblatt, 1989).

An alternative explanation for health inequalities lies in the process of social selection. According to this argument, social class differences in health result from healthy people moving up the social ladder and unhealthy people moving down it (Stern, 1983). After all, one would imagine that the healthy would be in a better position to hold down jobs, own their own homes and so on. Though intuitively attractive, there is little evidence to support this theory (Goldblatt, 1989).

A third alternative explanation focuses on the behaviour of individuals within the social classes. The lower social classes, according to this explanation, adopt less healthy lifestyles. In particular, their drinking, smoking and eating habits are held to be responsible for much of their ill-health. While these factors may well be important, the behavioural explanation of health inequalities diverts attention from the social conditions within which individuals make choices. It is clear that individuals do not make choices within a vacuum: eating, smoking and drinking habits, for example, are shaped by class and income as well as personal whim.

Studies which have attributed health inequalities to material circumstances and social class structure have been rejected with hostility by the Conservative government. In 1980, the report of a DHSS Working Party (the Black report), which had been established by the previous Labour government to explore health inequalities, was treated with contempt by Conservative ministers for putting this case forward (DHSS, 1980; Townsend, Davidson, Whitehead, 1988).

In 1987 an updated version of the Black report, by the Health Education Council, received a similar response (Whitehead, 1987). This report, entitled *The Health Divide*, confirmed that inequalities in health had persisted into the 1980s, and pointed out that in some respects the situation had worsened. Increasing homelessness (which, even according to official figures, almost doubled during the 1980s), greater income inequality, poverty and mass unemployment lay behind these trends. The report pointed out a particularly disturbing increase in child poverty and criticised the lack of a co-ordinated strategy to tackle the social roots of ill-health.

☐ *Where is the strategy?*

Although supporting specific prevention initiatives, the Thatcher government made little attempt to co-ordinate action on public health. At the top, departments within central government were often seen to be in conflict on public health issues. For example, in the late 1980s the Ministry of Agriculture and the Department of Health took different views on a number of issues, such as salmonella in eggs (Doig, 1990).

Even where clear public health initiatives had been adopted by central government, they were not fully implemented. This was largely because DHAs were not allocated specific funds for such programmes, and their performance was not properly monitored (House of Commons, 1986a). As a result, health authorities varied considerably in their commitment to public health initiatives. Particular criticism was levelled at the uneven development of heart disease prevention strategies at local level (House of Commons, 1989d; National Audit Office, 1989c).

Other failures of public health strategy were uncovered by public inquiries into two serious outbreaks of infectious disease during the mid-1980s. The first of these involved an outbreak of food poisoning at the Stanley Royd Hospital in Wakefield, which resulted in nineteen deaths (Cmnd 9716, 1986). The other incident concerned an outbreak of Legionnaires disease at Stafford General Hospital where thirty-nine people died (Cmnd 9772, 1986). Both cases exposed failures of public health planning at a local level and a shortage of medical expertise in environmental health.

The concern raised by these reports, along with the continuing problems faced by community physicians mentioned earlier in this chapter, led to the establishment of a further inquiry by the Chief Medical Officer (then Sir Donald Acheson) into the problems of public health function in England. The Acheson report suggested a number of changes (which will be discussed later), which provided the basis for a more sharply-focused approach to public health (Cm 289, 1988).

It was perhaps not surprising to find a lack of co-ordination between government departments and those concerned with public health at a local level, given the Thatcher government's refusal to adopt a coherent plan or strategy aimed at tackling the major causes of ill-health. Increasingly this seemed out of step with other countries. The UK was formally committed to the World Health Organisation's 'Health For All' initiative, which set objectives to be achieved by the year 2000. These included the achievement of equity in health, the development of public policies acknowledging the health dimension, reducing accidents, improving food safety and so on. In addition, other more specific targets – such as a 25 per cent reduction in alcohol consumption – were also set by the World Health Organisation for European countries (see Exhibit 11.1). On top of this, the European Community began to take a growing interest in tackling public health problems (House of Lords, 1985). This included imposing a common set of health warnings on tobacco products in member countries – moves which were vigorously and unsuccessfully opposed by the UK. This was followed by moves to ban tobacco advertising entirely.

For most of the 1980s the UK government acknowledged these international developments, but failed to formulate its own national strategy. Many local authorities bypassed central government and set up their own strategies for health. Many built on the experience of the World Health Organisation's 'Healthy Cities' initiative. This programme sought to establish a comprehensive strategy to improve the health of local people. It was targeted at cities with the worst health and social problems. The cities in the UK which participated in the programme were Liverpool, Belfast, Glasgow and the London Borough of Camden.

**Exhibit 11.1   World Health Organisation: Health for All
by the Year 2000**

Regional targets for Europe (base year 1980)

1. By the year 2000, the real differences in health status between countries and groups should be reduced by at least 25 per cent.
2. By the year 2000 people should have the basic opportunity to develop and use their health potential to live socially and economically fulfilling lives.
3. By the year 2000 disabled persons should have the physical, social and economic opportunities that allow for a socially and economically fulfilling and mentally creative life.
4. By the year 2000 the average number of years that people live free from major disease and disability should be increased by at least 10 per cent.
5. Life expectancy at birth in the region should be at least 75 years by the year 2000.
6. By the year 2000 there should be no indigenous measles, poliomyelitis, neonatal tetanus, congenital rubella, diphtheria, congenital syphilis or indigenous malaria in the region.
7. Infant mortality in the region should be less than 20 per 1000 live births by the year 2000.
8. Maternal mortality in the region should be less than 15 per 100 000 live births by the year 2000.
9. Mortality in the region from diseases of the circulatory system in people under 65 should be reduced by at least 15 per cent by the year 2000.
10. Mortality in the region from cancer in people under 65 should be reduced by at least 15 per cent by the year 2000.
11. Deaths from accidents in the region should be reduced by at least 25 per cent by the year 2000.
12. By the year 2000, the current rising trends in suicides should be reversed.
13. National policies in all member states should ensure that by 1990 legislative, administrative and economic mechanisms provide broad intersectoral support and resources for the promotion of healthy lifestyles and ensure effective participation of the people at all levels of such policy-making.
14. All member states should by 1990 have specific programmes which enhance the major role of the family and other social groups in developing and supporting healthy lifestyles.
15. Educational programmes in all states by 1990 should enhance the knowledge, motivation and skills of people to acquire and maintain health.
16. In all states by 1995 there should be significant increases in positive health behaviour, such as balanced nutrition, non-smoking, appropriate physical activity and good stress management.
17. In all states by 1995 there should be significant decreases in health-damaging behaviour, such as the overuse of alcohol and pharmaceutical products, use of illicit drugs, and dangerous chemical substances, dangerous driving and violent social behaviour.

18. By 1990 member states should have multisectoral policies that effectively protect the human environment from health hazards, ensure community awareness and involvement, and effectively support international efforts to curb such hazards.
19. By 1990 member states should have adequate machinery for the control of environmental hazards.
20. By 1990 people should have adequate supplies of safe drinking water. By 1995 pollution of rivers, lakes and seas should pose no threat to human health.
21. By 1995 the people should be protected from air pollution.
22. By 1990 states should have significantly reduced risk from food contamination and should have implemented measures to control harmful additives.
23. By 1995 member states should have eliminated major risks associated with hazardous waste.
24. By 2000 all the people of the region should have a better opportunity of living in houses which provide a healthy environment.
25. By 1995 people should be protected against work-related health risks.
26. By 1990 states should have developed health care systems based on primary care.
27. By 1990 states should ensure that health care resources are delivered according to need, and that services are accessible and acceptable to all.
28. By 1990 the primary care system should provide a wide range of services to meet basic health needs and give special attention to high risk, vulnerable and underserved groups and individuals.
29. By 1995 primary care systems should be based on co-operation and teamwork between health care workers, individuals, families and community groups.
30. By 1990 all states should have the means of co-ordinating all sectors related to health at the community level within the primary care system.
31. By 1990 all states should have effective mechanisms for ensuring the quality of patient care.
32. Before 1990 all states should have a research strategy to support 'Health for All' (HFA).
33. Before 1990 all states should ensure that health policies are in line with HFA.
34. Before 1990 all states should ensure that management and resource allocation processes are in harmony with HFA and health development priorities.
35. Before 1990 all states should have information systems to support HFA strategy.
36. Before 1990 all states should have staff training and deployment policies in line with HFA and the emphasis on primary care.
37. Before 1990 all states should ensure that staff in all sectors related to health have adequate information about HFA policies and programmes.
38. Before 1990 all states should have systems for assessing health technologies.

Some health authorities also paid attention to the 'Health for All' initiative. By 1990 around three-quarters of health authorities had established local priorities in line with 'Health for All' (Disken, 1990). Even so, this initiative had a relatively low priority. Less than a third of health authorities had specifically allocated resources to 'Health for All', and only half had appointed an individual to take responsibility for the initiative.

Elsewhere in the UK the picture was different. In Wales, attempts were made in the late 1980s to develop a clear health strategy along the lines of 'Health for All'. The NHS Welsh Health Planning Forum began to look at the development of such a strategy during 1988. It identified ten problem areas including heart and circulatory disease, respiratory illness, and healthy environments. Resources were then geared to tackling these specific problems with a view to increasing life expectancy and the quality of life (Health Promotion Authority for Wales, 1990). Other parts of the UK also seemed to be giving greater emphasis to health promotion and health targets. In Scotland, plans were drawn up setting attainment targets for improving health in the under-65s by the year 2000 (Scottish Office, 1991), while in Northern Ireland a consultation document was published on the subject of health promotion (Northern Ireland Health Promotion Agency, 1990).

■ A health strategy for England

□ The emergence of a health strategy

Public health issues were almost a permanent feature of the political agenda in the late 1980s: AIDS, drug and alcohol abuse, smoking, food poisoning, environmental pollution and so on. The government at first responded to these issues in a piecemeal fashion, but following the Acheson report, mentioned earlier, a more coherent response appeared to be developing.

The Acheson report on public health led to a number of administrative changes. These included the establishment of a public health unit within the Department of Health. The government also placed upon health authorities a new responsibility for the health of their resident populations. Health authorities were required to appoint directors of public health to monitor the health of the local population. The government also envisaged that, in future, improvements in the health of the local population would be used as an indicator of health authority performance.

Following the departure of Margaret Thatcher as Prime Minister in November 1990, it became clear that the government was thinking seriously of a much broader national strategy for health. After months of speculation, the government set out its ideas for such a strategy in a Green Paper entitled *The Health of the Nation* (Cm 1523, 1991). After a period of consultation, the government finalised its plans in the form of a White Paper (Cm 1986, 1992) a year later.

☐ *The health of the nation*

The goal of the government's strategy is to secure continuing improvement in the health of the population in two main senses. First, by adding years to life, which means increasing life expectancy and reducing premature death. Second, by adding life to years, which means increasing the quality of life and minimising illness. In accepting these goals, the government explicitly accepted the general thrust of the 'Health for All' approach.

At the heart of the government's strategy for health is the selection of key areas for action. The criteria for choosing key areas were as follows: that the health problem must be a major cause of premature death or avoidable ill-health; it must be responsive to effective intervention; and it must enable the setting of objectives, targets and monitoring.

The Green Paper had earlier set out a number of possible key areas from which a selection of priorities could be made. These included causes of substantial mortality such as coronary heart disease, stroke, cancers and accidents. Causes of substantial ill-health such as mental health problems, diabetes and asthma were also included, as were factors contributing to both mortality and morbidity, such as smoking, alcohol consumption and lack of exercise. Areas where there was clear room for improvement were also considered relevant. These included the health of the elderly; the health of pregnant women; dental health; the health of infants and children; rehabilitation of the physically disabled; back pain; drug misuse; and environmental quality. Finally, a number of other health problems were identified where there was great potential for harm, such as HIV/AIDS, other communicable diseases such as hospital-acquired infections, and food safety.

The White Paper narrowed these possibilities down to five key areas. Some potential key areas were discarded because the government believed them to be already sufficiently well-developed. These included childhood immunisation, maternal and child health, and food safety. Other areas were not designated as key areas because, according to the government, further research and development were required before national targets could be set. These included rehabilitation, the health of the elderly, asthma, back pain and drug misuse. Three other potential key areas – diabetes, hospital-acquired infections and breastfeeding were acknowledged by the government as being important but nevertheless did not qualify for key area status.

The remaining five priorities – cancer; heart disease and stroke; mental illness; HIV/AIDS and sexual health; and accidents – were considered to be suitable key areas for the setting of targets. Two types of targets were identified. First, main targets, setting out reductions in the incidence of illness and mortality in various key areas. Second, risk factor targets, aimed at tackling some of the causes of these illnesses. These targets as set out by the White Paper are detailed in Exhibits 11.2 and 11.3.

☐ *Implementing the strategy*

The government is seeking to implement the health targets in several ways: through central government policy; the NHS; local authorities; the Health Education Authority; voluntary organisations; the media; and the workplace.

Central government's main contribution is to co-ordinate the work of the various departments of state in line with the health strategy. The government established a ministerial cabinet committee (involving ministers drawn from eleven government departments) to oversee the implementation of the strategy for England and to co-ordinate UK-wide issues affecting health. Supporting this ministerial committee are three additional working groups: the 'Wider Health Working Group' (chaired by a Health Minister); the 'Health Priorities Working Group' (chaired by the Government's Chief Medical Officer); and the 'Working Group on Implementation in the NHS' (chaired by the NHS Chief Executive). The government also announced its intention to produce guidance on policy appraisal and health, with the aim of assessing all government policies in terms of their consequences for health.

The NHS is expected to operate within the framework of the national health strategy. Health authorities, in accordance with earlier guidance from the Department of Health mentioned above, are expected to monitor the health of their populations, and to plan services in relation to needs. Health authorities are also expected to collaborate with other agencies in an attempt to tackle the main health problems identified by the national strategy. Regional co-ordinators have been appointed subsequently, to assist with the implementation process by ensuring the dissemination of good practice. The NHSME has also established 'focus groups' for each of the key areas, to emphasise their importance within the NHS.

Exhibit 11.2   *The health of the nation: main targets*

Coronary heart disease and stroke

Targets
- To reduce death rates in the under 65 age group for both coronary heart disease (CHD) and stroke by 40 per cent by the year 2000 (from a 1990 baseline).
- To reduce death rate for CHD in people aged 65–74 by at least 30 per cent by the year 2000 (from a 1990 baseline).
- To reduce death rate for stroke in people aged 65–74 by at least 40 per cent by the year 2000 (1990 baseline).

Cancer

Targets
- To reduce the death rate from breast cancer in the screened population by at least 25 per cent by the year 2000 (1990 baseline).
- To reduce the incidence of invasive cervical cancer by at least 20 per cent by the year 2000 (1986 baseline).
- To reduce the death rate for lung cancer under the age of 75 by at least 30 per cent in men and by at least 15 per cent in women by 2010 (1990 baseline).
- To halt the year-on-year increase in skin cancer by 2005.

Mental health

Targets
- To improve significantly the health and social functioning of mentally ill people.
- To reduce the overall suicide rate by at least 15 per cent by the year 2000 (1990 baseline).
- To reduce the suicide rate of severely mentally ill people by at least 33 per cent by the year 2000 (1990 baseline).

HIV/AIDS and sexual health

Targets
- To reduce the incidence of gonorrhoea by at least 20 per cent by 1995 (1990 baseline) as an indicator of HIV/AIDS trends.
- To reduce by at least 50 per cent the rate of conceptions among the under-16s by the year 2000 (1989 Baseline).

Accidents

Targets
- To reduce the death rate for accidents among children aged under 15 by at least 33 per cent by 2005 (1990 baseline).
- To reduce the death rate for accidents among young people aged 15–24 by at least 25 per cent by 2005 (1990 baseline).
- To reduce the death rate for accidents among people aged 65 and over by at least 33 per cent by 2005 (1990 baseline).

Source: *The Health of the Nation*, Cm 1986, 1992, pp. 18–19.

Exhibit 11.3 The health of the nation: risk factor targets

Diet and nutrition

Targets
- To reduce the proportion of men drinking more than 21 units of alcohol (roughly 10.5 pints of beer) per week, and the proportion of women drinking more than 14 units per week, by 30 per cent by 2005 (1990 baseline).
- To reduce the proportion of obese men and women in the 16–64 age group by 25 per cent and 33 per cent respectively by 2005 (baseline, 1986/7).
- To reduce the average percentage of food energy derived by the population from saturated fat by at least 35 per cent by 2005 (baseline, 1990).
- To reduce the average percentage of food energy derived from total fat by the population by at least 12 per cent by 2005 (baseline, 1990).

Smoking

Targets
- To reduce the proportion of men and women smoking cigarettes to no more than 20 per cent by the year 2000 – a reduction of around a third (baseline, 1990).
- To reduce the consumption of cigarettes by 40 per cent by the year 2000 (baseline, 1990).
- To reduce the prevalence of smoking among 11–15 year olds by at least 33 per cent by 1994 (baseline, 1988).
- To reduce smoking among women at the start of pregnancy by at least 33 per cent by the year 2000.

Blood pressure

Target
- To reduce mean systolic blood pressure in the adult population by at least 5mm Hg by 2005 (baseline to be established by a new national survey).

HIV/AIDS

Target
- To reduce the percentage of injecting drug misusers who report sharing injecting equipment in the previous 4 weeks from 20 per cent in 1990 to no more than 10 per cent by 1997 and no more than 5 per cent by the year 2000.

Source: *The Health of the Nation*, Cm 1986, 1992, p. 20.

Collaboration is a central theme of the government's strategy. Local authorities are regarded as being important collaborators, given their role in protecting environmental health. Other agencies, such as the Health Education Authority, the voluntary sector, the media and employers have also been identified as having a role in relation to the strategy. They are expected to co-operate and collaborate with government agencies.

The government has envisaged the formation of 'healthy alliances' to improve health in certain key areas. Several settings have been identified as possible areas where healthy alliances could emerge. These are 'healthy cities', 'healthy schools', 'healthy hospitals', 'healthy homes', 'healthy workplaces', 'healthy prisons' and 'healthy environments'. These settings provide a focal point for collaborative action and the achievement of the key area targets.

The government also announced a series of measures directed at improving the information base. These included more surveys of health and illness, a public health information strategy, and new research and development priorities to reflect the health strategy.

☐ Criticism of the government's strategy

The overall aims set out in the Green Paper and White Paper attracted wide support, yet there have been a number of specific criticisms of the government's programme which deserve consideration.

First, there are worries about the usefulness of targets as a focus of activity. One of the main problems with targets is that they focus attention on what can be measured. This downgrades health problems that may be serious but which cannot easily be quantified (Faculty of Public Health Medicine, 1991b). Moreover, according to some, the justification for many of the targets is based on inadequate scientific evidence (Akehurst *et al.*, 1991). It has also been argued that some of the targets are not as tough as they appear, and may be achieved at least in part by current trends in these illnesses, rather than by additional efforts (Mooney and Healey, 1991).

A second criticism of the government's strategy is that it is rather vague about how the objectives and targets are going to be achieved (Akehurst *et al.*, 1991). There is as yet little indication that the government will use its considerable legislative and financial powers to promote health. For example, since the publication of the White Paper, the government has resisted strong pressure, from within Britain as well as from the European Community, to ban tobacco advertising. This is in spite of recent evidence, from the Department of Health itself, that such a ban might be effective in reducing smoking (DoH, 1992b).

Third, although the government has emphasised that everyone has a role to play in achieving the targets, it has said little about how public views are to be incorporated into health strategy. Indeed, the targets appear to reflect a medical rather than a social perspective, as the Radical Statistics Health Group has observed (1991). The focus of the strategy is upon specific diseases and habits, not on neglected groups within the population and their multiple problems. As a result, many of the targets relate to the prevention of disease rather than the promotion of health.

A further point is that the development of a health strategy sits rather at odds with the internal market in health care (Moran, 1989). True, the purchasing authorities may have an incentive to 'purchase' services more relevant to public health if they perceive that prevention is more cost-effective than cure (Ham and Mitchell, 1990), but there is no guarantee they will actually do this. A lot depends on the extent to which purchasers are willing to collaborate with each other in the setting of priorities and the achievement of common objectives. In addition, much depends on the availability of new resources for public health initiatives, since the diversion of budgets away from caring and curing services is likely to result in considerable opposition to a purchasing strategy based on prevention.

The final criticism of the government's health strategy has been levelled at its failure to consider the role of inequality and social deprivation in ill-health. In the Appendix to the Green Paper the government admitted that the WHO's regional target of reducing health inequalities by at least 25 per cent by the year 2000 would probably not be achieved. The relationship between poverty and ill-health is not explicitly discussed by either the Green or White Paper. Other aspects of deprivation are also given short shrift: a section illustrating the relationship between housing and ill-health, which allegedly appeared in an earlier, leaked, draft was omitted from the final published version of the Green Paper. In the White Paper, healthy homes are identified as a 'setting' on which to focus, but no clear commitments are made to improving poor housing conditions or reducing homelessness. The government merely states that it will 'continue to pursue its policies to promote choice and quality in housing, having regard to health and other benefits' (Cm 1986, 1992, p. 28).

■ Conclusion

The public health approach has returned. There are many factors behind its revival: the growing awareness of public health and environmental issues during the 1980s; the governing party's support for certain prevention policies; international pressures to conform, to name just a few. The Conservative government's recent conversion to a health strategy can be seen as a product of these forces.

There is now a widespread consensus on the benefits of such an approach. Important differences remain, however, over the contents of the health strategy and how it should be implemented. There are also powerful interests ranged against it. These include industrial interests (such as alcohol and tobacco), who risk long-term damage to their profits if consumption of their products falls. Also, there may be opposition from professional interests in the NHS, namely those involved in curative services. In the face of these formidable obstacles, the creation of a health strategy is really only the end of the beginning (Baggott, 1991).

■ *Chapter 12*

Conclusion

■ The challenges

As earlier chapters have shown, the British health care system faces a number of significant challenges at the present time, arising mainly from new and newly-perceived demands on services. These include the growth of the elderly population; the increasing burden of chronic illness; the toll of premature death; the extent of mental illness; the growing importance of new infectious diseases; and the persistence of variations in health status according to social class, geographical location, gender and ethnicity.

There are a number of important strategic, resource and accountability issues that must be resolved if these health challenges are to be tackled effectively.

First, it is vital that the health care system has a clear purpose in the face of these challenges. Its component parts must collaborate effectively to achieve stated objectives. Furthermore, as a great deal of illness is shaped by social, economic and environmental trends, a broad perspective incorporating these factors should be adopted when setting objectives.

Second, the availability and allocation of health care resources has to be considered in the light of changing needs. In particular, the adequacy of public funding for health care must be properly assessed. It is also important to establish a consensus about the most appropriate mix of private and public health care. In addition, given the scarcity of resources relative to need, it is vital that funding from whatever source is allocated as efficiently, as effectively and as fairly as possible.

Third, there has to be improved accountability in health care. Financial accountability, with full responsiblity taken for resources by those who commit and employ them, is of course important. There also has to be greater accountability to the user of health services. This is necessary in order to improve the responsiveness of services to those with increasingly complex needs. In addition, within the NHS itself accountability has to be clarified, particularly with regard to the relationship between central government and local management, so that everyone knows who is responsible for what.

■ The ideas

Britain is not alone in contemplating these issues. Almost all health care systems in the developed world face a similar situation, and many have undertaken a search for policy solutions. Proposals vary between countries but there have been a number of common themes. First, a growing interest in managed competition between providers of health care; second, more emphasis on the monitoring of the effectiveness, the cost and the quality of health care; third, greater encouragement of primary care, and care in the community more generally; and, finally, a sharper focus on public health strategies.

These themes are clearly identifiable in the programme of health care reform undertaken in Britain in the 1980s and 1990s. In a broad sense Britain has not been out of step with other countries, yet the approach of the British government to health care reform since 1979 can be contrasted sharply with that of previous governments, both Labour and Conservative. During the post-war period the problems facing the health care system were countered mainly by reorganisation and restructuring. By and large such changes were cautious and incremental. New structures were either grafted on to existing ones, or bore strong similarities to those they replaced. New planning, management and resource allocation systems introduced in the 1970s appeared more radical in design, but were implemented in an incrementalist fashion and in practice represented marginal rather than radical reform.

The Conservative government under Margaret Thatcher appeared to be more open to radical proposals. Its policies reflected many aspects of the economic critique of health care outlined in Chapter 3, viewing the NHS as an inefficient, public sector bureaucracy, largely unaccountable for the resources it consumed, and dominated by self-interested professionals. The Thatcher government favoured more evaluation, greater financial and managerial accountability, a greater role for markets and the private sector, and an emphasis on the patient as a consumer of health care. It also drew on other critiques of health care and of orthodox medicine. The public health model was viewed sympathetically because it enabled the government to place greater emphasis upon individual responsibility for health and it also raised the possibility of saving costs through prevention. There was also an element of technological pessimism in the government's approach, again mainly on cost grounds.

Unwittingly perhaps, the government's antagonism towards the medical profession had some affinity with the anti-medical thesis of Illich (1975). Needless to say, other critiques at the opposite end of the political spectrum – Marxism and feminism – received short shrift. The Thatcher government refused to admit that poor social and economic conditions lead to ill-health, though in the late 1980s it began to accept the importance of environmental factors, such as pollution, as causes of illness. Although the government has rejected the central arguments of the feminist perspective, it has responded to some concerns identified by women. It expanded some health services specifically for women, such as breast and cervical cancer screening services. The Department of Health has backed efforts to make health services more sympathetic to women, particularly in the area of maternity services. It has also expressed concern about the small proportion of senior women doctors and introduced a package of measures to improve the training and retention of female doctors.

■ The reforms and their impact

So much for the ideas underlying health policy during the 1980s. But to what extent did these ideas filter into practice? Marsh and Rhodes (1992) have argued that in many areas of policy there has been an implementation gap between the government's professed intention and the actual policy outcome. For them, the Thatcherite revolution was more a matter of rhetoric than political impact. Similarly, Wistow (1992), looking specifically at health policy, has observed that the basic principles of the NHS have survived the Thatcher government.

Certainly, the Thatcher government learned at an early stage that NHS reform should be handled carefully. Following the political uproar over allegations of a dramatic privatisation of health care, there was a return to a more cautious and pragmatic approach. Private health care and contracting-out were encouraged, and a more 'businesslike' management style was pursued within the NHS. But the pace of reform was gradual, reflecting the political sensitivity of health care. The reforms also led to greater centralisation. Despite the rhetoric about devolving management responsibility in the NHS, the government found itself taking an even closer interest in the detailed operation of health services. Meanwhile, it continued to spend large amounts of public money on health care, and even boasted about its commitment to the NHS to placate the electorate.

The prospects for radical change improved following the announcement of the NHS review in 1988. Though disappointing to many on the right because a tax-funded system of health care was retained, the new scheme that emerged was nevertheless radical in intent. The subsequent White Paper abandoned caution by replacing direct budget allocations with a system of contracting between budget-holding 'purchasers' of health care and service providers. However, the unpopularity of the reforms before the General Election, combined with the practical problems of introducing the reforms quickly, meant that it was necessary to implement the changes in a gradual manner. Following the Conservative victory at the 1992 General Election, it is possible that the market will be allowed to operate more freely, revealing the true radicalism of the scheme. However, for reasons to be discussed later in this chapter, further attempts to regulate and intervene in the internal market cannot be ruled out.

The Conservative government's health policy has addressed other concerns, such as the need to emphasise public health and to expand primary and community care. Policies in these areas have mirrored elements of the government's guiding principles, yet here too there has been a considerable degree of pragmatism and in some cases a departure from these principles. The government's approach to community care produced a massive increase in public spending on residential care. It was later to accept that local authorities should have the lead role in relation to community care, despite central government's hostility towards these authorities. Radical proposals in primary care, such as comprehensive cash limits and health care shops were either dropped or diluted. The government also changed its mind and produced a national health strategy, a move it had previously criticised as being too interventionist.

☐ *A better health care system?*

Is the health care system now better equipped to deal with the challenges it faces? Some developments over the past decade have been positive. The Conservative government has placed a greater emphasis on primary care, community care and public health than did its predecessors, and these reforms, while flawed in several respects, have at least focused attention on these neglected backwaters of health policy.

The government's encouragement of the voluntary sector over the past decade has also been a positive development. Voluntary organisations can make an important supplementary contribution to health care, although, as some have warned, there is a danger that voluntary services may be used as a means of bypassing, or even replacing, statutory services.

The concern with management and efficiency in health care has emphasised issues too long neglected. While the systems of management and cost-control introduced by the government have continued to attract criticism from various quarters, the reforms have nevertheless stimulated debate about important issues such as the measurement of costs, the monitoring of service quality, the assessment of health needs, and the importance of setting clear objectives for health services.

To some extent, the management reforms, and other influences such as the internal market, have provided a countervailing force to the medical profession. Given the various criticisms of the profession's dominance of health care (from across the political spectrum), this may also be seen in a positive light. In future doctors will be more accountable, both for their clinical actions and for the resources they use. This could tie medical practice more closely than previously to the needs and objectives of the health care system. As we saw in Chapter 2, the medical profession will retain a powerful position in relation to health care, though doctors may in future have to share power to a greater extent with the new managerial élite.

The internal market in health care has potential benefits, although it will be some time before its impact can properly be evaluated. The division between purchasers and providers is likely to produce a more judicious use of health care resources. The internal market also contains great potential for improving the responsiveness of health services to patients' needs, provided that purchasers act on behalf of patients and heed the views of the public.

☐ *Problems with markets*

There are also significant risks which may offset such benefits. The government's faith in markets as an allocative mechanism for health care has surely been misplaced. Markets have a poor record in relation to health care. There are very real dangers that internal markets may well generate many of the problems found in private health care markets. Without tough safeguards, 'high-risk' individuals, those who need health services the most, and users of 'unprofitable' services, are likely to be marginalised.

As a means of rationing scarce health care resources, markets are a crude device. Because purchasing power does not necessarily correlate with need, even in an internal market, services may be inappropriately allocated. This could also lead to greater variations in access and service quality. The result could be a less efficient, less comprehensive and more fragmented system of care resembling that which existed prior to the creation of the NHS.

The internal market also involves administrative and regulatory costs. Some of these costs are associated with the establishment of the market, but others – such as the employment of staff to monitor and operate the market – are ongoing. The cost of the market could offset any efficiency gains generated, in the short term and possibly also in the longer term.

Moreover, the internal market is unlikely to perform adequately without extra funding. Although public expenditure has risen, Britain spends much less on health care than comparable countries. As we saw in Chapter 7, there is evidence of underfunding relative to the growing need for care and in relation to the rising cost of health services.

There is some scope for bridging this gap by improving efficiency. Indeed, the government has constantly emphasised this approach as a means of securing extra resources for patient care. However, there is a limit to the amount of money which can be produced by efficiency gains. Worse still, crude cost-cutting can cause inefficiency if it inhibits the development of services which in the long run may be more cost-effective.

☐ *Private health care*

The British government has tried to encourage the private sector, both as a source of new finance and as an alternative mode of provision. Although the NHS remains the dominant agency in the health care system, the private sector has grown enormously in importance since 1979. It now has a market share of around 15 per cent, and in some sectors (abortions, minor surgery, residential care) and in some regions (the South and London) is even more significant.

Supporters of private medicine claim that it is a kind of safety valve for the NHS. Its opponents criticise the expansion of private health care for enabling widespread rationing by price for non-emergency treatments, which are increasingly difficult to secure on the NHS. In this way, it is alleged that the private sector underpins a 'two-tier system', with different standards of care depending on ability to pay. The private sector is also seen as a drain on NHS resources by employing doctors and nurses trained at public expense. Finally, it is argued that the growth of the private sector has been unplanned, haphazard and is unrelated to health needs.

The interdependence between the private and public sectors of health care has to be addressed. It is possible that the two can co-exist in their mutual interest. Joint arrangements are on the increase, as we have seen, and will probably expand further. Future arrangements between the two sectors must, however, be monitored carefully to ensure that public funding is being used appropriately and efficiently. In addition service developments within the private sector should perhaps operate inside a broader framework of regulation and planning. This would help to ensure that the activities of the private sector are consistent with health care objectives, policies and standards at local and national level.

The introduction of such 'rules of the game' may well attract support from the private sector. It has been noted with some irony that the commercialisation of the NHS could present a serious challenge to the private sector in the future. The creation of an internal market in health care means that the trust hospitals will be in a position to compete with the private sector. Similarly, the long-term shift in purchasing power away from residential care within the social care 'market' is likely to cast a shadow over private provision in this sector. The likelihood is that the private sector will actively lobby for regulations preventing the public sector from undertaking activities that may threaten its market share.

☐ Management and accountability

We turn now to the management reforms of the past decade. Despite the intentions behind the Griffiths report, local initiative has been constrained by a centralised management structure and ministers have continued to interfere with the detailed operation of the NHS. The formal separation of policy and management is unlikely to reduce ministerial interference, though it may help ministers to distance themselves from many of the problems faced by health authorities and providers at a local level.

The net effect of this has been to reduce the public accountability of the NHS. Health authorities and providers, despite the rhetoric of the market, are not directly accountable to the public. The new rules on health authority membership mean that they are no longer obliged to contain local representatives. The analysis of their composition undertaken in Chapter 6 revealed their membership to be unrepresentative. The same argument applies to self-governing trusts, and perhaps also to GP fundholders. Although fundholders are closer to the patient than health authorities and trusts, they do not operate in a clear framework of public accountability.

The management reforms and other initiatives such as the Patient's Charter have not as yet ensured that services are responsive to patients. Moreover, it is by no means clear that services will be more responsive in future. Instead of being dominated by doctors, the patient might well be at the mercy of managers. Indeed, management represents a new élite, alongside senior clinicians. The patient, on the other hand, has no real source of power with which to challenge either of these interests.

☐ Primary care, community care and public health

As stated earlier, the emphasis upon community care, primary care and public health is welcome. Yet the specific reforms introduced here can also be viewed in a negative light. The primary care reforms have been criticised as being too narrow, too closely geared to the activities of the family practitioner professions (in particular GPs), and too managerialist. They also sit uneasily with some of the internal market reforms, such as GP fundholding, which serves to undermine the ability of FHSAs to plan and manage primary care services. Meanwhile, specific reforms such as the introduction of charges for optical and dental checks have revealed the government's agenda: to increase wherever possible the scope for private expenditure on health care. The government has also angered the family practitioner professions – whose co-operation is essential – by introducing new contracts without considering fully the implications for remuneration, workload and quality of service.

The primary care reforms have been poorly integrated with other key reforms in community care and public health. The deplorable level of collaboration between the NHS and other agencies in primary and community care has been well documented. Critics of the government's community care policy have also attacked the repeated delays which have prevented the kind of long-term planning which is urgently needed if community care is to be properly developed. Both primary care and community care policies have been criticised for encouraging commercial provision in areas where its contribution is to say the least unproven. In the case of community care, there has been particular criticism of the increasing reliance on informal carers in the absence of an adequate framework of support services.

The public health reforms are regarded by some as being fairly mild, in the light of the government's reluctance to tackle the social roots of ill-health and health inequalities. It is also difficult to see how national health objectives, such as those listed in *The Health of the Nation* White Paper, will override the preoccupation with market forces. The health strategy requires proper planning and implementation. Despite attempts to incorporate the strategy within the planning process, it is difficult to see how it can be be reconciled with a fragmented system of health care, where purchasers and providers have a degree of freedom and independence to enter into contracts. In particular, GP fundholding in its present form is recognised as a serious obstacle to a coherent strategy on public health.

☐ *The impact on the public*

It is important to try and evaluate the impact of recent changes in health care upon the patients' experience and on public opinion. This is not easy, as these changes have often had an uneven and in some respects a contradictory effect.

The general public has always had a strong commitment to the NHS. Despite the well-publicised problems of the 1980s, the public's commitment to the fundamental principles of the NHS – a comprehensive service, available to all and free at the point of use – became stronger (Jowell *et al.*, 1992). But at the same time, paradoxically, there was a greater willingness to use the private sector, which in some respects undermines these principles.

During the 1980s the public also became more critical of the performance of the NHS. As we noted in Chapter 8 complaints about the NHS and about doctors increased during this decade. Attitude surveys have also detected increasing dissatisfaction with services provided. The British Social Attitudes survey, for example, calculated that the overall level of public dissatisfaction with the NHS increased from a quarter of the population to almost a half between 1983 and 1990. This survey also found high levels of dissatisfaction with particular NHS services such as out-patient and GP appointment systems, and with long waiting lists.

While the public have been more critical of the NHS, they have also reacted cautiously to the government's reform programme, in particular towards internal markets. Between a half and three-quarters of the public were opposed to this policy at the time of its introduction. Opposition has perhaps softened slightly since, but a substantial portion of the British public continues to express concern about the changes.

Attitude surveys give an impression of the general public's view. But what of the impact of the reforms on patients? Of course, some of the changes in health care experienced by patients have arisen independently of the government's policies. These include technological advances of the kind discussed in Chapter 3. Many of these applications have had a dramatic impact on the experience of patients. The development of minimally invasive therapies, for example, has helped to reduce hospital stays in recent years, and will further enhance this trend in the future.

The government's reforms have had an impact on patient care over and above such changes in therapy. It is perhaps too early to make any final judgements on the impact of these reforms. Up to now the impact has been mixed: some patients will have benefited from the shorter waiting times which accompanied the introduction of the internal market, although, as was noted in Chapter 8, this improvement largely resulted from increased funding in the run-up to the 1992 General Election. Since this time, funding has been relatively less generous and waiting lists have begun to grow once again.

Some patients have definitely benefited from the introduction of GP fundholding. They appear to have enjoyed a quicker, more responsive service for a range of non-emergency treatments covered by the scheme. But the patients of non-fundholders have not as yet benefited to the same degree, and there are strong suspicions that they may even have been disadvantaged by fundholding.

Something that all patients will have noticed is the improved public relations profile of the NHS. Glossy brochures and leaflets abound. Marketing strategies and Patient's Charters may for a time convince patients and the wider public that all is well, but they will not in the long run obscure the perception of real service standards if these begin to deteriorate relative to public expectations.

■ The future

In 1988 the Social Services committee commented that 'any new system of funding or delivering health care must be broadly agreed between the major parties. If it is not, it may not stand the test of time' (House of Commons, 1988b, p. lx). The ultimate test of any reform is its ability to withstand a change of government. The experience of national health insurance and the creation of the NHS illustrates not only that it is possible to introduce durable reform, but also that such changes can last even where there is significant opposition.

In recent years the health policies of the opposition parties have differed considerably from those of the government, in several respects. Both the Labour and Liberal parties have argued strongly that the NHS has been underfunded, and have called for an increase in public spending on health. These parties have also disagreed with the government over aspects of community care, primary care and public health policies.

The main bone of contention between the opposition parties and the government has been over the internal market in health care. Both opposition parties set out plans to abolish the market prior to the General Election in 1992 (Labour Party, 1992b; Liberal Democrats, 1992). Yet they have had to accept many of the changes introduced by the Conservative government since it came to power in 1979. Both now support the idea of a division between purchasers and providers of health care, although in their schemes, markets and contracts would be replaced with planning and performance agreements.

The opposition parties know that as trust status and fundholding are extended, and as contracts become more specific and detailed, it may be difficult, if not impossible, for a future government to abolish the market and start afresh. There will be practical difficulties associated with unravelling contractual obligations and reversing the organisational changes that have followed reform, such as mergers between hospitals or health authorities.

Attempts to replace the market will also give rise to political difficulties. The creation of the market has set in motion the development of a new managerial culture within the NHS, which will inhibit any future moves to reverse the reforms. The market has also created new vested interests – fundholding GPs, provider units having a monopoly position, the bureaucrats who regulate and operate the market. These groups will resist a movement away from the system that benefits them. Indeed, the trusts and fundholders have already established new associations to campaign and lobby on their behalf.

Abolition of the market is unlikely, even with a change of government in the future. Further reform, to plan and regulate the market for health care is, however, a strong possibility. Even the Conservative government, should it continue its long period in office, may have to intervene in the future, despite its present commitment to detachment from the health market. There are a number of reasons why this is likely.

The operation of the internal market in the absence of improved funding will produce tougher and probably more explicit rationing decisions. Purchasing authorities are already deciding not to fund certain treatments deemed to be 'non-urgent'. Patients will then be faced with either purchasing these operations privately or continuing to suffer discomfort. Unlike the old form of rationing by waiting list, there will be no guarantee of NHS treatment for such patients, even in the longer term. The rationing process also creates incentives for purchasers to discriminate against certain 'high cost' patients, and the elderly and those with disabilities. If this does result in treatment being denied, the media interest in the victims of rationing is likely to be considerable and the government will be under great pressure to intervene.

The government will also find it difficult to stand back over allegations of poor and varying standards of care, as well as problems of access. It is true that the standard of care in the NHS has never been uniform. Yet the creation of an internal market and the encouragement of the private sector has produced a strong movement towards greater fragmentation of services that implies wider rather than narrower variations in the standards of care. Allegations of a two-tier or multi-tier system of care have in the past touched a raw nerve within the government: hence the introduction of the Patients' Charter standards, and the codes of practice on admission criteria to block 'queue-jumping' (see Chapter 8). Despite attempts to distance itself from responsibility for local services, central government will find it very difficult in future not to intervene in the face of such allegations.

Closure of health care facilities, such as hospitals in London, is also likely to continue to cause political problems for the government. Although some rationalisation is necessary to adjust the balance of care between primary and hospital care, politicians may find this difficult to justify in the face of public protests. These protests will increase if the closure of hospitals is not preceded by an expansion of new primary care facilities. The plans will be implemented in an incremental, low-key manner, or even diluted, to make them more palatable. Increasingly the talk will be of hospital mergers rather than closures.

There are other areas of controversy that might cause problems for the government in the future. The community care arrangements, which began in April 1993, will involve considerable upheaval as the system moves out of its 'steady state'. There has been a great deal of concern already about the level of funding for the introduction of the new system, which many feel to be inadequate. There are also doubts about the willingness and ability of some local authorities to perform their new responsiblities, and the quality of joint working arrangements between local government and the NHS. It also seems likely that the social care 'market' introduced by the community care reforms will raise (largely unforeseen) problems, as happened with the implementation of the internal market in health care. Indeed, as we noted in Chapter 10, some are already coming to light – such as the consequences of needs assessment, for example. The initial shortcomings of the new scheme – 'the poisoned chalice' – will probably be laid at the door of local government. However, an accumulation of problems over time will place the focus of responsibility squarely back on central government, which designed and introduced the new system and which provides a large part of the funding.

A further area of political conflict is likely to occur in relation to the government's health strategy. There are two possible scenarios here. The strategy will either wither on the vine, a casualty of conflict between government departments (indeed, there were reports that it would be killed off after the Conservatives, victory in the 1992 election, a rumour which turned out to be 'much exaggerated'), or the government will have to contemplate interventionist measures to tackle the social, economic and environmental roots of ill-health in order to achieve its longer-term objectives. This latter course will bring the Conservative government into conflict with its own right-wing supporters and the powerful industrial interests which fund the party.

One thing is clear: health issues will remain on the political agenda as we move towards the next century. The Conservative government's implicit aim – to take health care out of politics by turning it into a management problem or an economic commodity – has not succeeded so far and is unlikely to meet with greater success in the future. Because, to quote Sir Douglas Black (1987, p. 38), 'it is not possible, as some wish, to take the health service out of politics – both the amount of money involved, and the sensitivity of anything to do with health, will keep the health service a major political preoccupation'.

Further Reading

☐ *Chapter 1*

Concepts of health are explored by Aggleton (1990). Sources on the health of the British population include surveys by Blaxter (1990) and the General Household Survey (OPCS, 1988, 1990, 1992). International comparisons of health can be found in WHO (1992), while Phillips (1990) provides a good, up-to-date analysis of health and health care in the Third World. Johnson *et al.* (1989) provide a cogent analysis of the problems posed by the ageing population. The evidence of health inequalities is compiled in Townsend, Davidson and Whitehead (1988). Ethnic differences in health and illness are explored by Rathwell and Phillips (1986). A number of good sources now cover women's health, including Miles (1991), Jenkins (1985) and Roberts (1992).

☐ *Chapter 2*

Inglis (1965) gives a good account of the history of medicine. The role of the medical profession in relation to health, illness and health care is explored critically by Gould (1987), Inglis (1981), Illich (1975) and Kennedy (1981). The cultural aspects of medicine are examined by Payer (1989) and Helman (1990). Recent work on alternative medicine includes Saks (1992) and Sharma (1992). The restatement of the public health model by McKeown (1979) is still perhaps the best starting place for those interested in this area. The politics of the medical profession is examined by Watkins (1987), while Moran and Wood (1992) provide a good analysis of the politics of professional regulation. An official history of the BMA is found in Grey-Turner and Sutherland (1982).

The sociology of medicine is explored by Freidson (1988) and Turner (1987). Parry and Parry (1976) give an account of the rise of the medical profession. Lay beliefs about health are discussed by Calnan (1987). The best account of the role and status of nurses is given by Salvage (1985). Deep-rooted interprofessional rivalries and political conflict between midwives and doctors are analysed by Donnison (1988).

☐ *Chapter 3*

Economists' perspectives on health care can be found in Culyer *et al.* (1990) and Mooney *et al.* (1986). Weale (1988) explores the economic, moral and political dilemmas involved in the resourcing and rationing of health care, while Honigsbaum (1992) examines the Oregon case. The implications of high technology in medicine are discussed by Jennett (1986). The Marxist perspective on health care is set out by Doyal (1979). Doyal's book also discusses the feminist critique. Oakley's (1980, 1984) work provides evidence by analysing the case of women and childbirth.

☐ *Chapter 4*

A number of sources discuss the pre-NHS system of health care (Honigsbaum, 1979; Hodgkinson, 1967; Abel-Smith, 1964). The creation of the NHS is comprehensively analysed by Webster (1988) and Honigsbaum (1989). The history of the NHS and its problems since inception are covered by a number of books including Allsop (1984), Klein (1983, 1989b) and Haywood and Alaszewski (1980). Perhaps the best work on Thatcherism is Hugo Young's *One of Us* (1991). The health policies of the Thatcher government are discussed by Iliffe (1988) and Wistow (1992).

☐ *Chapter 5*

Field (1989) provides a useful overview of health care systems. A number of OECD publications (1987, 1990) outline the problems facing health care systems in industrialised countries. Health care reforms in a number of countries are discussed by Ham, Robinson and Benzeval (1990). Ginzberg (1990) is perhaps the best contemporary work on the US system of health care. Policy-making in the NHS is covered by a number of books including Ham (1993), Klein (1989b) and Small (1989). Fowler (1991) and Currie (1990) give some insight into the work of health ministers, while Stowe (1989) contains the reflections of a former senior civil servant in the health department. Ham (1991) provides a handy guide to the structure of the NHS.

☐ *Chapter 6*

The evolving role of the health service manager is discussed by Harrison (1988). The impact of the Griffiths management reforms is assessed by Strong and Robinson (1990) and Harrison *et al.* (1992). Loveridge and Starkey (1992) also examine the organisational and managerial aspects of the NHS post-Griffiths. Organisational change in health authorities is explored by Pettigrew *et al.* (1991). The impact of new management systems at hospital level is examined by Packwood *et al.* (1991) and Perrin (1988).

☐ *Chapter 7*

Jones and Prowle (1987) give a good account of health service finance before the introduction of the internal market. Appleby (1992) provides a comprehensive analysis of financial issues in the NHS today. The role of the private sector is discussed by Higgins (1988). Ascher (1987) provides a good account of the introduction of competitive tendering. Recent health expenditure trends are summarised by Robinson (1991).

☐ *Chapter 8*

Timmins (1988) provides a journalist's view of the unfolding crisis in the NHS during the late 1980s. The NHS review is discussed by Paton (1992), while the implementation of the reforms is well covered by Butler (1992). The implications of the internal market are thoroughly discussed by Le Grand and Bartlett (1993) and McLachlan (1990). The problems of health care in London are analysed by Benzeval *et al.* (1991).

☐ *Chapters 9 and 10*

Hicks (1976) provides a comprehensive, though perhaps now a little dated, overview of primary care. An analysis of the government's primary care reforms is given by Marks (1988). A useful summary of the current state of general practice is given by Roberts (1991b). The Audit Commission (1992a) provides a useful background to debates about the future of community health services.

Higgins (1989) explores the meaning of community care. Hunter and Wistow (1987a and b) examine the development of community care policies. The problems of inter-agency collaboration are discussed in Challis *et al.* (1988). The problems of specific client groups are covered by Butler (1993) (mental illness) and Ryan and Thomas (1980) (mental handicap). Contrasting predictions about the future of community care are given by Langan (1990) and Levick (1992).

☐ *Chapter 11*

The new public health is discussed by Ashton and Seymour (1988) and by Draper (1991). Wohl (1984) explores Victorian public health while Baggott (1991) compares the period with today. Specific public health issues are covered by the following sources: smoking (Taylor, 1984); alcohol (Baggott, 1990); AIDS (Blaxter, 1991); food and health (Cannon, 1987); environment and health (Hall, 1990); and housing and health (Lowry, 1991).

Bibliography

Abel-Smith, B. (1960) *History of the Nursing Profession* (London, Heinemann).

Abel-Smith, B. (1964) *The Hospitals 1800–1948* (London, Heinemann).

Adams, B. (1991) 'Health care data briefing: unpaid care', *Health Service Journal*, 7 February, 26.

Adam Smith Institute. (1989) *Extending Care* (London, Adam Smith Institute).

Adler, M. (1987) 'ABC of AIDS: Development of the Epidemic', *British Medical Journal*, vol. 294, 1083–5.

Aggleton, P. (1990) *Health* (London, Routledge).

Akehurst, R., Godfrey, J., and Robertson, E. (1991) *Health of the Nation: An Economic Perspective on Target Setting* (University of York, Centre for Health Economics).

Alchian, A. and Allen, W. (1974) *University Economics* (London, Prentice-Hall).

Alford, R. (1975) *Health Care Politics* (Chicago, Ill., University of Chicago Press).

Allen, I. (1988) *Is There Any Room at The Top?* (London, Policy Studies Institute).

Allsop, J. (1984) *Health Policy and the NHS* (London, Longman).

Allsop, J. (1986) 'Primary Health Care – The Politics of Change', *Journal of Social Policy* vol. 20(2), 489–96.

Allsop, J. and May, A. (1986) *The Emperor's New Clothes. Family Practitioner Committees in the 1980s* (London, King's Fund Institute).

Appleby, J. and Adams, B. (1989) 'Health Care Data Briefing: Inflation in the Health Service', *Health Service Journal* 4 October, 1215.

Appleby, J. (1992) *Financing Health Care in the 1990s* (University Press, Buckingham).

Appleby, J., Robinson, R., Ranade, W., Little, V. and Salter, J. (1990) 'The Use of Markets in the Health Service: The NHS Reforms and Managed Competition', *Public Money and Management*, vol. 10 (4), 27–33.

Armstrong, D. (1990) 'Medicine as a Profession: Times of Change', *British Medical Journal*, vol. 301, 691–3.

Ascher, K. (1987) *The Politics of Privatisation: Contracting out Public Services* (London, Macmillan).

Ashburner, L. and Cairncross, L. (1992) 'Just Trust Us', *Health Service Journal*. 14 May, 20–2.

Ashmore, M., Mulkay, M. and Pinch, T. (1989) *Health and Efficiency: A Sociology of Health Economics* (Buckingham, Open University Press).

Ashton, J. and Seymour, H. (1988) *The New Public Health* (Milton Keynes, Open University Press).

Association of Community Health Councils (1992) *A Health Standards Inspectorate* (London, Action for Victims of Medical Accidents).

Audit Commission (1986) *Making a Reality of Community Care* (London HMSO).

Audit Commission (1989) *Developing Community Care for Adults with a Mental Handicap* (London, HMSO).

Audit Commission (1990) *A Short Cut to Better Services: Day Surgery in England and Wales* (London, HMSO).

Audit Commission (1991) *Report and Accounts* (London, HMSO).

Audit Commission (1992a) *Homeward Bound: A New Course for Community Health* (London, HMSO).

Audit Commission (1992b) *All in a Day's Work: An Audit of Day Surgery in England and Wales* (London, HMSO).

Audit Commission (1993a) *Their Health: Your Business: The Role of the District Health Authority* (London, HMSO).

Audit Commission (1993b) *Practices Make Perfect: The Role of the FHSA* (London, HMSO).

Baggott, R. (1990) *Alcohol, Politics and Social Policy* (Aldershot, Avebury).

Baggott, R. (1991) 'Looking Forward To The Past? The Politics of Public Health', *Journal of Social Policy*, vol. 20 (2), 191–213.

Bakwin, H. (1945) 'Pseudoxia Pediatrica', *New England Journal of Medicine* 232, 691–7.

Balarajan, R. (1989) 'Inequalities in Health within the Health Sector', *British Medical Journal*, vol. 299, 822–5.

Balarajan, R. (1991) 'Ethnic Differences: Mortality from Ischaemic Heart Disease and Cerebrovascular Disease in England and Wales', *British Medical Journal*, vol. 302, 560–4.

Barclay, S. (1989) 'Smear Campaign', *The Listener*, 2 November, 14.

Barnard, K., Lee, K., Mills, A. and Reynolds, J. (1979) *Towards a New Rationality: A Study of Planning in the NHS* (University of Leeds, Nuffield Centre for Health Studies).

Bartlett, W. (1991) 'Quasi-Markets and Contracts: A Market and Hierarchies Perspective on NHS Reform', *Public Money and Management*, vol. 11 (3), 53–62.

Beardshaw, V. (1988) *Last on the List: Community Services for People with Physical Disabilities* (London, King's Fund Institute).

Bell, R. S. and Loop, J. W. (1971) 'The Utility and Futility of Radiographic Skull Examination for Trauma', *New England Journal of Medicine* 287, p. 236–9.

Benzeval, M., Judge, K. and New, B. (1991) 'Health and Health Care in London', *Public Money and Management* 11 (1), 25–32.

Berwick, D. M., Enthoven, A. and Bunker, J. P. (1992) 'Quality Management in the NHS: The Doctors' Role', *British Medical Journal*, vol. 304, 235–9.

Best, G., Douglas, R. and Webb, N. (1988) 'Performance Review and General Management, in H. Koch, *General Management in the Health Service* (London, Croom Helm).

Bevan, G., Holland, W., Maynard, A. and Mays, N. (1988) *Reforming UK Health Care to Improve Health: The Case for Research and Experiment* (University of York, Centre for Health Economics).

Bhat, A. Carr-Hill, R. and Ohri, S. (1988) *Britain's Black Population* (Aldershot, Gower).

Birch, S. (1986) 'Increasing Patient Charges in the NHS: A Method of Privatising Primary Care' *Journal of Social Policy*, vol. 15 (2), 163–84.

Birch, S. and Maynard, A. (1988) *Performance Indicators* (Oxford, Policy Journals).

Bjorkman, J. W. (1989) 'Politicising Medicine and Medicalising Politics: Physician Power in the United States' in Freddi, G. and Bjorkman, J. W. *Controlling Medical Professionals: The Comparative Politics of Health Governance* (London, Sage), 28–73.

Black, D. (1984) *An Anthology of False Antitheses* (London, Nuffield Provincial Hospitals Trust).

Black, D. (1987) *Recollections and Reflections* (London, British Medical Journal Publications).

Blane, D., Smith, G. D. and Bartley, M. (1990) 'Social Class Differences in Years of Potential Life Lost: Size, Trends and Principal Causes', *British Medical Journal*, vol. 301, 29–32.

Blaxter, M. (1990) *Health and Lifestyles*, (London, Tavistock/Routledge).

Blaxter, M. (1991) *Aids, World-wide Policies and Problems* (London, Office of Health Economics).

BMA (British Medical Association) (1929) *A General Medical Service for the Nation* (London, BMA).

BMA (British Medical Association) (1942) *Draft Interim Report of the Medical Planning Commission* (London, BMA).

BMA (British Medical Association) (1962) *Report of the Medical Services Review Committee* (The Porritt Report) (London, BMA).

BMA (British Medical Association) (1986a) *Diet, Nutrition and Health* (London, BMA).

BMA (British Medical Association) (1986b) *Alternative Therapy* (London, British Medical Association).

BMA (British Medical Association) (1987) *Deprivation and Ill-Health* (London, BMA).

BMA (British Medical Association) (1993) *Complementary Medicine: New Approaches to Good Practice* (Oxford University Press).

Bond, J., Cartlidge, A. M. and Gregson A. B. (1987) 'Inter-Professional Collaboration in Primary Care', *Journal of the Royal College of General Practitioners*, vol. 37, 158–61.

Bosanquet, N. (1975) *A New Deal for the Elderly* (London, Fabian Society).

Bosanquet, N. (1986) 'GPs as Firms: Creating an Internal Market for Primary Care', *Public Money and Management*, vol. 6 (1), 53–62.

Bosanquet, N. (1992) 'Interim Report: The National Health' in Jowell, R., Brooke, L., Prior, G., Taylor, B. *British Social Attitudes: The 9th Report, 1992/93 edition* (Aldershot, Social and Community Planning Research, Dartmouth).

Bradshaw, J. and Gibbs, I. (1988) *Public Support for Residential Care* (Aldershot, Avebury).

Brand, J. L. (1965) *Doctors and the State: The British Medical Profession and Government Action on Public Health: 1870–1912* (Baltimore, Md. Johns Hopkins University Press).

Brazier, M., Lovecy, J., Moran, M. and Potton, M. (1993) 'Falling from a Tightrope? Doctors and Lawyers between the Market and State', *Political Studies*, vol. 41 (2), 197–213.

Brent Borough Council (1984) *A Child in Trust: Report of a Panel of Inquiry into Circumstances Surrounding the Death of Jasmine Beckford* (London, Brent Borough Council).

Brenton, M. (1985) *The Voluntary Sector in British Social Services* (London, Longman).

Brewin, T. (1985) 'Orthodox and Alternative Medicine', *Scottish Medical Journal*, vol. 30, 203–5.

British Cardiac Society (1987) *Report of the British Cardiac Society Working Group on Coronary Disease Prevention* (London, British Cardiac Society).

Brittain, J. M. (1992) 'The Emerging Market for Information Professionals in the UK National Health Service', *International Journal of Information Management*, vol. 12, 261–7.

Brittan, L. (1988) *A New Deal for Health Care* (London, Conservative Political Centre).

Brown, G. W. and Harris, T. (1982) 'Social Class and Affective Disorder', Ihsan Al-Issa (ed.), *Culture and Psychopathology* (Baltimore, Md. University Park Press).

Brown, M., Fallon, M., Favell, T., Forth, E., Hamilton, N., Heathcoat-Amory, D., Howarth, G., Jones, G., Leigh, E., Redwood, J., Stewart, A., Twinn, I. (1988) *The NHS: A Suitable Case for Treatment* (London, Conservative Political Centre).

Buck, N., Devlin, B. and Lunn, J. N. (1987) *Report of a Confidential Inquiry into Perioperative Deaths* (London, Nuffield Hospitals Provincial Trust).

Burke, C. and Goddard, A. (1990) 'Internal Markets: The Road to Inefficiency?' *Public Administration*, vol. 68 (3), 389-96.

Butler, E. and Pirie, M. (1988) *The Health Alternatives* (London, Adam Smith Institute).

Butler, J. (1992) *Patients, Policies and Politics: Before and After 'Working for Patients'* (Buckingham Open University Press).

Butler, T. (1993) *Changing Mental Health Services* (London, Chapman and Hall).

Byrne, P. S. and Long, B. E. (1976) *Doctors Talking to Patients* (London, HMSO).

Calnan, M. (1987) *Health and Illness* (London, Tavistock).

Cameron, H. M. and McCoogan, E. (1981) 'A Prospective Study of 1152 Hospital Autopsies', *Journal of Pathology*, vol. 133, 273–85.

Campbell, E. J. M., Scadding, J. G., Roberts, R. S. *et al.* (1979) 'The Concept of Disease', *British Medical Journal*, vol. 2, 757–62.

Camplin, E. A., Lunn, J. A., Devlin, H. B. (1992) *The National Confidential Enquiry into Perioperative Deaths*, (London, NCEPOD).

Cannon, G. (1987) *The Politics of Food* (London, Century Hutchinson).

Carr-Hill, R. (1987) 'The Inequalities in Health Debate: A Critical Review of the Literature', *Journal of Social Policy*, vol. 16 (4), 509–42.

Carr-Hill, R. (1991) 'Allocating Resources to Health Care: Is the Qaly a Technical Solution to a Political Problem?' *International Journal of Health Services*, vol. 21 (2), 351–63.

Castle, B. (1990) *The Castle Diaries: 1974–6* (London, Macmillan).

Cataldo, J. K. (1985) 'Obesity: A New Perspective on an Old Problem', *Health Education Journal*, vol. 44, 213–16.

Cd 4499 (1909) *Royal Commission on the Poor Laws and Relief of Distress*, Minority Report (London, HMSO).

Central Statistical Office. (1992) *Social Trends* (London, HMSO).

Chadwick, E. (1842) *Report on the Sanitary Condition of the Labouring Population of Great Britain* (London, Poor Law Commission).

Challis, L., Klein, R. and Webb, A. (1988) *Joint Approaches to Social Policy: Rationality and Practice* (Cambridge University Press).

Chaplin, N. W. (1982) *Getting it Right: The 1982 Reorganisation of the NHS* (London, Institute of Health Service Administrators).

Cmd 693 (1920) *Interim Report on the Future Provision of Medical and Allied Services* (The Dawson Report) (London, HMSO).

Cmd 2596 (1926) *Report of the Royal Commission on National Health Insurance* (London, HMSO).

Cmd 6404 (1942) *Social Insurance and Allied Services* (The Beveridge Report) (London, HMSO).

Cmd 6502 (1944) *A National Health Service* (London, HMSO).

Cmd 9663 (1956) *Report of the Committee of Inquiry into the Cost of the National Health Service* (The Guillebaud Report) (London, HMSO).

Cmnd 1604 (1962) *A Hospital Plan for England and Wales* (London, HMSO).

Cmnd 1973 (1963) *Health and Welfare: The Development of Community Care. Plans for the Health and Welfare Services of the Local Authorities in England and Wales*, (London, HMSO).

Cmnd 4683 (1971) *Better Services for the Mentally Handicapped* (London, HMSO).

Cmnd 5055 (1972) *National Health Service Reorganisation: England* (London, HMSO).

Cmnd 6018 (1975) *Report of the Committee of Inquiry into the Regulation of the Medical Profession* (London, HMSO).

Cmnd 6233 (1975) *Better Services for the Mentally Ill* (London, HMSO).

Cmnd 7047 (1977) *Prevention and Health* (London, HMSO).

Cmnd 7615 (1979) *Report of the Royal Commission on the NHS* (The Merrison Commission) (London, HMSO).

Cmnd 8173 (1981) *Growing Older* (London, HMSO).

Cmnd 9716 (1986) *Report of the Committee of Inquiry into an Outbreak of Food Poisoning at Stanley Royd Hospital* (London, HMSO).

Cmnd 9771 (1986) *Primary Health Care: An Agenda for Discussion* (London, HMSO).

Cmnd 9772 (1986) *First Report of the Committee of Inquiry into the Outbreak of Legionnaire's Disease in Stafford, April 1985* (London, HMSO).

Cm 249 (1987) *Promoting Better Health* (London, HMSO).

Cm 289 (1988) *Public Health in England*, Report of the Acheson Committee of inquiry into the Future Development of the Public Health Function (London, HMSO).

Cm 555 (1989) *Working for Patients* (London, HMSO).

Cm 849 *(1989) Caring for People* (London, HMSO).

Cm 1343 (1990) *The Government's Plans for the Future of Community Care*, (London, HMSO).

Cm 1523 (1991) *The Health of the Nation: A Consultative Document for Health in England* (London, HMSO).

Cm 1867 (1992) *Budgetary Reform* (London, HMSO).

Cm 1986 (1992) *The Health of the Nation: A Strategy for Health in England* (London, HMSO).

Coburn, D. (1992) 'Freidson Then and Now. An Internalists' critique of Freidson's Past and Present Views of the Medical Profession', *International Journal of Health Services*, vol. 25(3), 497–512.

Cochrane, A. L. (1971) *Effectiveness and Efficiency: Random Reflections on Health Services* (London, Nuffield Provincial Hospital Trust).

Cochrane, M., Ham, C., Heginbotham, C. and Smith, R. (1992) 'Rationing: At the Cutting Edge', *British Medical Journal*, vol. 303, 1039–42.

Coid, J. (1984) 'How many Psychiatric Patients in Prison?', *British Journal of Psychiatry*, vol 145, 78–86.

Collier, J. (1989) *The Health Conspiracy* (London, Century Hutchinson).

Collins, E. and Klein, R. (1988) 'Equity and the NHS: Self-Reported Mobility, Access and Primary Care', *British Medical Journal*, vol. 282, 1111–5.

Conservative Party (1987) *The Next Moves Forward: The Conservative Manifesto of 1987* (London, Conservative Central Office).

Conway, J. (1988) *Prescription for Poor Health: The Crisis for Homeless Families* (London, London Food Commission and Others).

Council for Science and Society (1982) *Expensive Medical Technologies: Report of a Working Party* (London, Council for Science and Society).

Crisp, R. (1989) 'Deciding Who Will Die. Qualys and Political Theory', *Politics*, vol. 9 (1), 31–5.

Crossman, R. (1977) *The Diaries of a Cabinet Minister Volume Three, Secretary of State for Social Services 1968–70* (London, Hamilton Cape).

Culyer, A. (1991) 'The Promise of a Reformed NHS: An Economist's Angle', *British Medical Journal*, vol. 302, 1253–6.

Culyer, A. J., Brazier, J. E. and O'Donnell, O. (1988) *Organising Health Service Provision. Drawing on Experience* (London, Institute for Health Service Management).

Culyer, A., Maynard, A., Posnett, J. (1990) *Competition in Health Care. Reforming the NHS* (London, Macmillan).

Currie, E. (1990) *Life Lines: Politics and Health 1986–88* (London, Pan Books).

Daily Telegraph (1993) 'GPs' £200 million health drive is a flop', 19 July, 7.

Dally, A. (1991) *Women Under the Knife* (London, Hutchinson).

Davies, B., Bebbington, A. and Charnley, H. (1990) *Resources, Needs and Outcomes in Community-Based Care* (Aldershot, Avebury).

Davison, A. (1988) *General Management at District Level*, in H. Koch, *General Management in the Health Service* (London, Croom Helm).

Day, P. (1985) 'Regulating the Private Sector of Welfare', *Political Quarterly*, vol. 56 (3), 282–5.

Day, P. and Klein, R. (1985) 'Central Accountability and Local Decision Making', *British Medical Journal*, vol. 290, 1676–78.

Day, P. and Klein, R. (1987) *Accountabilities: Five Public Services* (London, Tavistock).

Day, P. and Klein, R. (1991) 'Variations in Budgets of Fundholding Practices', *British Medical Journal*, vol. 303, 168–70.

Deakin, N. (1991) 'Government and the Voluntary Sector in the 1990s', *Policy Studies*, vol. 12 (3), 11–21.

Delamothe, T. (1991) 'Social Inequalities in Health', *British Medical Journal*, vol. 303, 1046–50.

Department of Social Security (1992) *Households Below Average Income*, 3rd Edition (London, HMSO).

DHSS (Department of Health and Social Security) (1970) *National Health Service. The Future Structure of the National Health Service in England* (London, HMSO).

DHSS (Department of Health and Social Security) (1971) *National Health Service Reorganisation: A Consultative Document* (London, DHSS).

DHSS (Department of Health and Social Security) (1976a) *Priorities for Health and Personal Social Services in England: A Consultative Document* (London, HMSO).

DHSS (Department of Health and Social Security) (1976b) *Report of the Regional Chairmen's Enquiry into the Working of the DHSS, in Relation to Regional Health Authorities* (London, DHSS).

DHSS (Department of Health and Social Security) (1976c) *Prevention and Health: Everybody's Business* (London, HMSO).

DHSS (Department of Health and Social Security) (1977) *The Way Forward* (London, HMSO).

DHSS (Department of Health and Social Security) (1979) *Patients First* (London, HMSO).

DHSS (Department of Health and Social Security) (1980) *Report on the Working Group on Inequalities in Health* (London, DHSS).

DHSS (Department of Health and Social Security) (1981a) *Report of a Study on Community Care* (London, DHSS).

DHSS (Department of Health and Social Security) (1981b) *The Primary Care Team: Report of a Joint Working Group* (The Harding Report) (London, HMSO).

DHSS (Department of Health and Social Security) (1981c) *Care in Action* (London, HMSO).

DHSS (Department of Health and Social Security) (1981d) *Community Care* (London, DHSS).

DHSS (Department of Health and Social Security) (1982) *The NHS Planning System* (London, DHSS).

DHSS (Department of Health and Social Security) (1983) *NHS Management Inquiry* (The Griffiths Mangement Report) (London, DHSS).

DHSS (Department of Health and Social Security) (1985) *Working Group on Joint Planning. Progress in Partnership* (London, DHSS).

DHSS (Department of Health and Social Security) (1986a) *NHS Management Board. A National Strategic Framework for Information Management in the Hospital and Community Services* (London, DHSS).

DHSS (Department of Health and Social Security) (1986b) *Neighbourhood Nursing: A Focus for Care. Report of the Community Nursing Review* (The Cumberlege Report) (London, HMSO).

DHSS (Department of Health and Social Security) (1988a) *Health Services Development: Resources Assumptions and Planning Guidelines* (London, HMSO).

DHSS (Department of Health and Social Security) (1988b) *Community Care: Agenda for Action* (The Griffiths Community Care report) (London, HMSO).

DHSS (Department of Health and Social Security) Fitton, F. and Acheson, H. (1979) *Doctor–Patient Relationships* (London, HMSO).

Disken, S. (1990) 'Health for All and All For One', *Health Service Journal*, 10 May, 691.

DoH (Department of Health) (1989) *Health Service Management Resource Assumptions and Planning Guidelines* Circular HC (89) 24 (London, Department of Health).

DoH (Department of Health) (1990a) *Developing Districts* (London, HMSO).

DoH (Department of Health) (1990b) *Contracts for Health Services: Operating Contracts* (London, HMSO).

DoH (Department of Health) (1990c) *NHS Trusts: A Working Guide* (London, HMSO).

DoH (Department of Health) (1990d) *The NHS Reforms and You* (London, Central Office of Information).

DoH (Department of Health) (1990e) *Improving Prescribing* (London, Department of Health).

DoH (Department of Health) (1991) *The Patients' Charter* (London, HMSO).

DoH (Department of Health) (1992a) *On the State of The Public Health 1991. The Annual Report of the Chief Medical Officer* (London, HMSO).

DoH (Department of Health) (1992b) *Effect of Tobacco Advertisements on Tobacco Consumption. A Discussion Document Reviewing the Evidence* (London, Department of Health, Economics and Operational Research Division).

DoH (Department of Health) (1992c) *Health and Social Service Statistics 1992* (London, HMSO).

DoH (Department of Health) (1993) *Making London Better* (London, Department of Health).

DoH and OPCS (Department of Health) (1993a) *Health Survey for England, 1991* (London, HMSO).

DoH and OPCS (Department of Health and Office of Population Censuses and Surveys) (1993b) *Departmental Report* (London, HMSO).

Doig, A. (1990) 'Routine Crisis and Muddle: Mishandling the Egg Crisis', *Teaching Public Administration*, vol. 10 (1), 15–26.

Doll, R. and Peto, R. (1981) 'The Causes of Cancer', *Journal of the National Cancer Institute*, vol. 66, 1191–1308.

Donnison, J. (1988) *Midwives and Medical Men: A History of Interprofessional Rivalries and Women's Rights* (London, Heinemann).

Doyal, L. (1979) *The Political Economy of Health* (London, Pluto).

Draper, P. (ed.). (1991) *Health Through Public Policy. The Greening of Public Health* (London, Merlin).

Dubos, R. (1959) *The Mirage of Health* (New York, Harper & Row).

Duncan, C., Sams, K. and White, P. (1989) 'The House of Commons and the NHS', *Political Quarterly*, vol. 60 (3), 365–73.

Dunnigan, M. G. (1993) 'The Problem with Cholesterol', *British Medical Journal*, vol. 306, 1355–6.

Eckstein, H. (1960) *Pressure Group Politics: The Case of the BMA* (London, George Allen & Unwin).

Economist (1991) 'Dithering Over Community Care', 20 April, 27.

Elcock, H. and Haywood, S. (1980) 'The Centre Cannot Hold', *Public Administration*, Bulletin, vol. 36, 53–62.

Engel, G. I. (1977) 'The Need for a New Medical Model: A Challenge for Biomedicine', Science, vol. 196, 129–36.

Enthoven, A. C. (1985) *Reflections on the Management of the National Health Service* (London, Nuffield Provincial Hospitals Trust).

Faculty of Public Health Medicine (1991a) *Alcohol and the Public Health* (London, Macmillan).

Faculty of Public Health Medicine (1991b) *UK Levels of Health* (London, Faculty of Public Health Medicine).

Field, F. (1988) 'Thoughts on Reforming the Health Service', *Catholic Herald*, 12 February.

Field, M. G. (ed.). (1989) *Success and Crisis in National Health Systems* (London, Routledge).

Fitzherbert, L. (1992) *Charity and NHS Reform* (London, Directory of Social Change).

Fitzherbert, L. and Giles, S. (1990) *Charity and The National Health: A Report on the Extent and Potential of Charitable Funds within the NHS* (London, The Directory of Social Change).

Fitzpatrick, R. (1984) 'Lay Concepts of Illness' in R. Fitzpatrick *et al. The Experience of Illness* (London, Tavistock).

Fitzpatrick, R., Hinton, S., Newman, S., Scambler, G., Thompson, G. (1984) *The Experience of Illness* (London, Tavistock, 11–31) .

Flanagan, H. (1989) 'Effective or Efficient Management of Health Care?', *Health Services Management*, December 1989, 266–69.

Flynn, R. (1992) *Structures of Control in Health Management* (London, Routledge).

Foot, M. (1975) *Aneurin Bevan* (London, Paladin Granada).

Foucault, M. (1973) *The Birth of the Clinic* (London, Tavistock).

Fowler, N. (1991) *Ministers Decide: A Personal Memoir of the Thatcher Years* (London, Chapman).

Fox, J. (ed.). (1989) *Health Inequalities in European Countries* (Aldershot, Gower).

Freddi, G. and Bjorkman, J. W. (1989) *Controlling Medical Professionals: The Comparative Politics of Health Governance* (London, Sage).

Freemantle, N. (1992) 'Spot the Flaw', *Health Service Journal*, 9 July, 122–3.

Freidson, E. (1988) *Profession of Medicine* (London, University of Chicago Press).

Fuchs, V. R. (1974) *Who Shall Live?* (New York, Basic Books).

Fulder, S. (1992) 'Alternative Therapists in Britain' in Saks, M .P. (ed.) *Alternative Medicine in Briiain* (Oxford, Clarendon), 166–82.

Gaines, A. D. (1979) 'Definitions and Diagnoses: Cultural Implications of Psychiatric Help Seeking and Psychiatrists' Definitions of the Situation in Psychiatric Emergencies', *Culture, Medicine and Psychiatry*, vol. 3 (4), 381–428.

Gamble, A. (1988) *The Free Economy and the Strong State. The Politics of Thatcherism* (London, Macmillan).

Garrow, J. (1991) 'The Importance of Obesity', *British Medical Journal*, vol. 303, 704–6.

George, S. (1976) *How the Other Half Dies: The Real Reasons for World Hunger* (Harmondsworth, Penguin).

Ginzberg, E. (1990) *The Medical Triangle: Physicians, Politicians and the Public* (Cambridge, Mass.Harvard University Press).

Gladstone, D. (1992) *Opening up the Medical Monopoly: Consumer Choice Versus Professional Power* (London, Adam Smith Institute).

Glennerster, H., Owens, P. and Matsaganis, M. (1992) *A Foothold for Fundholding* (London, Kings Fund Institute).

Godt, P. (1987) 'Confederation, Consent and Corporation: State Strategies and the Medical Profession in France, Great Britain and West Germany', *Journal of Health Politics, Policy and Law*, vol. 12 (3), 459–80.

Goffman, E. (1968) *Stigma: Notes on the Management of Spoiled Identity* (Harmondsworth, Penguin).

Goldacre, M. J. and Harris R. T. (1980) 'Mortality, Morbidity, Resource Allocation and Planning: A Consideration of Disease Classification', *British Medical Journal*, vol. 281, 1515–19.

Goldblatt, P. (1989) 'Mortality by Social Class 1971–85', *Population Trends, (London, HMSO)*.

Goldsmith, M. and Willetts, D. (1988) *Managed Health Care Organisations: A New System for a Better Health Service* (London, Centre for Policy Studies).

Gould, D. (1987) *The Medical Mafia* (London, Sphere).

Graham, H. (1984) *Women, Health and the Family* (Brighton, Wheatsheaf).

Grant, C. (1985) *Private Health Care in the UK: Review*. Economist Intelligence Unit, Special Report no. 207 (London, *Economist*).

Green, D. G. (1986) 'Joint Finance: An Analysis of the Reasons for its Limited Success', *Policy and Politics*, vol. 14 (2), 209–20.

Green, D. G. (1988) *Everyone a Private Patient* (London, Institute for Economic Affairs).

Green, D. G., Neuberger, J., Lord Young and Burstall, M. L. (1990) *The NHS Reforms: What Happened to Consumer Choice?* (London, Institute for Economic Affairs).

Green, D. S. (1987) *The New Right: The Counter Revolution in Political, Economic and Social Thought* (Brighton, Wheatsheaf).

Green, H. (1988) *General Household Survey 1985: Series GHS15A – Informal Carers* (London, HMSO).

Grey-Turner, E. and Sutherland, F. M. (1982) *History of the BMA Part 2, 1932–81* (London, BMA).

Griffiths, D. (1971) 'Inequalities and Management in the NHS', *The Hospital*, July 1971, 229–33.

Griggs, E. (1991) 'The Politics of Health Care Reform in Britain', *Political Quarterly*, vol. 62 (4), 419–30.

Groves, T. (1990) 'The Future of Community Care', *British Medical Journal*, vol. 300, 923–4.

Guardian. (1992) 'Carers made ill by strains of duties', 22 May, 4.

HM Treasury *Government Expenditure Plans 1988/9*, London HMSO 1988.

Hall, J. (1990) 'How We Won the Contracts Race', *Health Service Journal*, 17 June, 846–7.

Hall, R. H. (1990) *Health and the Global Environment* (Oxford, Polity).

Ham, C. (1981) *Policy Making in the National Health Service* (London, Macmillan).

Ham, C. (1986) *Managing Health Services: Health Authority Members in Search of a Role* (University of Bristol, School of Applied Urban Studies).

Ham, C. (1991) *The New NHS* (Oxford, Radcliffe Medical Press).

Ham, C. (1992) *Locality Purchasing* (Birmingham, Health Services Management Centre).

Ham, C. (1993) *Health Policy in Britain* (London, Macmillan).

Ham, C. and Heginbotham, C. (1991) *Purchasing Together* (London, King's Fund).

Ham, C. and Matthews, T. (1991) *Purchasing with Authority: The New Role of DHAs* (London, King's Fund College Paper).

Ham, C., and Mitchell, J. (1990) 'A Force to Reckon With', *Health Service Journal*, 1 February, 164–5.

Ham, C., Robinson, R. and Benzeval, M. (1990) *Health Check: Health Care Reforms in an International Context* (London, King's Fund).

Hambleton, R. (1983) 'Health Planning – A Second Chance', *Policy and Politics*, vol. 11 (2), 198–201.

Hampton, J.R. (1983) 'The End of Clinical Freedom', *British Medical Journal*, vol. 287, 1237–8.

Hancock, G. and Carim, E. (1987) *AIDS: The Deadly Epidemic* (London, Gollancz).

Harrison, S. (1988a) *Managing the National Health Service: Shifting the Frontier* (London, Chapman and Hall).

Harrison, S. (1988b) 'The Workforce and the New Managerialism', in R. Maxwell (ed.), *Reshaping the NHS* (Oxford, Policy Journals), pp.141–52.

Harrison, S. and Schulz, R.I. (1989) *Clinical Autonomy in the UK and the US: Contrasts and Convergence* in Freddie, G. and Bjorkman, J.W. (eds), *Controlling Medical Professionals* (London, Sage) pp. 198–209.

Harrison, S. and Wistow, G. (1992) 'The Purchaser/Provider Split in English Health Care: Towards Explicit Rationing?', *Policy and Politics*, vol. 20 (2), 123–30.

Harrison, S., Hunter, D.J., Marnoch, G. and Pollitt, C. (1992) *Just Managing: Power and Culture in the National Health Service* (London, Macmillan).

Hart, N. (1982) 'Is Capitalism Bad For Your Health?', *British Journal of Sociology*, vol. 33, 435–43.

Harvard Medical Practice Study (1990) *Patients, Doctors and Lawyers: Medical Injury Malpractice and Patient Compensation in New York* (Boston, Harvard Medical Practice Study).

Hashemi, K. and Merlin, M. (1987) 'Are Routine Bacteriological Cultures Necessary in an Accident and Emergency Department?', *British Medical Journal*, vol. 294, 1462–3.

Hayward, S. and Fee, E. (1992) 'More in Sorrow than in Anger: The British Nurses' Strike of 1988', *International Journal of Health Services*, vol. 22 (3), 397–416.

Haywood, S. (1987) 'Not What the Ministers Ordered', *The Times*, 22 April, 12.

Haywood, S. (1990) 'Efficiency and the NHS', *Public Money and Management*, vol. 10 (2), 51–4.

Haywood, S. and Alaszewski, A. (1980) *Crisis in the Health Service* (London, Croom Helm).

Haywood, S. and Ranade, W. (1985) 'Health Authorities: Tribunes or Prefects?', *Public Administration Bulletin*, vol. 47, 39–52.

Health Advisory Service (1987) *Annual Report* (Sutton, HAS).

Health Education Council, (1992) *Allied Dunbar National Fitness Survey. A Report on Activity Patterns and Fitness Levels* (London, Sports Council and HEA).

Health Promotion Authority for Wales (1990) *Health for All in Wales: Health Promotion Challenges for the 1990's* (Cardiff, HPAFW).

Helman, C. (1990) *Culture, Health and Illness* (2nd edn) (London, Wright).

Henderson, J., Goldacre, M. J., Graveney, M. J. and Simmons, H. M. (1989) 'Use of Medical Record Linkage to Study Re-Admission Rates', *British Medical Journal*, vol. 299, 709–13.

Hennessy, P. (1988) *Whitehall* (London, Secker & Warburg).

Herzlich, C. and Pierret, J. (1985) 'The Social Construction of the Patient: Patients and Illnesses in Other Ages', *Social Science and Medicine*, vol. 25, 1019–32.

Hibbard, J. H. and Weekes, E. C. (1987) 'Consumerism in Health Care: Prevalence and Predictors', *Medical Care*, vol. 25 (11), 1019–32.

Hicks, D. (1976) *Primary Health Care: A Review* (London, HMSO).

Higgins, J. (1988) *The Business of Medicine: Private Health Care in Britain* (London, Macmillan).

Higgins, J. (1989) 'Defining Community Care: Realities and Myths', *Social Policy and Administration* vol. 23(1), 3–16.

Hill, J. D., Hampton, J. R. and Mitchell, J. R. A. (1978) 'A Randomised Trial of Home versus Hospital Management for Patients with Suspected Myocardial Infarction', *The Lancet*, 22 April, 837–841.

Hirsch, J. and Leibel, R. (1988) 'New Light on Obesity', *New England Journal of Medicine*, vol. 318, 509–10.

Hodgkinson, R. (1967) *The Origins of the NHS: The Medical Services of the New Poor Law* (London, Wellcome Foundation).

Hoffenberg, R. (1987) *Clinical Freedom* (London, Nuffield Hospital Provincial Trust).

Honigsbaum, F. (1979) *The Division in British Medicine* (London, Kogan Page).

Honigsbaum, F. (1989) *Health, Happiness and Security: The Creation of the NHS* (London, Routledge and Chapman & Hall).

Honigsbaum, F. (1990) 'The Evolution of the NHS', *British Medical Journal*, vol. 301, 694–9.

Honigsbaum, F. (1992) *Who Shall Live? Who Shall Die?*, Oregon's Health Financing Proposals (London, King's Fund College Papers).

House of Commons (1984) (HC 209) *1st Report 1983/4. Griffiths NHS Management Inquiry Report*, Social Services Committee (London, HMSO).

House of Commons (1985) (HC 13) *2nd Report. Community Care with Special Reference to Adult Mentally Ill and Mentally Handicapped People*, Social Services Committee (London, HMSO).

House of Commons (1986a) (HC 413) *44th Report 1985/6. Preventive Medicine*, Public Accounts Committee (London, HMSO).

House of Commons (1986b) (HC 387) *4th Report 1985/6 Public Expenditure in the Social Services*, Social Services Committee (London, HMSO).

House of Commons (1987) (HC 37) *1st Report 1986/7. Primary Health Care*, Social Services Committee (London, HMSO).

House of Commons (1988a) (HC 264) *1st Report 1987/8. Resourcing the NHS: Short Term Issues*, Social Services Committee (London, HMSO).

House of Commons (1988b) (HC 613) *5th Report 1987/8. The Future of the NHS*, Social Services Committee (London, HMSO).

House of Commons (1988c) (HC 494) *8th Report 1987/8 Civil Service Reform: The Next Steps*. Treasury and Civil Committee (London, HMSO).

House of Commons (1989a) (HC 214–II) *5th Report 1988/9. Resourcing the NHS: The Government's White Paper 'Working for Patients'*, Social Services Committee (London, HMSO).

House of Commons (1989b) (HC 214–III) *8th Report 1988/9. Resourcing the NHS: The Government's Plans for the Future of the NHS*, Social Services Committee (London, HMSO).

House of Commons (1989c) (HC 108) *1st Report 1988/9. Salmonella in Eggs*, Select Committee on Agriculture (London, HMSO).

House of Commons (1989d) (HC 249) *26th Report. 1988/9 Coronary Heart Disease*, Public Accounts Committee (London, HMSO).

House of Commons (1990a) (HC 397) *18th Report 1989/90. Hospital Building in England*, Public Accounts Committee (London, HMSO).

House of Commons (1990b) (HC 380) *35th Report 1989/90. Maternity Services*, Public Accounts Committee (London, HMSO).

House of Commons (1990c) (HC 163) *The NHS and the Independent Hospitals 1989/90*, Public Accounts Committee (London, HMSO).

House of Commons (1990d) (HC 410) *5th Report 1989/90. Community Care: Carers*, Social Services Committee (London, HMSO).

House of Commons (1990e) (HC 444) *6th Report 1989/90. Choice for Service Users*, Social Services Committee (London, HMSO).

House of Commons (1990f) (HC 580) *8th Report 1989/90. Community Care: Planning and Co-operation*, Social Services Committee (London, HMSO).

House of Commons (1990g) (HC 558) *9th Report 1989/90. Community Care: Quality*, Social Services Committee (London, HMSO).

House of Commons (1990h) (HC 664) *11th Report 1989/90. Community Care: Services for People with Mental Handicap and People with Mental Illness*, Social Services Committee (London, HMSO).

House of Commons (1991) (HC 614) *3rd Report 1990/1. Public Expenditure on Health and Personal Social Services*, Health Committee (London, HMSO).

House of Commons (1992) (HC 321) *1st Report 1992/3. NHS Trusts: Interim Conclusions and Proposals for Future Enquiries*, Health Committee (London, HMSO).

House of Commons (1993) (HC 309) *3rd Report 1992/3. Community Care: Funding from April 1993*, Health Committee (London, HMSO).

House of Lords (1985) (HL 211) *13th Report of the European Communities Select Committee 1984/5. Co-operation at Community Level on Health-Related Problems*, (London, HMSO).

Hudson, B. (1992) 'Quasi-Markets in Health and Social Care in Britain. Can The Public Sector Respond?', *Policy and Politics*, vol. 20 (2), 131–42.

Hughes, D. (1990) 'Same Story, Different Words', *Health Service Journal*, 22 March, 432–4.

Hughes, D. and Dingwall, R. (1990) 'What's in a Name?', *Health Service Journal*, 29 November, 1770–1.

Hunter, D. J., Judge, K. and Price, S. (1988) *Community Care. Reacting to Griffiths (Briefing No. 1)* (London, King's Fund Institute).

Hunter, D. J. and Webster, C. (1992) 'Here We Go Again', *Health Services Journal*, 5 March, 26–7.

Hunter, D. J. and Wistow, G. (1987a) *Community Care in Britain. Variations on a Theme*, (London, King's Fund).

Hunter, D. J., and Wistow, G. (1987b) 'The Paradox of Policy Diversity in a Unitary State: Community Care in Britain', *Public Administration*, vol. 65 (1), 3–24.

Huntington, J. (1993) 'From FPC to FHSA To ... Health Commission?', *British Medical Journal*, vol. 306, 33–6.

IHSM/NAHA (Institute of Health Services Management/National Association of Health Authorities), (1989) *Efficiency in the NHS* (London, King's Fund).

Iliffe, S. (1988) *Strong Medicine: Health Service Politics for the 21st Century* (London, Lawrence & Wishart).

Illich, I. (1975) *Limits to Medicine*, (Harmondsworth, Penguin).

Illsley, R. (1986) 'Occupational Class Selection and the Production of Inequalities in Health', *Quarterly Journal of Social Affairs*, vol. 2 (2), 151–65.

Independent Scientific Committee on Smoking and Health, (1988) *4th Report* (London, HMSO).

Independent, (1988), 'NHS Tenders', 15 June, 6.

Independent, (1991) 'Advisers on cutting costs paid £500 000 by health authority', 15 April, 2.

Independent, (1991) 'Hospital to begin two-tier service', 3 May, 2.

Independent, (1991) 'Surgeons refuse to put patients on waiting list', 6 November, 4.

Independent, (1993) 'Wessex wasted £20 million on computer scheme', 11 February, 2.

Inglis, B. (1965) *A History of Medicine* (London, Weidenfeld and Nicolson).

Inglis, B. (1981) *The Diseases of Civilisation* (London, Hodder & Stoughton).

Institute for Economic Affairs (1989) *Empowering the Elderly* (London, IEA).

Institute of Health Service Management (IHSM) (1988) *The Potential Role of Private Health Insurance* (London, IHSM).

Jacobson, B. (1981) *The Lady-killers* (London, Pluton).

Jacobson, B. (1983) 'Smoking and Health: A New Generation of Campaigners', *British Medical Journal*, vol. 287, 483–4.

Jenkins, J. (1985) *Caring for Women's Health* (London, Search Press).

Jenkins, P. (1987) *Mrs Thatcher's Revolution: The Ending of the Socialist Era* (London, Jonathan Cape).

Jennett, B. (1986) *High Technology Medicine* (Oxford University Press).

Johnson, N. (1989) 'The Privatisation of Welfare', *Social Policy and Administration*, vol. 23 (2), 17–30.

Johnson, P., Conrad, C. and Thomson, D. (1989) *Workers versus Pensioners* (London, Centre for Economic Policy Research).

Johnson, T. J. (1972) *Professions and Power* (London, Macmillan).

Joint NHS Privatisation Unit (1990) *The Privatisation Experience* (London, JNPU).

Jones, I. and Higgs, P. (1990) 'Putting People before Logic', *Health Service Journal*, 31 May, 814–5.

Jones, T. and Prowle, M. (1987) *Health Service Finance: An Introduction* (London, Certified Accountants Educational Trust).

Jönsson, B. (1990) 'What can Americans Learn from Europeans?' in OECD *Health Care Systems in Transition* (Paris, OECD).

Jowell, R., Witherspoon, F. and Brook, L. (1989) *British Social Attitudes Survey* (London, Social and Community Planning Research).

Jowell, R., Brooke, L., Prior, G., Taylor, B. (1992) *British Social Attitudes: The 9th Report*, 1992/3 edn, Social and Community Planning Research (Aldershot, Dartmouth).

Kavanagh, D. (1990) *Thatcherism and British Politics* (Oxford University Press).

Kennedy, I. (1981) *The Unmasking of Medicine* (London, Allen & Unwin).

King, D.S. (1987) *The New Right: Politics Markets and Citizenship* (London, Macmillan).

Klein, R. (1980) *Between Nationalism and Utopia in Health Care*, Lecture, Yale University, New Haven (Unpublished).

Klein, R. (1982) 'Reflections of an Ex-AHA Member', *British Medical Journal*, vol. 284, 992–4.

Klein, R. (1983) *The Politics of the National Health Service* (London, Longman) 1st edn.

Klein, R. (1989a) 'The Role of Health Economics', *British Medical Journal*, vol. 299, 275–6.

Klein, R. (1989b) *The Politics of the NHS* (London, Longman) 2nd edn.

Klein, R. (1990a) 'The State and the Profession: The Politics of the Double Bed', *British Medical Journal*, vol. 301, 700–2.

Klein, R. (1990b) 'What Future for the Department of Health?', *British Medical Journal*, vol. 301, 481–4.

Klein, R. and Day, P. (1992) 'Constitutional and Distributional Conflict in British Medical Politics: The Case of General Practice 1911–1991', *Political Studies*, vol. 40 (3), 462–78.

Kleinman, A. (1978) 'Concepts and a Model for the Comparison of Medical Systems as Cultural Systems', *Social Science and Medicine*, vol. 12 (2B), 85–93.

Labour Party (1992a) *No Previous Experience Required: A Survey of 3rd Wave Trusts* (London, Labour Party).

Labour Party (1992b) *Your Good Health* (London, Labour Party).

Laing, W. (1989) *Laing's Review of Private Health Care 1989/90* (London, Laing & Buisson).

Laing, W. (1990) *Laing's Review of Private Health Care 1990/1* (London, Laing & Buisson).

Langan, M. (1990) 'Community Care in the 1990s. The Community Care White Paper "Caring for People"', *Critical Social Policy*, vol. 29, 58–71.

Larkin, G. (1983) *Occupational Monopoly and Modern Medicine* (London, Tavistock).

Lawson, N. (1992) *The View from Number 11. Memoirs of a Tory Radical* (London, Bantam Press).

Leadbeater, P. (1990) *Partners in Health: The NHS and the Independent Sector* (Birmingham, National Association of Health Authorities and Trusts).

Leavey, R., Wilkin, D. and Metcalfe, D. (1989) 'Consumerism and General Practice', *British Medical Journal*, 298, 737–9.

Leeson, J. and Gray, J. (1978) *Women and Medicine* (London, Tavistock).

Le Grand, J. (1978) 'The Distribution of Public Expenditure and the Case of Health Care', *Economica*, vol. 45, 125–42.

Le Grand, J. and Bartlett, W. (1993) *Quasi-Markets and Social Policy* (London, Macmillan).

Leichter, H. M. (1979) *A Comparative Approach to Policy Analysis: Health Care Policy in Four Nations* (London, Cambridge University Press).

Levick, P. (1992) 'The Janus Face of Community Care Legislation: An Opportunity for Radical Possibilities', *Critical Social Policy*, vol. 34, 75–92.

Lewis, J. (1987) *What Price Community Medicine?* (Brighton, Wheatsheaf).

Ley, P. (1982) 'Satisfaction, Compliance and Communication', *British Journal of Clinical Psychology*, vol. 21, 241–54.

Liberal Democrats (1992) *Restoring the Nation's Health*, Federal Paper Number 5 (London, Liberal Democrats).

Light, D. (1990a) 'Bending the Rules', *Health Service Journal*, 11 October 1513–14.

Light, D. (1990b) 'Biting Hard on the Research Bit', *Health Service Journal*, 25 October, 1604–5.

Loewy, E. H. (1980) 'Cost Should Not Be A Factor In Medical Care', *New England Journal of Medicine*, vol. 302, 697.

Lord President of the Council (1991) *Action Against Alcohol Misuse* (London, HMSO).

Loveridge, R. and Starkey, K. (1992) *Continuity and Crisis in the NHS* (Buckingham, Open University Press).

Lowry, S. (1988) 'Focus on Performance Indicators', *British Medical Journal*, vol. 296, 992–4.

Lowry, S. (1991) *Housing and Health* (London, British Medical Journal Publications).

Mann, G. V. (1974) 'The Influence of Obesity on Health' *New England Journal of Medicine*, vol. 291, 178–85.

Mann, J. (ed.) (1993) *Aids in the World: A Global Report* (Cambridge University Press, Harvard).

Marks, L. (1988) *Promoting Better Health: An Analysis of the Government's Programme for Improving Primary Care*, Briefing Paper no. 7 (London King's Fund Institute).

Marmot, M. G., Adelstein, A. and Bulusu, L. (1984) *Immigrant Mortality in England and Wales 1970–78*, OPCS Studies of Medicine and Population Subjects 47 (London HMSO).

Marmot, M. G., Davey-Smith, G., Stansfield, S., Patel, C., North, F., Head, J., White, I., Brunner, E., Feeney, A. (1991) 'Health inequalities among British Civil Servants: the Whitehall II Study', *The Lancet*, vol. 337, 1387–93.

Marsh, D. and Rhodes, R. (1992) *Implementing Thatcherite Policies* (Buckingham, Open University Press).

Martin, C. (1992) 'Attached, Detached or New Recruits?', *British Medical Journal*, vol. 305, 348–50.

Martin, J. (1984) *Hospitals in Trouble* (Oxford, Blackwell).

Maxwell, R. (1981) 'On Ministers of Health', *The Lancet*, vol. 1, 1412–14.

Maxwell, R. (1993) 'Other Cities, Same Problems', *British Medical Journal*, vol. 306, 199–201.

May, A. (1989) 'A Guru Vexed by his Disciples', *Health Service Journal*, 21 September, 1150

May, A. (1990) 'Who Guards the Money?', *Health Service Journal*, 10 May, 696–7.

May, A. (1991) 'Turning Round the Aircraft Carrier' *Health Service Journal*, 20 June, 14.

Mays, N. and Bevan, G. (1987) *Resource Allocation in the Health Service* (London, Bedford Square Press).

McAuley, R. G. and Henderson, H. W. (1984) 'Results of the Peer Assessment Programme of the College of Physicians and Surgeons at Ontario', *Canadian Medical Association Journal*, vol. 131, 557–61.

McCormick, S. S. (1989) 'Cervical Smears: A Questionable Practice?', *The Lancet*, vol. 2, 207.

McCullough, S. (1989) 'Useless Smear Campaign', *The Spectator*, 11 February, 20–1.

McDonnell, R. and Maynard, A. (1985) 'The Costs of Alcohol Misuse', *British Journal of Addiction*, vol. 80, 27–35.

McGregor, G. (1990) 'Privatisation on Parade', *Health Service Journal*, 3 May, 670–1.

McKeown, T. (1979) *The Role of Medicine: Dream, Mirage or Nemesis?* (Oxford, Blackwell).

McKinlay, J. B. (1979) 'Epidemiological and Political Developments of Social Policies Regarding the Public Health', *Social Science and Medicine*, vol. 13A, 541–8.

McLachlan, G. (1990) *What Price Quality? The NHS in Review* (London, Nuffield Provincial Hospitals Trust).

McPherson, K., Strong, P. M. and Epstein, A. (1981) 'Regional Variations in the Use of Common Surgical Procedures: Within and Between England and Wales, Canada and the USA', *Social Science and Medicine*, vol. 15A, 273–88.

Mechanic, D. (1961) 'The Concept of Illness Behaviour', *Journal of Chronic Diseases*, vol. 15, 189–94.

Mercer, J. and Talbot, I. C. (1985) 'Clinical Diagnosis: A Post Mortem Assessment of Accuracy in the 1980s', *Post Graduate Medical Journal*, vol. 61, 713–16.

Miles, A. (1988) *Women and Mental Illness: The Social Context of Female Neurosis* (Brighton, Wheatsheaf).

Miles, A. (1991) *Women, Health and Medicine* (Buckingham, Open University Press).

Millstone, E. (1986) *Food Additives* (Harmondsworth, Penguin).

Milne, R. (1987) 'Competitive Tendering in the NHS: An Economic Analysis of the Early Implementation of HC(83)18', *Public Administration*, vol. 65 (2), 145–60.

Milne, R. (1989) 'Tender Topics for the NHS', *Health Service Journal*, 5 January, 16–17.

Ministry of Health (1954) *Report of the Committee on Economic and Financial Problems of Old Age (The Phillips Report) (London, HMSO)*.

Ministry of Health (1959) *Report of the Committee on Maternity Services* (The Cranbrook Report) (London, HMSO).

Ministry of Health (1963) *The Field of Work of the Family Doctor* (The Gillie Report) (London, HMSO).

Ministry of Health (1968) *The National Health Service. The Administrative Structure of the Medical and Related Services in England and Wales* (London, HMSO).

Mohan, J. (1986) 'Private Medical Care and the British Conservative Government. What Price Independence?', *Journal of Social Policy*, vol. 15 (3), 337–60.

Mooney, G.H. and Healey, A. (1991) 'Strategy full of good intentions', *British Medical Journal*, vol. 303, 1119-20.

Mooney, G.H., Russell, E.M. and Weir, R.D. (1986) *Choices for Health Care: A Practical Introduction to the Economics of Health Provision* (London: Macmillan).

Moore, J., Phipps, K. and Marcer, D. (1985) 'Why Do People Seek Treatment by Alternative Medicine', *British Medical Journal*, vol. 290, 28–9.

Moore, W. (1988) 'Two Authorities Overruled over In-house Contracts', *Health Service Journal*, 4 August, 869.

Moran, G. (1989) 'Public Health at Risk', *Health Service Journal*, 1 June, 668–9.

Moran, M. (1991) *Welfare State, Health Care State*, Paper given at the Political Studies Annual Conference, Lancaster.

Moran, M. and Wood, B. (1992) *States, Regulation and the Medical Profession* (Buckingham, Open University Press).

Morley, V. (1993) 'Empowering GP's as Purchasers', *British Medical Journal*, vol. 306, 112–14.

Morris, J.N. (1980) 'Are Health Services Important to People's Health?', British Medical Journal, vol. 280, 167–8.

Nairne, P. (1984) 'Parliamentary Control and Accountability', in R. Maxwell and R. Weaver (eds) *Public Participation in Health* (London, King Edward's Hospital Fund for London), 33–51.

NAHA (National Association of Health Authorities and National Council for Voluntary Organisations) (1987) *Partnerships for Health* (Birmingham, NAHA).

NAHAT (National Association of Health Authorities and Trusts) (1990) *Healthcare Economic Review* (Birmingham, NAHAT).

NAHAT (National Association of Health Authorities and Trusts) (1992) *Implementing The Reforms. A Second National Survey of District General Managers* (Birmingham, NAHAT).

NAHAT (National Association of Health Authorities and Trusts) (1993) *The Financial Survey 1992/3* (Birmingham, NAHAT).

NAO (National Audit Office) (1986) (HC 12) *Value for Money Developments in the NHS* (London, HMSO).

NAO (National Audit Office) (1987) (HC 108) *Community Care Developments 1987/88* (London, HMSO).

NAO (National Audit Office) (1988a) (HC 498) *Management of Family Practitioner Services* (London, HMSO).

NAO (National Audit Office) (1988b) (HC 736) *Quality of Clinical Care in NHS Hospitals* (London, HMSO).

NAO (National Audit Office) (1989a) (HC 106) *The NHS and the Independent Hospitals* (London, HMSO).

NAO (National Audit Office) (1989b) (HC 566) *Financial Management in the NHS* (London, HMSO).

NAO (National Audit Office) (1989c) (HC 208) *NHS: Coronary Heart Disease* (London, HMSO).

NAO (National Audit Office) (1990) (HC 297) *Maternity Services* (London, HMSO).

NAO (National Audit Office) (1991) (HC 306) *Use of NHS Operating Theatres in England. A Progress Report* (London, HMSO).

Nath, U. R. (1986) *Smoking: Third World Alert* (Oxford, University Press).

National Consumer Council (1992) *Quality Standards in the NHS. The Consumer Focus* (London, NCC).

National Institute for Social Work (1988) *Residential Care: A Positive Choice Report of the Independent Review of Residential Care* (The Wagner Report) (London, HMSO).

Navarro, V. (1978) *Class Struggle, The State and Medicine.* (Oxford, Robertson).

Newbiggin, R. and Lister, J. (1988) *Private Health Care: The Record of Private Companies in NHS Support Services* (London, Association of London Health Authorities).

Newbrander, W. and Parker, D. (1992) 'The Public and Private Sectors in Health and Economic Issues', *International Journal of Health Planning and Management,* vol. 7, 37–49.

NHSME (NHS Management Executive) (1990) *NHS Priorities in 1991/92* (London, Department of Health).

NHSME (NHS Management Executive) (1991a) *Priorities and Planning Guidance for the NHS for 1992/93* (London, Department of Health).

NHSME (NHS Management Executive) (1991b) *A Review of the Management Executive* (London, Department of Health).

NHSME (NHS Management Executive) (1991c) *NHS Reforms. The First Six Months* (London, Department of Health).

NHSME (NHS Management Executive) (1992a) *Priorities and Planning Guidance 1993/94* (Leeds, NHSME).

NHSME (NHS Management Executive) (1992b) *NHS Trusts: The First 12 Months* (London, Department of Health)..

NHSME (NHS Management Executive) (1992c) *Local Voices* (London, Department of Health).

Nicholl, J. P., Beeby, N. R. and Williams B. T. (1989a) 'Comparison of the Activity at Short Stay Independent Hospitals in England and Wales, 1981 and 1986', *British Medical Journal,* vol. 298, 239–42.

Nicholl, J. P., Beeby, N. R. and Williams B. T. (1989b) 'Role of the Private Sector in Elective Surgery in England and Wales', *British Medical Journal,* vol. 298, 243–7.

Nikolaides, K., Barnett, A. H., Spiliopoulos, A. J. and Watkins, P. J. (1981) 'West Indian Diabetic Population of a Large Inner City Diabetic Clinic', *British Medical Journal,* vol. 283, 1374.

Noppa, H., Bengtsson, C., Wedel, H. and Wilhemson, L. (1980) 'Obesity in Relation to Morbidity and Mortality from Cardio-Vascular Disease', *American Journal of Epidemiology,* vol. 111, 682–92.

Normand, C. (1991) 'Economics, Health and the Economics of Health', *British Medical Journal*, vol. 303, 1572–7.

Northern Ireland Health Promotion Agency (1990) *Health Promotion in Northern Ireland. A Discussion Paper* (Belfast, NIHPA).

Noyce, J., Snaith, A. and Trickey, A. (1974) 'Regional Variations in the allocation of financial resources to the Community Health Services', *The Lancet*, vol. 1, 554–7.

Oakley, A. (1980) *Women Confined*, (Oxford, Martin Robertson).

Oakley, A. (1984) *The Captured Womb: A History of the Medical Care of Pregnant Women* (Oxford, Blackwell).

O'Connor, J. (1973) *The Fiscal Crisis of the State* (New York, St Martin's Press).

O'Donnell, O., Propper, C. and Upward, R. (1991) *An Empirical Study of Equity in the Finance and Delivery of Health Care in Britain*, Discussion Paper No. 85 (*Centre for Health Economics*, University of York).

OECD (Organisation for Economic Co-operation and Development) (1987) *Financing and Delivering Health Care: A Comparative Analysis of OECD Countries* (Paris, OECD).

OECD (Organisation for Economic Co-operation and Development)(1990) *Health Care Systems in Transition: The Search for Efficiency*. Paris, OECD.

Offe, C. (1984) *The Contradictions of the Welfare State* (London, Hutchinson).

Office for Public Management (1991) *The Rubber Windmill One Year On: Assuring Health Gain* (Cambridge, East Anglian Regional Health Authority).

Office of Health Economics (1984) *Compendium of Health Statistics* (London, Office of Health Economics).

OPCS (Office of Population Censuses and Surveys) (1986) *Occupational Mortality: decennial supplement 1979–80 and 1982–3* (London, HMSO).

OPCS (1988) *(Office of Population Censuses and Surveys) OPCS Surveys of Disability in Great Britain: The Prevalence of Disability Among Adults* (London, HMSO).

OPCS (Office of Population Censuses and Surveys) (1990) *General Household Survey 1988* (London, HMSO).

OPCS (Office of Population Censuses and Surveys) (1992) *General Household Survey 1990* (London, HMSO).

Owen, D. (1988) *Our NHS* (London, Pan).

Owens, P. and Glennerster, H. (1990) *Nursing in Conflict* (London, Macmillan).

Packwood, T., Keen, J. and Buxton, M. (1991) *Hospitals in Transition. The Resource Management Experiment* (Buckingham, Open University Press).

Pamuk, E. R. (1985) 'Social Class Inequality in Mortality from 1971–72 in England and Wales', *Population Studies*, vol. 39, 17–31.

Parker, P. (1988) 'A Free Market in Health Care', *The Lancet*, vol. 1, 1210–14.

Parkin, D. (1989) 'Comparing Health Service Efficiency across Countries', *Oxford Review of Economic Policy*, vol. 5 (1), 75–88.

Parry, N. and Parry, J. (1976) *The Rise of the Medical Profession* (London, Croom Helm).

Parsons, T. (1951) *The Social System* (New York, Free Press of Glencoe).

Paton, C. (1992) *Competition and Planning in the NHS. The Danger of Unplanned Markets* (London, Chapman and Hall).

Payer, L. (1989) *Medicine and Culture* (London, Gollancz).

Perkin, H. (1989) *The Rise of Professional Society* (London, Routledge).

Perrin, J. (1988) *Resource Management in the NHS* (London, Chapman & Hall).

Petchey, R. (1987) 'Health Maintenance Organisations: Just What the Doctor Ordered?', *Journal of Social Policy*, vol. 16 (4), 489–507.

Pettigrew, A., Ferlie, E., FitzGerald, L. and Wensley, R. (1991) *Research in Action Authorities in the NHS* (University of Warwick, Centre for Corporate Strategy and Change).

Phillips, A. and Rakusen, J. (1989) *The New 'Our Bodies Ourselves'*, (Harmondsworth, Penguin)

Phillips, D.R. (1990) *Health and Healthcare in the Third World* (London, Longman).

Phillips, M. (1985) 'Tools of the the Party', *British Medical Association News Review*, January, 3.

Political and Economic Planning (1937) *Report on the British Health Services* (London, Political and Economic Planning).

Pollitt, C. (1985) 'Measuring Performance: A New System for the NHS', *Policy and Politics*, vol. 13 (1), 1–15.

Pollitt, C. (1992) 'The Struggle for Quality: The Case of the NHS', Paper given at Political Studies Association Annual Conference, Queens University, Belfast.

Pollock, A.M. and Whitty, P.M. (1990) 'Crisis in our hospital kitchens: ancillary staffing during an outbreak of food poisoning in a long stay hospital', *British Medical Journal*, vol. 300, 383–5.

Powell, M. (1990) 'Need and Provision in the NHS: An Inverse Care Law?', *Policy and Politics*, vol. 18, 31–8.

Powell, M. (1992) 'A Tale of Two Cities: a Critical Evaluation of the Geographical Provision of Health Care Before the NHS', *Public Administration*, vol. 70 (1), 67–80.

Powles, J. (1973) 'On the Limitations of Modern Medicine', *Science, Medicine and Man*, vol. 1, 1–30.

Pritchard, C. (1992) 'What Can We Afford for the NHS?', *Social Policy and Administration*, vol. 26 (1), 40–54.

Pritchard, P. (1978) *Manual of Primary Care: Its Nature and Organisation*, (Oxford University Press).

Public Health Alliance (1988) *Beyond Acheson* (Birmingham, PHA).

Radical Statistics Health Group (1977) *RAWP Deals: A Critique of 'Sharing Resources for Health in England'*, (London, Radical Statistics Health Group).

Radical Statistics Health Group (1991) 'Let Them Eat Soap', *Health Service Journal*, 14 November, 25–7.

Radical Statistics (1992) 'NHS Reforms: The First 6 Months. Proof of Progress or Statistical Smokescreen?', *British Medical Journal*, vol. 304, 705–9.

Ranade, W. (1985) 'Motives and Behaviour in District Health Authorities', *Public Administration*, vol. 63 (2), 183–200.

Rathwell, T. and Phillips, D. (1986) *Health, Race and Ethnicity* (London, Croom Helm).

Rayner, G. (1986) 'Health Care as a Business?', *Policy and Politics*, vol. 14 (4), 439–59.

Redwood, J. (1988) *In Sickness and in Health: Management Change in the NHS* (London, Centre for Policy Studies).

Regan, D. E. and Stewart, J. (1982) 'An Essay in the Government of Health: The Case for Local Authority Control', *Social Policy and Administration*, vol. 16 (1), 19–42.

Reiser, J. (1978) *Medicine and the Reign of Technology* (Cambridge University Press).

Richman, J. (1987) *Medicine and Health* (London, Longman).

Riddell, P. (1991) *The Thatcher Era and its Legacy* (Oxford, Blackwell).

Robb, B. (1967) *Sans Everything* (London, Nelson).

Roberts, H. (ed.) (1992) *Women's Health Matters* (London, Routledge).

Roberts, J. (1991a) 'Navigating the Seas of Change', *British Medical Journal*, vol. 302, 34–7.

Roberts, J. (1991b) 'General Practice: Feeling Fine, Getting Better', *British Medical Journal*, vol. 302, 97–100.

Robinson, D. (1971) *The Process of Becoming Ill* (London, Routledge).

Robinson, R. (1990) *Competition and Health Care: A Comparative Analysis of UK Plans and US Experience* (London, King's Fund Institute).

Robinson, R. (1991) 'Health Expenditure: Recent Trends and Prospects for the 1990s', *Public Money and Management*, vol. 11 (4), 19–24.

Royal College of General Practitioners (1986) *Alcohol: A Balanced View*, Reports from General Practice, (London, RCGP).

Royal College of Nursing (1990) *Memorandum to the House of Commons Social Services Committee 5th Report 1989/90. Community Care: Carers* (London, RCN).

Royal College of Physicians (1981) *Medical Aspects of Dietary Fibre* (London, Pitman).

Royal College of Physicians (1983a) 'Obesity', *Journal of the Royal College of Physicians*, vol. 17, 5–64.

Royal College of Physicians (1983b) *Health or Smoking?* (London, Pitman).

Ryan, J. and Thomas, F. (1980) *The Politics of Mental Handicap* (Harmondsworth, Penguin).

Sagan, L. A. (1987) *The Health of Nations* (New York, Basic Books).

Saks, M. P. (1990) 'Power, Politics and Alternative Medicine', *Teaching Politics*, vol. 3 (2), 68–72.

Saks, M. P. (ed.) (1992) *Alternative Medicine in Britain* (Oxford, Clarendon).

Salter, B. (1992) 'Heart of the Matter', *Health Service Journal*, 1 October, 28–30.

Sandler, G. (1979) 'Cost of Unnecessary Tests', *British Medical Journal*, vol. 2, 21.

Savage, R. and Armstrong, D. (1990) 'Effect of a GP's Consulting Style on Patients' Satisfaction: A Controlled Study', *British Medical Journal*, vol. 301, 968–70.

Salvage, J. (1985) *The Politics of Nursing* (Oxford, Heinemann).

Scottish Health Services Council (1966) *Administrative Practice of Hospital Boards in Scotland* (The Farquharson-Lang Report) (Edinburgh, HMSO).

Scottish Office (1991) *Health Education in Scotland* (Edinburgh, HMSO).

Scrivens, E. and Henneh, A. (1989) 'Working for Patients: Making the Internal Market Effective', *Public Money and Management*, vol. 9 (4), 53–7.

Scull, A. T. (1979) *Museums of Madness: The Social Organisation of Insanity in Nineteenth Century England* (London, Allen Lane).

Sharma, U. (1992) *Complementary Medicine Today* (London, Routledge).

Shearer, A. (1991) *Who Calls the Shots?* (London, King's Fund).

Shimmin, S., McNally, J. and Liff, S. (1981) 'Pressures on Women Engaged in Factory Work', *Employment Gazette*, August, 344–9.

Skinner, P.W., Riley, D. and Thomas, E.M. (1988) 'The Use and Abuse of Performance Indicators', *British Medical Journal*, vol. 292, 1256–9.

Small, N. (1989) *Politics and Planning in the NHS* (Milton Keynes, Open University Press).

Smith, A. (1987) 'Qualms about QALYs', *The Lancet*, vol. 1, 1134–6.

Smith, A. and Jacobson, B. (1988) *The Nation's Health: A Strategy for the 1990s* (London, King Edward's Hospital Fund).

Smith, F.B. (1979) *The People's Health* (London, Croom Helm).

Smith, G.D., Bartley, M. and Blane, D. (1990) 'The Black Report on Socio-economic Inequalities in Health: 10 Years On', *British Medical Journal*, vol. 301, 373–7.

Smith, R. (1987) *Unemployment and Health* (Oxford University Press).

Social Services Inspectorate (1988) *Certain Standards: Inspection for the Implementation of the 1984 Registered Homes Act*, (London, DHSS).

Stacey, M. (1989) 'The General Medical Council and Professional Accountability', *Public Policy and Administration*, vol. 4 (1), 12–27.

Stanway, A. (1986) *Alternative Medicine* (Penguin, Harmondsworth).

Starey, N., Bosanquet, N. and Griffiths, J. (1993) 'General Practitioners in Partnership with Management: An Organisational Model for Debate', *British Medical Journal*, vol. 306, 308–10.

Steel, K., Gertman, P., Crescenzi, C. and Anderson, J. (1981) 'Iatrogenic Illness on a General Medical Service at a University Hospital', *New England Journal of Medicine*, vol. 304, 638–42.

Steele, K. (1992) 'Patients as Experts: Appraisal of Health Services', *Public Money and Management*, vol. 12 (4), 31–8.

Stern, J. (1983) 'Social Mobility and the Interpretation of Social Class Mortality Differentials', *Journal of Social Policy*, vol. 12(1), 27–49.

Stocking, B. (1988) *Expensive Medical Technologies* (Oxford University Press).

Stocking, B. and Morrison, S.L. (1978) *The Image and the Reality: A Case Study of the Impact of Medical Technology* (London, Nuffield Provincial Hospitals Trust).

Strong, P. and Robinson, J. (1990) *The NHS: Under New Management* (Buckingham, Open University Press).

Stowe, K. (1989) *On Caring for the National Health* (London, Nuffield Provincial Hospitals Trust).

Szasz, T.S. and Hollender, M.H. (1956) 'A Contribution to the Philosophy of Medicine: The Basic Models of the Doctor–Patient Relationship', *American Medical Association, Archives of Internal Medicine*, vol. 97, 585–92.

Szreter, S. (1988) 'The Importance of Social Intervention in Britain's Mortality Decline C1850–1914', *Social History of Medicine*, vol. 1 (1), 1–38.

Taylor, D. (1988) 'Primary Care Services', in Maxwell, R. (ed.) *Reshaping the National Health Service* (Oxford, Policy Journals), 2–47.

Taylor, M. (1988) *Into the 1990s: Voluntary Organisations and the Public Sector* (London, National Council for Voluntary Organisations, Royal Institute of Public Administration).

Taylor, P. (1984) *The Smoke Ring: Tobacco, Money and Multi-National Politics* (London, Bodley Head).

Thain, C. and Wright, M. (1992) 'Planning and Controlling Public Expenditure in the UK (Part 1 The Treasury's Public Expenditure Survey)', *Public Administration*, vol. 70 (1), 3–24.

Thane, P. (1987) 'The Growing Burden of an Ageing Population', *Journal of Public Policy* vol. 7(4), 373–87.

Thatcher, M. (1982) Speech to Conservative Party Conference, Brighton, 8 October.

The Times (1989) 'Public wants acupuncture on NHS, poll says', 13 November, 15.

Thompson, J. (1984) 'Compliance' in R. Fitzpatrick *et al.* (1984) *The Experience of Illness* (London, Tavistock).

Thwaites, B. (1988) *The Grand Dilemmas of a National Health Service* (Leeds, Nuffield Institute).

Timmins, N. (1988) *Cash, Crisis and Cure: The Independent Guide to the NHS Debate* (Oxford, Alden Press).

Tomlinson, B. (1992) *Report of the Inquiry into London's Health Service* (London, HMSO).

Townsend, P., Davidson, N. and Whitehead, M. (1988) *Inequalities in Health* (Harmondsworth, Penguin).

Tucket, D., Bolton, M., Olson, C. and Williams, A. (1985) *Meetings Between Experts: An Approach to Sharing Ideas in Medical Consultation* (London, Tavistock).

Tudor-Hart, J. (1971) 'The Inverse Care Law', *The Lancet*, 27 February, 405–12.

Tudor-Hart, J. (1981) 'A New Kind of Doctor', *Journal of the Royal Society of Medicine*, vol. 74, 871–83.

Turner, B. (1987) *Medical Power and Social Knowledge* (London, Sage).

Twaddle, A. C. (1974) 'The Concept of Health Status', *Social Science and Medicine*, vol. 8 (1), 29–38.

Vayda, E. (1973) 'A Comparison of Surgical Rates in Canada and England and Wales', *New England Journal of Medicine*, vol. 289, 1224–9.

Vayda, E., Mindell, W. R. and Rutkow, I. M. (1982) 'A Decade of Surgery in Canada, England and Wales and the US', *Archives of Surgery*, vol. 117, 846–53.

Waitzkin, M. (1983) *The Second Sickness: Contradictions of Capitalist Health Care* (New York, Free Press).

Waller, D., Agass, M., Mant, D., Coulter, A., Fuller, A. and Jones, L. (1990) 'Health Checks in General Practice: Another Example of Inverse Care?', *British Medical Journal*, vol. 300, 1115–8.

Warr, P. and Parry, G. (1982) 'Paid Employment and Women's Psychological Well Being', *Psychological Bulletin*, vol. 91, 498–516.

Watkins, S. (1987) *Medicine and Labour. The Politics of a Profession* (London, Lawrence and Wishart.

Weale, A. (ed.) (1988) *Cost and Choice in Health Care* (London, King Edward's Hospital Fund for London).

Webb, A. and Wistow, G. (1983) 'Public Expenditure and Policy Implementation: The Case of Community Care', *Public Administration*, vol. 61 (1), 21–44.

Webster, C. (1988) *Health Services Since the War, Volume I: Problems of Health Care. The National Health Service before 1957* (London, HMSO).

Weiner, J. P. and Ferriss, D. M. (1990) *GP Budget Holding in the UK: Lessons from America* (London, King's Fund).

Weller, M. (1989) 'Psychosis and Destitution at Christmas 1985–88', *The Lancet*, vol. 2, 1509–1.

West, R. R. and Lowe, C. R. (1976) 'Regional Variations in Need for and Provision and Use of Child Health Services in England and Wales', *British Medical Journal*, vol. 2, 843–6.

Whitehead, M. (1987) *The Health Divide* (London, Health Education Council).

Whitehead, M. (1989) *Swimming Upstream: Trends and Prospects in Health Education*, Research Report No. 5 (London, King's Fund).

Whitney, R. (1988) *National Health Crisis: A Modern Solution* (London, Shepherd-Walwyn).

WHO (World Health Organisation) (1946) *Constitution: Basic Documents* (Geneva, WHO).

WHO (World Health Organisation) (1978) *Alma Ata 1977: Primary Health Care* (Geneva, WHO/UNICEF).

WHO (World Health Organisation) (1985) *Targets for Health for All: Targets in Support of the European Regional Strategy for Health for All* (Copenhagen, WHO Regional Office for Europe).

WHO (World Health Organisation) (1986) *Health and the Environment* (Geneva, WHO).

WHO (World Health Organisation) (1988) *Healthy Nutrition. Preventing Nutrition-Related Disease in Europe* (Copenhagen, WHO).

WHO (World Health Organisation) (1990) *World Health Statistics Annual, 1989* (Geneva, WHO).

WHO (World Health Organisation) (1992) *World Health Statistics Annual, 1991* (Geneva, WHO).

Widgery, D. (1988) *The National Health: A Radical Perspective* (London, Hogarth).

Wilding, P. (1982) *Professional Power and Social Welfare* (London, Routledge).

Wilding, P. (1992) 'The British Welfare State: Thatcherism's Enduring Legacy', *Policy and Politics*, vol. 20 (3), 201–12.

Wilkinson, R. G. (1992) 'Income Distribution and Life Expectancy', *British Medical Journal*, vol. 304, 165–8.

Williams, A. (1985) 'The Cost of Coronary Artery Bypass Grafting', *British Medical Journal*, vol. 291, 326–9.

Williams, A. (1988) 'Health Economics: The End of Clinical Freedom?', *British Medical Journal*, vol. 297, 183–8.

Williamson, O. (1975) *Markets and Hierarchies* (New York, Free Press).

Wilsford, D. (1991) *Doctors and the State: The Politics of Health Care in France and the United States* (London, Duke University Press).

Wilson, D. (1983) *The Lead Scandal* (London, Heinemann).

Wilson, M. (1975) *Health is for People* (London, Darton, Longman & Todd).

Windsor, P. (1986) *Introducing Körner: A Critical Guide to the Work and Recommendations of the Steering Group on Health Service Information* (Weybridge, British Journal of Health Care Computing).

Winkler, F. (1987) 'Consumerism in Health Care: Beyond the Supermarket Model', *Policy and Politics*, vol. 15 (1), 1–8.

Winn, L. (ed.) (1990) *Power to the People: The Key to Responsive Services in Health and Social Care* (London, King's Fund).

Wistow, G. (1990) *Community Care Planning: A Review of Past Experience and Future Imperatives* (London, Department of Health).

Wistow, G. (1992) 'The National Health Service' in D. Marsh and R. Rhodes (eds), *Implementing Thatcherite Policies* (Buckingham, Open University Press).

Wistow, G., Hardy, B. and Turrell, A. (1990) *Collaboration Under Financial Constraint: Health Authorities' Spending of Joint Finance* (Aldershot, Avebury).

Wohl, A. S. (1984) *Endangered Lives: Public Health in Victorian Britain* (London, Unwin Methuen).

Wood, B. (1990) 'Policy Failure: The Non-Reform of American Health Care', *Public Policy and Administration*, vol. 5. (3), 19–36.

Woolhandler, S. and Himmelstein, D. U. (1991) 'The Deteriorating Administrative Efficiency of the US Health Care System', *New England Journal of Medicine*, vol. 324, 1253–8.

Young, H. (1991) *One of Us* (London, Macmillan) final edn.

Zola, I. K. (1975) 'Medicine as an Institution of Social Control', in G. Cox and A. Mead (eds) *A Sociology of Medical Practice* (London, Collier Macmillan).

Index